HIV-RELATED ISSUES

BACKGROUND PAPER

11

ADVERSE REACTIONS TO HIV VACCINES: MEDICAL, ETHICAL, AND LEGAL ISSUES

CONGRESS OF THE UNITED STATES

OFFICE OF TECHNOLOGY ASSESSMENT

Recommended Citation: U.S. Congress, Office of Technology Assessment, *Adverse Reactions to HIV Vaccines: Medical, Ethical, and Legal Issues,* OTA-BP-H-163 (Washington, DC: U.S. Government Printing Office, September 1995).

For sale by the U.S. Government Printing Office
Superintendent of Documents, Mail Stop: SSOP, Washington, DC 20402-9328
ISBN 0-16-048257-7

Foreword

AIDS researchers are investigating new vaccines that would prevent infection with HIV and reduce the spread of AIDS. Some have argued that product liability concerns have discouraged investment in HIV vaccine research and development. The purpose of this OTA background paper is to describe the current state of development of HIV vaccines, and to discuss what is known about adverse reactions that may occur. The background paper provides an overview of ethical issues that arise in the conduct of HIV vaccine trials. The report also discusses alternatives to the current product liability system to encourage the development of HIV vaccines and to fairly compensate those who are harmed as a result of adverse reactions to the vaccine.

This background paper was prepared in response to a request from the Subcommittee on Health of the House Ways and Means Committee. It is eleventh in OTA's series of studies on HIV-related issues. The preceding papers in this series were:

- Do Insects Transmit AIDS? (9/87),
- AIDS and Health Insurance: An OTA Survey (2/88),
- How Effective is AIDS Education? (6/88),
- The Impact of AIDS on the Kaiser Permanente Medical Care Program (Northern California Region) (7/88),
- How Has Federal Research on AIDS/HIV Disease Contributed to Other Fields? (4/90),
- The Effectiveness of Drug Abuse Treatment: Implications for Controlling AIDS/HIV Infection (9/90),
- HIV in the Health Care Workplace (11/91),
- The CDC's Case Definition of AIDS: Implications of the Proposed Revisions (8/92),
- Difficult-to-reuse Needles for the Prevention of HIV Infection Among Injecting Drug Abusers (10/92), and
- External Review of the Federal Centers for Disease Control and Prevention's HIV Prevention Programs (9/94).

Other OTA reports addressing AIDS-related issues include:

- Blood Policy and Technology (1/85),
- Review of the Public Health Service's Response to AIDS (technical memorandum, 1/85),
- The Cost of AIDS and Other HIV Infections: Review of the Estimates (staff paper, 5/87),
- Medical Testing and Health Insurance (8/88),
- Adolescent Health (11/91), and
- The Continuing Challenge of Tuberculosis (9/93).

ROGER C. HERDMAN
Director

Project Staff

Clyde J. Behney
Assistant Director, OTA

Sean Tunis
Health Program Director

ADMINISTRATIVE STAFF

Louise Staley
Office Administrator

Carolyn Martin
Word Processing Specialist

Monica Finch
Word Processing Specialist

Charlotte Brown
Word Processing Specialist

Carolyn Swann
PC Specialist

PRINCIPAL PROJECT STAFF

Robert S. McDonough
Study Director

Jay Randolph
Research Analyst[1]

Thomas McDaniels, Jr.
Research Assistant[2]

PRINCIPAL CONTRACTORS

David T. Karzon
Vanderbilt University Medical Center

Wendy Mariner
Boston University School of Public Health and School of Medicine

CONTRACTORS

Nancy Kass
Johns Hopkins University
School of Hygiene and Public Health

David Schwartz
Johns Hopkins University
School of Hygiene and Public Health

Robert Stein
Blicker & Stein

PUBLISHING STAFF

Mary Lou Higgs
Manager

Arna Lane
Production Editor

Bonnie Sparks
Electronic Publishing Specialist

Christine Onrubia
Senior Graphic Designer

---

[1]Through September 1994
[2]From September 1994

Workshop Participants

ISSUES IN THE DEVELOPMENT AND MARKETING OF AN AIDS VACCINE—*April 6, 1994*

Lawrence Miike, *Chairman*
Health Care Administration Division
Department of Human Services
State of Hawaii
Honolulu, HI

Don Des Jarlais
Research Director
Chemical Dependency Institute and Grants Management Research Support
Beth Israel Medical Center
New York, NY

Christine Grady
Research Associate
National Institute of Nursing Research
National Institutes of Health
Bethesda, MD

Derek Hodel
Director of Treatment and Research Issues
AIDS Action Council
Washington, DC

Rodney Hoff
Chief, Vaccine Trials
Vaccine Trials and Epidemiology Branch
Division of AIDS
National Institute of Allergy and Infectious Diseases
National Institutes of Health
Bethesda, MD

Michael Horowitz
Senior Fellow
Manhattan Institute
Washington, DC

Peter Barton Hutt
Partner
Covington & Burling
Washington, DC

David T. Karzon
Professor of Pediatrics, Microbiology and Immunology
Division of Pediatric Infectious Diseases
Vanderbilt University Medical Center
Nashville, TN

Nancy Kass
Assistant Professor
Program in Law, Ethics, and Health
Department of Health Policy and Management
School of Hygiene and Public Health
Johns Hopkins University
Baltimore, MD

Wendy Mariner
Professor of Health Law
Health Law Department
Boston University School of Public Health and School of Medicine
Boston, MA

Tom Matthews
Associate Professor of Experimental Surgery
Department of Surgery
Duke University School of Medicine
Durham, NC

David Schwartz
Assistant Professor
Department of Immunology and Infectious Diseases
School of Hygiene and Public Health
Johns Hopkins University
Baltimore, MD

John Siegfried
Associate Vice President for Medical Affairs
Pharmaceutical Research and Manufacturers Association
Washington, DC

Robert Stein
Partner
Blicker & Stein
Washington, DC

Tom Vernon
Executive Director
Medical, Scientific, and Public Health Affairs
Merck Vaccine Division
Bluebell, PA

Roy Widdus
Consultant
National Vaccine Program Office
Washington, DC

Note: OTA appreciates and is grateful for the valuable assistance and thoughtful critiques provided by the participants in OTA's workshop on April 6, 1994. The workshop participants do not, however, necessarily approve, disapprove, or endorse this background paper. OTA assumes full responsibility for the background paper and the accuracy of its contents.

Contents

APPENDICES

Overview of Findings and Executive Summary 1

OVERVIEW OF FINDINGS

Potential and Risks of HIV Vaccines

- Although the human immunodeficiency virus (HIV) that causes acquired immunodeficiency syndrome (AIDS) is the most intensively studied virus of all time, a successful preventive vaccine lies at least several years ahead. In addition, we have yet to define the immune response elements necessary for protection from HIV infection.
- HIV is endowed with an unusual set of capacities that enables it to evade or manipulate normal immune responses. Because of these unique capacities, a model for an effective HIV vaccine is much more complicated than the model for other vaccines.
- More than 1,400 volunteers have participated in U.S. trials of HIV vaccines since 1988. Most vaccinees have received envelope-based vaccines (proteins present on the surface of the virus). Adverse reactions following immunization with HIV vaccines have been minimal.
- Of the more than 1,400 individuals who have participated in U.S. trials, 17 have become infected with HIV. There is no evidence that the experimental vaccines increased susceptibility to HIV infection or increased the rate of disease progression in these individuals.
- A number of vaccines are being developed that use new strategies, and each of these strategies may carry special risks.

"Each of the HIV vaccine strategies may carry special risks."

1. Vaccines using *live vectors*, such as the vaccinia virus shown to be attenuated in laboratory animals, may prove to be inadequately attenuated, producing the disease caused by the unattenuated vector:
2. *Naked DNA* vaccines have been shown to create potent immune responses, but there are theoretical reasons to be concerned that they might produce tumors or autoimmune diseases, or be transmitted from mother to fetus.
3. Although *inactivated whole virus* vaccines have generally been successful in protecting from infection with other viral diseases, it would be difficult to assure that all HIV particles in such a vaccine were inactivated.
4. *Live attenuated virus* vaccines have also been successful in protecting from other viral diseases, but there is the potential for the viruses to be inadequately attenuated, for an adequately attenuated viral vaccine to cause disease in immunocompromised individuals, and for an adequately attenuated virus to revert to virulence. There is also concern that a live attenuated HIV vaccine could induce tumors.

- A number of *social harms*—nonmedical adverse consequences—may result from vaccination:

1. Vaccines may cause a false-positive HIV screening test, making the diagnosis of HIV infection more difficult. This vaccine-induced positivity on HIV screening tests may result in discrimination against vaccine recipients in, for example, military service, health insurance, life insurance, employment, and travel.
2. Participation in an HIV vaccine trial, in itself, may result in stigmatization, as others may assume that all vaccine trial participants are members of groups, such as injection drug users and men who have sex with men, who are at increased risk for HIV infection.
3. Vaccinees, relying on the protection afforded by an experimental vaccine, may engage in behaviors that increase their risk for HIV infection.

- In June 1994, the AIDS Research Advisory Committee (ARAC) of the National Institute of Allergy and Infectious Diseases (NIAID) recommended that Phase III clinical trials with envelope vaccines should not proceed in the United States. Factors contributing to the decision included scientific, political, and ethical issues, and the significant level of scientific uncertainty about the wisdom of immediate trials. Phase I and Phase II clinical trials of HIV vaccines will continue.

Ethical Issues in HIV Vaccine Development

- Procedures must be in place to ensure the confidential handling of research data, given the sensitive nature of the information collected in the trial.
- Community involvement with the trial is important to ensure sensitivity to trial participants concerns and to better protect the rights of trial participants.
- Pregnant women should not be excluded from HIV vaccine trials because the efficacy of vaccines to prevent transmission of HIV from an infected mother to her fetus can only be demonstrated in pregnant women.
- It may be ethically acceptable to recruit persons who have little control over their ability to avoid exposure to HIV, such as women whose high-risk male partners refuse to wear condoms, because such persons may be targeted for HIV vaccination, once it is approved.
- Vaccine efficacy trials will target for enrollment individuals from high-risk groups, many of whom may be involved in illegal behaviors (such as injection drug user, prostitution, and, in certain jurisdictions, male-to-male sex). These individuals may increase their risk of detection as a result of trial participation. Assurances of confidentiality are essential to ensure their participation.

- In addition to the general requirements for informed consent, potential subjects of HIV vaccine trials need to be informed of the potential social harms of participation.
- Investigators have an ethical obligation to ensure that research subjects are counseled about avoidance of risk behaviors because some subjects will be randomly assigned to receive placebo vaccine, there is no assurance that the experimental vaccine will be effective, and no vaccine is completely effective.
- If potential subjects are to be screened for HIV infection, there should be an informed consent process for this screening, in addition to the informed consent process for participation in the vaccine trial.
- Investigators have an ethical obligation to provide subjects with documentation of their trial participation, and to make available sophisticated tests necessary to distinguish vaccine-induced false positivity from true HIV infection.
- Trial participants should agree not to be tested for HIV outside of the study; participant's knowledge of their assignment may bias study results.
- Vaccine trials also need to be conducted in developing countries because AIDS is a devastating problem in these countries, and because the circulating strains in each part of the world differ, so that findings from vaccine trials in developed countries may not be generalizable to the developing world.
- Local representatives should be consulted at all stages of vaccine trials in developing countries. Both Western requirements and local requirements for informed consent must be met. Efforts must be made to ensure that potential subjects have an adequate understanding of the study's risks, and the importance of avoiding risk behaviors in order to provide informed consent, but potential subjects and investigators need not have a completely shared understanding of disease causation.
- Investigators have the ethical obligation to ensure that the trial does not interfere with other health care or public health efforts.
- To ensure fairness in the distribution of benefits and burdens, the vaccine must be made available to the communities where trials were conducted. In poorer communities, this may require that the vaccine be made available either at cost or free of charge.
- Although vaccine sponsors have no legal obligation to provide compensation to subjects for injuries incurred as a result of their participation, there is an ethical obligation to do so.

Liability and Compensation for Adverse Reactions

- Any system that limits compensation to injuries from one specific cause, like an HIV vaccine, raises questions of fairness to people with similar injuries from a different vaccine. A compensation system limited to persons with adverse reactions to an HIV vaccine invites the question why people living with injuries from other vaccines or from other causes should not be compensated as well.
- More companies are engaged in HIV vaccine research than in research for any other type of vaccine. Potential liability may have discouraged some companies, but it has not stopped HIV vaccine development.
- Some have argued that drug and vaccine makers should be exempt from liability because their products confer significant benefits and their designs and labeling are approved by the Food and Drug Administration (FDA). Supporters of liability argue that no exemption should be granted because not all drugs provide significant social benefits, and that manufacturers should be held to at least the same standards as manufacturers of ordinary consumer goods because consumers are vulnerable to undetectable risks in pharmaceutical and biological products.

- Physicians are more likely than vaccine manufacturers to be the target of complaints that patients were not informed of vaccine risks. The "learned intermediary" rule permits the maker of prescription drugs or vaccines to warn only the prescribing physician, and not the patient who receives the product. Physicians have an independent legal obligation to obtain their patients' informed consent to immunization.
- Although the legal basis for liability is the same, both the likelihood of claims and the probability that any such claims would succeed in practice is far lower with respect to investigational vaccines than with marketed vaccines.
- For a number of reasons, there has been little concern about liability for adverse reactions to therapeutic vaccines, in contrast to preventive vaccines.
- Liability claims based on low levels of effectiveness have not been brought against existing vaccines. The likelihood of success of a claim of lack of effectiveness of an HIV vaccine is speculative, but probably small as long as those who take the vaccine are warned of its limited efficacy and advised to take precautions against exposure to HIV infection.
- The likelihood of a successful claim of liability for enhanced susceptibility to infection of disease progression would depend upon whether the manufacturer knew or should have known that the vaccine was capable of causing the reaction, and whether the plaintiff could prove that the vaccine was the only cause of the reaction in his or her case.
- Given the need for an HIV vaccine, it appears unlikely that a manufacturer would be held responsible for distributing a vaccine with a risk of development of cancer that could not be verified at the time it was released.
- The decision whether or not to invest in the development of a vaccine depends on complex financial considerations of a number of factors, including the scientific obstacles to vaccine development, the potential market for the vaccine, the price at which the vaccine could be sold, and the potential liability for vaccines. The major factor influencing vaccine development is the expected return on investment or profitability, and the major obstacles to developing an HIV vaccine are scientific.
- Evidence that liability may deter some companies from developing an HIV vaccine comes from anecdotal reports that several companies interrupted HIV vaccine research or testing and sought immunity from liability before they would consider proceeding. Other factors, however, including scientific problems with the candidate vaccine, inadequate financing, poor market predictions, patent problems, and internal corporate restructuring, may also explain their decisions about whether to pursue testing.
- Nonrecombinant vaccines that use killed, inactivated, or attenuated virus may be unappealing to vaccine makers because of the consequences of the failure of the manufacturing process to inactivate a virus that could cause active infection. Companies may not wish to pursue a type of vaccine that might produce HIV infection, regardless of exposure to liability, especially if they believe that they cannot eliminate the risk of a manufacturing error.
- Vaccine manufacturers are not likely to be responsible for harms resulting from the bigotry of others. Physicians who administer HIV vaccines may be the more likely targets for any claim that a vaccine recipient was not adequately warned about possible discrimination.
- Preventive vaccines may be more susceptible to claims of liability than most drugs and biologics, primarily because they are used in large numbers of healthy people. The rate of actual liability, however, has been quite low.
- Since liability is so rarely imposed for vaccines, the fear of liability may be more accurately described as the fear of having to litigate at all. Complaints about the litigation process, however, are not limited to cases involving

HIV vaccines, so that any alternative that is intended to remedy tort litigation's inefficiencies would have application beyond HIV vaccines.

- Tort reform proposals have sought to change the substantive grounds for liability, the procedures or evidence used in litigation, or the amount of compensation payable. Similar proposals to reform the law of medical malpractice and product liability have been the subject of considerable debate. If considered for HIV vaccines, they may have to be considered for other types of injuries.
- Voluntary agreements between companies and individuals to provide compensation for an adverse reaction without the necessity of litigation reduce the time and expense of resolving claims. Voluntary agreements are unlikely to work well with new HIV vaccines, because the company and the vaccinee do not have the relationship necessary for contract, and because there are likely to be substantial unresolved issues about whether the injury was caused by the vaccine.
- Government-funded excess insurance would limit the amount of financial exposure companies face from liability payments, but the primary difficulties are in estimating the amount of excess insurance needed for a new vaccine and determining the amount of liability expenditures that should be considered excessive for manufacturers. In addition, an excess insurance program might set a precedent for government reinsurance of liability expenses for other types of tort claims.
- Vaccine-related injuries could be compensated through government disability insurance programs. A more general expansion of disability insurance to cover injuries regardless of cause avoids questions of justice to persons with injuries from other causes and the costs of such a program would be more predictable than the costs of a program that compensates only those injuries caused by new HIV vaccines. But a government disability insurance program would be costly.
- No-fault compensation programs eliminate the need to prove negligence or legal responsibility for injury, so that administrative costs can be lower than those of litigation. No-fault compensation systems that are limited to injuries from a specific cause, like adverse reactions to vaccines, require proof of causation, which is often difficult, time-consuming, and expensive, especially where the scientific evidence is uncertain or conflicting. No-fault compensation programs also have the disadvantage of treating one group of people differently from others with similar injuries or needs. Also, no-fault compensation systems may generate more, rather than less, costs and typically compensate more people than would recover compensation in tort law.
- The National Vaccine Injury Compensation Program may provide a model for a no-fault system of compensation for adverse reactions to HIV vaccines. Adding HIV vaccines to the program would expand its scope beyond children's vaccines, but it would also avoid the need for creating a new administrative structure to provide compensation.
- By themselves, compensation programs cannot guarantee that any vaccine is developed. Alternative methods of encouraging vaccine development may be necessary, including tax incentives, expedited FDA review, purchase guarantees, expanded patent protection, and facilitation of collaborative efforts.

EXECUTIVE SUMMARY

AIDS researchers are investigating new vaccines that would prevent HIV infection and reduce the spread of AIDS. Some have claimed that potentially promising approaches to developing a vaccine against HIV have been deferred due to concerns about liability of vaccine manufacturers, and have urged legislation that would limit the liability of manufacturers of HIV vaccines. This study examines the current state of HIV vaccine development, the adverse reactions that may be associated with HIV vaccines, and proposals to reform product liability to encourage the development of an HIV vaccine. The findings of this study may be used in considering legislation that addresses HIV vaccine liability, and also have important implications for the reform of product liability in general.

The next three chapters address the medical, ethical, and legal issues in the development and marketing of an HIV vaccine. Chapter 2 addresses the potential safety problems that may emerge from vaccines for the prevention of HIV infection.[1] The chapter reviews the biological basis for development of a vaccine to prevent AIDS, the difficulties that must be overcome in developing an effective HIV vaccine, and the unique features of the virus and disease it produces that elude vaccine control. The chapter also reviews the adverse events that have occurred to date in clinical trials of HIV vaccines. The chapter explains the difficulties in predicting the types and rates of adverse reactions that may occur with HIV vaccines; this uncertainty has important implications for the design of a compensation scheme. The chapter concludes with a discussion of the important adverse social consequences of being vaccinated for HIV.

Chapter 3 provides an overview of the basic ethical principles that guide human subjects research, and shows how these ethical issues apply to each stage of HIV vaccine development. The chapter discusses ethical issues in the design of clinical trials, selection of research subjects, the informed consent process, compensation for trial-related injuries, and incorporation of HIV vaccines into clinical practice. The chapter also addresses special ethical issues that arise in clinical trials in developing countries.

Chapter 4 summarizes existing product liability law and relevant literature on liability for vaccine-related injury and analyzes how that law might apply to vaccines to prevent HIV infection or progression to AIDS. To gauge how liability might affect the vaccine industry's ability or willingness to develop and market new HIV vaccines, the report reviews other factors that influence such decisions, such as the feasibility of identifying an effective HIV vaccine and the attractiveness of the potential market. Although there is little basis for assuming that liability itself will halt HIV vaccine development, some highly risk-averse companies may avoid specific types of vaccine products that they fear may induce severe adverse reactions. Whether such products should be encouraged depends upon their safety and effectiveness compared with available alternatives.

Liability's effect on vaccine development does not answer the question whether society should endorse compensation for vaccine-related injuries, which may be desirable to achieve other social goals. For this reason, chapter 4 begins with a brief description of common reasons for compensating injuries and assigning responsibility (liability) to different entities for paying compensation. Finally, the chapter summarizes several types of compensation systems as a guide to issues that should be considered in any debate on the desirability of establishing a new compensation system for HIV vaccine-related injuries.

Appendix A provides a detailed technical discussion of adverse reactions that may, in theory, be predicted to occur. These include late-occurring reactions and rare adverse reactions that may not be detected until after an HIV vaccine has been approved for marketing. The appendix also assesses the strength of the support for these potential harms from HIV vaccines.

POTENTIAL FOR ADVERSE REACTIONS TO HIV VACCINES

Role of Vaccines in Control of Disease

One way to control the spread of AIDS is to vaccinate individuals against HIV infection. Vaccines have been credited with eliminating smallpox and of reducing the number of cases of measles, mumps, rubella, diphtheria, pertussis, tetanus, and other infectious diseases. Vaccines consist of

[1] In this report, the term HIV will refer to human immunodeficiency virus type 1 (HIV-1), unless otherwise indicated.

a microorganism or its components, in a safe form, which are administered to stimulate, or "prime," the body's immune system to generate protective defenses specifically directed against the microorganism. The portions of the microorganism that stimulate the body's immune system are called antigens.

The immune system has three response components: 1) antibody circulating in the bloodstream (humoral immunity); 2) a network of immune white cells in the blood and tissues (cellular immunity); and 3) a specialized system of antibody and immune cells located at mucous membranes (mucosal immunity), such as those covering the surface of the vagina, anus, and penile urethra (the routes of sexual transmission of HIV infection). Antibodies are produced by immune white cells called B lymphocytes. Each antibody is antigen-specific, and can neutralize virus particles that are free in the circulation, but cannot inactivate virus that is located inside infected cells. Another type of white cell, the T lymphocyte, participates in cellular immunity. Among the types of T lymphocytes are the CD4+ "helper" T lymphocytes, which are necessary for the development of mature functional lymphocytes, and the CD8+ "cytotoxic" T lymphocytes, which can kill cells undergoing active viral infection.

Vaccines in use today follow only a few basic designs. Most common are live attenuated vaccines, which are composed of a live virus or other pathogenic organism that has been altered to reduce or eliminate its potential to produce disease. Also common are inactivated virus vaccines, which use virus that has been killed (i.e., rendered unable to replicate). Two are protein subunit vaccines, which are composed of antigenic proteins from the pathogenic organism. And one vaccine, Hepatitis B, is prepared by recombinant biotechnology. The number of infectious agents for which we have failed to develop a satisfactory vaccine, however, is far greater than the number of those that have been successful.

Unique Features of HIV

Although HIV is the most intensively studied virus of all time, a successful vaccine lies several years ahead. Because of several unique features of HIV, a model for an effective HIV vaccine is much more complicated than the model for contemporary vaccines. HIV is endowed with an unusual set of capacities that enables it to evade or manipulate normal immune responses. These include the following:

- HIV is a "retrovirus" that integrates its genome into the human genome through a process called "reverse transcription." Once this happens, it cannot be detected and eliminated by the immune system.
- HIV is able to evade immune recognition through a process of rapid genetic mutation and selection.
- The virus selectively invades and can injure CD4+ lymphocytes and macrophages, the very cells that play central roles in immune defenses.
- The virus can spread through direct cell-to-cell contact, avoiding immune activation.
- During the years of apparent clinical wellness before the onset of HIV-related symptoms, the virus continues to multiply to high concentrations in lymphoid tissues of the body, and is silently transmissible.
- HIV is transmissible by three different routes (through sexual contact with mucous membranes, by direct inoculation into the bloodstream, or by transfer from mother to fetus or infant), which, in itself, can complicate the task of developing a vaccine that mounts an effective immune blockade.
- HIV can be transmitted as free virus as well as virus inside cells; it is more difficult to block the transmission of virus inside cells.
- Unlike other viral infections that are self-limited, there are few, if any, instances of recovery

from HIV infection to offer clues for understanding the key immune response elements necessary for protection from the virus.

- Primate models of human HIV infection have not yielded definitive guidance to the immune elements necessary for protection.

Animal Models of HIV Infection and Disease

Animal models of infection historically have contributed to the development of vaccines by helping to define the immune responses associated with control of infection, and to predict the behavior of a candidate vaccine in man. The chimpanzee is the only animal in which HIV will replicate. But in the chimpanzee, the virus causes a minimal persistent infection, waning over time, with no disease manifestations. Macaque monkeys can become infected with simian immunodeficiency virus (SIV), a retrovirus that is closely related to HIV. SIV is highly virulent in macaques, and causes a persistent infection leading to an AIDS-like syndrome within 6 to 24 months after infection. Thus, the HIV/chimpanzee system models HIV infection in humans, while the SIV/macaque system parallels HIV disease progression in humans.

There are examples of vaccine protection or partial protection in primates, largely under conditions that are optimal for protection, but do not mirror typical conditions. Also, large doses of antibody administered to the chimpanzee provide passive protection to infection with HIV for several hours, but no longer. Live attenuated vaccines show a high level of protection against SIV infection in macaques, but there are safety concerns that may have inhibited the development of live attenuated HIV vaccines for human use.

Development and Clinical Evaluation of HIV Vaccines

The U.S. Public Health Service has established a program of basic science and clinical research toward the development of a safe and effective preventive HIV vaccine. The effort is centered at the National Institutes of Health (NIH), with the National Institute of Allergy and Infectious Diseases as the lead institute. The NIAID Division of AIDS (DAIDS) has created an AIDS Vaccine Clinical Trial Network (AVCTN), which has several components. The AIDS Vaccine Evaluation Group (AVEG) includes six AIDS Vaccine Evaluation Unit (AVEU) trial sites at university research centers. Each unit has an associated Community Advisory Board. Other AVCTN elements include a Central Immunology Laboratory, a Mucosal Immunology Laboratory, a Data Coordinating and Analysis Center, and a Data and Safety Monitoring Board.

The process of testing a candidate vaccine in clinical trials is initiated by a sponsor, which presents preclinical data for review by the Food and Drug Administration's Center for Biologicals, Evaluation and Research (CBER). The FDA is also responsible for approval and oversight of experimental protocols as vaccines progress through clinical trials. The AIDS Vaccine Selection Group determines whether a vaccine will be entered into federally funded AVEG trials. Other major participants in HIV vaccine development include the National Cancer Institute, the Center for Disease Control and Prevention (CDC), vaccine manufacturers, the World Health Organization (WHO), and the Department of Defense, with capacities for research, product development, and conduct of clinical trials in the developed and developing world.

Promising candidate vaccines are selected for initial assessment of immune responses and safety in carefully monitored, randomized, controlled trials. The first phase (Phase I) of clinical trials of vaccine focuses on the safety and immunogenicity of the vaccine. The Phase I protocol involves 25 to 100 individuals at low risk for HIV infection, assigned to one or more experimental groups and to a placebo group for comparison. If immune responses and safety warrant further studies, the vaccine may undergo Phase II trials involving up to several hundred individuals. Phase II studies refine and enlarge on the database, may directly compare vaccine products or sequences, or may include individuals at higher risk of acquiring infection.

HIV vaccine sponsors have been, to a large extent, small biotechnology companies, private research institutions, and universities; some of the large pharmaceutical manufacturers in the United States are not represented among vaccine sponsors. A number of considerations influence corporate decisions to enter into the development of an HIV vaccine, including the opportunity costs of vaccine development relative to development of drugs, potential markets for HIV vaccines, the scientific feasibility of vaccine development, and the potential for liability for adverse reactions to HIV vaccines. Because of concerns about vaccine safety, manufacturers have primarily pursued the development of HIV vaccines composed of envelope protein subunits, proteins present on the surface of the virus, which have inherently more limited immune capability, but have fewer inherent safety risks, than vaccines composed of inactivated or live attenuated virus.

Adverse Reactions to HIV Vaccines

The standard of safety applied to preventive vaccines has been extremely high; even the rare occurrence of significant injuries to uninfected, healthy individuals has been considered unacceptable. Despite the inherent potential for injury from vaccines, currently licensed vaccines have been extremely safe, and have provided a highly cost-effective method for disease prevention.

Initial approaches to HIV vaccines have concentrated on gp120 and gp160, glycoproteins that are present in the membrane or "envelope" of the virus. Purified envelope proteins have been produced using recombinant biotechnology. A second method of immunization uses live vaccinia virus (derived from the strain used to prevent smallpox) as a delivery "vector, which has been genetically altered to express HIV gp160 on its surface. From the initiation of the AVEG program in 1988, more than 1,400 volunteers have participated in trials. Twelve envelope-based vaccine products have been used, prepared by five manufacturers, using three different strains of HIV.

Envelope vaccines have induced neutralizing antibody against strains of HIV that are homologous (identical) to strains used in vaccine preparation. The titers (concentrations) of antibody induced by envelope vaccines have been 5- to 10-fold lower than titers of antibody seen in HIV-infected individuals, and have fallen rapidly after each vaccine dose. Heterologous (nonidentical) strains of HIV were neutralized less well, and strains of HIV that were recently isolated in the community were entirely resistant to the vaccine. Envelope vaccines failed to generate cytotoxic T lymphocyte responses (cellular immunity).

Adverse reactions following immunization with envelope products have been minimal. Sequential measurements of biochemical, blood, and immune status, and kidney and liver function tests have shown no significant vaccine-related abnormal findings. Importantly, there has been no evidence of adverse effects on immune function.

Envelope vaccines that were combined with alum "adjuvant" (a substance used to enhance the vaccine's immunogenicity) were accompanied by local reactions at the injection site, consisting of mild pain, tenderness, redness, and swelling for 1 to 2 days after injection. Vaccinations with some of the newer adjuvants were accompanied by transient moderate to severe local reactions and febrile flu-like illnesses for one to three days after injection in a number of recipients.

Ten vaccinees developed a rash to several products, and one also developed joint pain. A few individuals developed a positive antinuclear antibody (ANA) test (which may at times be associated with autoimmune disease, such as rheumatoid arthritis). However, further testing ruled out any vaccine-related diseases. Despite careful screening and counseling, 14 pregnancies occurred during these trials. There was no evidence of vaccine-related adverse events to the fetus.

The trials permitted comparison of the side effects of an attenuated vaccinia/gp160 vector with the commercial vaccinia virus strain used to prevent smallpox. Reactions to the vaccine resembled those seen following classical smallpox vaccination. There were no differences in the development of pustules at the inoculation site, regional lymph node swelling, or level of systemic symptoms. The vaccinia virus vector did not appear to be adequately attenuated and thus could carry the risk of vaccinia complications known to occur with classical vaccination. With broad use of an HIV vaccine, substitution of a more attenuated virus vector, such as canarypox, is preferable.

As of May 1994, 10 neoplasms (tumors) were observed among participants in 9 vaccine trial protocols. One of the neoplasms was benign. Cases of malignancy tended to occur among older participants. Analysis by the Data Safety and Monitoring Board and an ad hoc expert committee found no evidence that the neoplasms were linked with any vaccine products. Because of the wide variety of tumor types, it was judged to be biologically implausible that the tumors had a causal relationship to the vaccine.

To date, 12 of the 1,400 individuals in AVEG trials since 1988 have become infected with HIV. Of the 12 infected vaccinees, three received a placebo vaccine, eight received an envelope protein vaccine, and one received a vaccinia/gp160 vaccine. Five of the infected vaccinees received one or two doses of vaccine, and only four infected vaccinees received an adequate series of three to four doses. Three additional "breakthrough cases" occurred in an intramural NIAID trial, and two others occurred in non-NIAID trials, so that a total of 17 infections have occurred in all HIV vaccine trials to date. Envelope vaccines of all participating manufacturers were involved. A number of breakthrough infections was to be expected because some volunteers received placebo, some volunteers had not completed a full dosage schedule, and the protective efficacy of the vaccines being tested is not known.

Envelope vaccines, in themselves, cannot cause HIV infection. The possibility that the vaccine may increase susceptibility to HIV infection or may increase the rate of disease progression (a phenomenon called "antibody-dependent enhancement") must be considered and investigated. Although there is laboratory evidence of an increase in growth of virus in cell cultures in the presence of antibodies from the serum of vaccinees, there is no evidence of enhancement with SIV or HIV in primate experiments.

There is concern that HIV vaccines have the potential to cause autoimmunity (an immune reaction against the bodies own tissues), because HIV shares several envelope proteins that are identical to proteins on human tissues. For example, there is a similarity between one HIV envelope protein region and a normal human blood-type protein. Autoimmunity has not been observed among vaccine recipients to date, although in theory, autoimmune phenomena could first appear months to years after vaccination.

New Generation Vaccines: Implications for Safety

Because of HIV's unique abilities to evade immune controls, all immune response elements may need to be invoked to provide protection, including humoral immunity, cellular immunity, and mucosal immunity. Vaccines using new strategies may be needed to fulfill these immune requirements for protection. Each vaccine formulation or variation on a formulation is regarded as a new product by the FDA and requires a separate evaluation. Each new approach may carry special risks, some unique to that strategy.

Proteins that duplicate viral antigenic proteins may be artificially synthesized. These "synthetic peptides" have been shown to induce cytotoxic T lymphocyte responses to SIV in macaques. In clinical trials, reactions to synthetic peptide vaccines have been benign.

Vaccines using a number of vectors (e.g., canarypox virus, adenovirus, Salmonella, Shigella, and attenuated poliovirus) are being studied. These live vectors are better able to induce cytotoxic T lymphocyte responses, and vectors that grow on body surfaces (e.g., adenovirus and Shigella) are better able to induce mucosal immune responses to HIV. Live vectors, however, carry inherent safety concerns. If they are inadequately or unstably attenuated, they may produce the disease caused by the unattenuated vector. They may result in unwanted spread to contacts and the community at large. And even an adequately attenuated vector may cause disease in individuals with impaired immunity.

Some new vaccines are composed of "naked DNA," pure viral genetic material. Persistent antibody and cytotoxic T lymphocyte responses have been induced in laboratory animals immunized with naked DNA. The mechanisms leading to the potent immune responses are not understood. Concerns about naked DNA involve the theoretical possibilities of tumor formation, production of autoimmune disease, or the transmission of DNA to the fetus.

Development of inactivated whole virus vaccines against HIV was seriously considered in early deliberations. Although inactivated whole virus vaccines have generally been successful in protecting from infection with other viruses, this strategy has not been applied to HIV by vaccine manufacturers because of inherent risks. The primary concern with these vaccines is the difficulty in assuring inactivation of all HIV particles. Of particular concern is whether cell cultures or animal models are sufficiently sensitive to detect minimal amounts of residual live virus capable of infecting humans.

Vaccines using live attenuated viruses have also been successful in protecting from other viral diseases. Live attenuated vaccines are capable of inducing a vigorous and broad antibody response, as well as inducing cellular immunity and mucosal immunity. Live attenuated SIV vaccines were able to protect monkeys against challenge with large doses of virulent virus. In addition, the attenuated virus used in these vaccines was shown to be stable, not reverting to a virulent form over an observation period of several years.

However, there are a number of concerns about the safety of attenuated viral vaccines. First, there is the potential for the viruses used to be inadequately attenuated, resulting in the induction of the disease that the vaccine was designed to prevent. By contrast, viruses that are overattenuated may not be able to induce protective immune responses. Second, even an adequately attenuated virus may be virulent in individuals whose immune system is impaired by immunosuppressive drugs, cancers, or other causes.

Third, there is concern about the "stability" of attenuation of the virus—the potential for an attenuated strain of virus to undergo genetic reversion to a more virulent form during replication in the vaccinee. Spread of the attenuated virus to contacts (secondary spread) provides the virus with further opportunities to revert to virulence. Fourth, live attenuated HIV may induce tumors. Other retroviruses have been shown to produce tumors, and in theory, the prolonged residence of an attenuated HIV strain in humans could allow the production of tumors. There is recent evidence that HIV has a direct role in the etiology of some T-cell lymphomas, a type of immune cell cancer.

Social Harms as Adverse Reactions to HIV Vaccines

Individuals may suffer social harms—non-medical adverse consequences—as a result of HIV vaccination. Vaccines may cause a "false-positive" screening test for HIV infection. The false-positive tests from envelope vaccines can only be distinguished from HIV infection by the Western blot test, which is widely used to confirm the results of positive screening tests. These false-positive screening tests could potentially result in discrimination against false-positive individuals, for example, in eligibility for military service, employment, health or life insurance, or restriction of travel. Volunteers in NIAID-sponsored trials have received identification documents certifying their participation in these trials, although AVEG personnel have had to provide validation of confounding Western blot confirmatory tests. This problem may be greater with new generation vaccines that include many more types of antigenic proteins than are currently used, which may render the Western blot tests incapable of distinguishing false-positive screening tests from HIV infection. Reliance must then be placed on more expensive and time-consuming polymerase chain reaction (PCR) tests and viral cultures.

Participation in an HIV vaccine trial, in itself, may engender social harms. Others may perceive that trial participation implies that the volunteer is a member of a group at special risk for acquiring HIV infection, resulting in stigmatization of that volunteer. Furthermore, volunteers immunized with one vaccine may be precluded from participation in clinical trials of subsequent, possibly more effective, vaccines. Also, trial participants, assuming that the vaccine protects them from infection, may increase their risk-taking behaviors. This may occur despite intensive counseling about the possibility of assignment to placebo vaccine and about the unknown efficacy of the experimental vaccine.

Clinical Trials in HIV-Infected Individuals

A number of vaccines to prevent transmission of HIV from an infected mother to her fetus or infant (maternal-fetal transmission) are being developed. Although pregnancy had been a cause for exclusion from Phase I and II clinical trials of HIV vaccines, Phase I clinical trials of HIV envelope vaccines, involving 23 infected pregnant women, are now in progress. Such trials are specifically designed to study safety and possible efficacy of vaccines in prevention of infection in the infant. No significant vaccine-related adverse events have occurred in the mothers or in the 20 infants that have been delivered thus far.

A number of vaccines are being developed to treat individuals with established HIV infection. Approximately 35 Phase I and Phase II trials of therapeutic HIV vaccines are being conducted in the United States and abroad. Thus far, there has been no clear evidence that these vaccines have delayed or prevented disease progression in infected individuals. Conversely, there is no evidence that these vaccines have accelerated or enhanced HIV infection in vaccinees.

Phase III Efficacy Trials

The purpose of Phase III efficacy trials of HIV vaccine is to determine its capability to protect against infection, and to provide a more definitive assessment of vaccine safety. Efficacy trials of HIV vaccines will be large, complex, lengthy, and expensive, involving several thousand volunteers per experimental group. Trials will be conducted among groups with a high incidence of HIV infection, such as injection drug users and men who have sex with men; members of these groups may feel disenfranchised and socially stigmatized, and may distrust government and scientific experimentation.

In anticipation of these large-scale efficacy trials, preparatory studies involving several thousand injection drug users and men who have sex with men with high HIV incidence are under study by the HIV Evaluation Network (HIVNET), sponsored by the NIAID, the CDC, and the National Institute of Drug Abuse. The purposes of these trials are multiple: to study the social and cultural factors affecting trial recruitment and retention; to measure the effect of trial participation, counseling, and unblinding on risk behaviors; to determine the basis for attitudes toward vaccine acceptance; to develop educational strategies and consent forms appropriate to the groups that will be targeted; and to study the dynamics of trial acceptance and feasibility. Information derived from such studies will help to prepare for full-scale HIV vaccine efficacy trials in the United States.

A number of criteria may be used to select vaccine candidates for Phase III efficacy trials: 1) evidence of the vaccine's safety and immunogenicity in Phase I and Phase II trials; 2) the ability of the vaccine to induce high and sustained titers of broadly reactive antibody capable of neutralizing strains circulating in the community; 3) the ability of the vaccine to induce cytotoxic T lymphocyte responses; 4) evidence of vaccine protection in primate models. Because of the scientific uncertainty, the relative emphasis given to each of these criteria have varied.

Two vaccines, Biocine SF2 with MF59 and Genentech MN with alum adjuvant, have completed Phase II efficacy trials. In June 1994, the NIAIDS AIDS Subcommittee and the AIDS Research Advisory Committee recommended that Phase III clinical trials with the envelope vaccines should not proceed in the United States at this time. Factors contributing to the decision included scientific, political, and ethical issues, as well as the significant level of scientific uncertainty about the wisdom of immediate efficacy trials. Phase I and Phase II clinical trials of HIV vaccines, however, will continue. New products recently entered into Phase I trials or in preclinical testing are designed to increase and improve the quality of the protective immune response to the vaccine. Additional vaccines should be available for consideration for Phase III trials within two to three years.

Long-term followup of large numbers of vaccine trial participants and controls allows for surveillance of events that are infrequent or occur after an interval of years. The trial participants constitute prospectively defined cohorts that are not easily duplicated once controlled efficacy trials are completed. Vaccinated cohorts from efficacy trials could be compared with unvaccinated cohorts currently under epidemiologic and virologic surveillance. Provision for long-term followup should be an integral part of trial efficacy design to allow surveillance for adverse events, such as enhanced infection, autoimmune disease, tumors, or reversion to virulence.

The NIAID and U.S. military are working with governments in the Americas, Africa, and Asia to establish sites for HIV vaccine trials. Trials of HIV vaccine in developing countries provide opportunities to study diverse population groups in highly endemic areas, including heterosexual and maternal-fetal transmission of HIV and a variety of cultural and health settings, and to test vaccines targeting a multiplicity of HIV subtypes.

ETHICAL ISSUES IN HIV VACCINE TRIALS

Ethical issues arise in all stages of vaccine development and marketing. A prophylactic vaccine for HIV infection raises some unique ethical issues.

Principles of Research Ethics

All biomedical research should be conducted in a manner that seeks not to violate three primary ethical principles: beneficence, respect for autonomy, and justice.

The principle of *beneficence* addresses one's obligations toward the well being of others. In clinical research, beneficence requires that the welfare of research subjects be protected. In vaccine trials, the investigators and vaccine sponsors are responsible for protecting research subjects from undue or excessive risks, and this responsibility cannot be avoided merely by informing subjects of those risks. There are certain risks that are too great for any altruistic volunteer to consent to, regardless of whether the volunteer understands the risks. In clinical trials, an external review board determines whether the risks of the trial are excessive.

Respect for autonomy obligates investigators to recognize research subjects as individuals who have the right to make their own decisions. The doctrine of informed consent is derived from this principle.

Justice requires fairness in the distribution of benefits and burdens. In research, this requires that no individuals or groups bear a disproportionate share of the risks of research without justification, and that all groups have equal access to the benefits of research participation.

Design of Clinical Trials

In designing clinical trials of HIV vaccines, a number of ethical issues should be addressed. First, investigators should determine whether a randomized trial is ethical. Random assignment to an experimental intervention is ethical only in cases of "clinical equipoise"—that is, where there is a lack of consensus in the medical or scientific community about whether the experimental intervention is beneficial. It is not ethical to randomly assign research subjects to vaccine and placebo control groups if there is consensus that the experimental vaccine is effective. Given the serious consequences of erroneous vaccine research findings, it is also unethical to base conclusions about vaccine efficacy on nonrandomized studies, because of the risk of bias. Thus, it is ethical to conduct randomized clinical trials to determine whether a vaccine is effective, but not to provide confirmatory data.

Second, investigators have an ethical obligation to ensure that research subjects are counseled about avoidance of risk behaviors. Behavioral counseling is ethically required in HIV vaccine trials because some subjects will be assigned to placebo vaccine, because there is no assurance that the experimental vaccine will be effective, and because no vaccine is completely efficacious. Also, it would be good to give research subjects some benefit in return for participation, if it can be provided at not at too great an expense.

Third, procedures should be in place to ensure the confidential handling of research data. Protection of confidentiality is important in any clinical research, but especially in HIV-related research, because of the sensitive nature of the information being collected. A number of practical measures should be taken to better ensure that confidentiality is maintained: each research subject should be assigned a unique identification number to be used, instead of full names, for labeling written forms, specimens, and any other information about the subject; all research data should be kept in locked storage cabinets or computer files with restricted access; only a select group of investigators should be allowed access to the "master key" that links subjects' names to their unique identifiers; all research staff should be educated in procedures that ensure the protection of research subjects' confidentiality.

Vaccine sponsors should pay for all trial-related medical procedures. Patient confidentiality may be threatened if investigators are allowed to bill the subject's insurer for medical procedures related to the trial.

Research subjects should be assured that they may have access to their own files upon completion of the trial, and that they may obtain documentation of their trial participation, even years later, if they need to demonstrate, for example, that the experimental vaccine was the source of a positive HIV antibody test.

Fourth, community involvement in the trial is important. A community board, usually composed of trial participants, meets with investigators periodically throughout the course of the trial to discuss plans, to review progress, and to make recommendations to the investigators. The community board can serve as a liaison between research subjects and investigators, and can help ensure that the rights of research subjects are protected. The research subjects' resultant greater involvement with and "ownership" of the research could improve retention and compliance.

Sample Selection

Research ethics has been concerned with protecting vulnerable populations from being enrolled in human subjects research without their (or their guardian's) knowledge and without adequate justification for their specific inclusion. More recently, there has also been a concern that vulnerable populations not be denied the benefit of participation in research.

Vulnerable" populations are those that are unable to provide valid informed consent, either because they do not have the mental capacity to provide consent (such as children or the mentally ill), or because they may not be able to provide consent voluntarily (such as prisoners or patients who are in a dependent relationship with the investigator). Such vulnerable populations should only be included if they will contribute knowledge that cannot be obtained from studying other, less vulnerable populations, and if the members of the vulnerable population (or their guardians) believe that the research will be beneficial.

Until recently, pregnant women have been excluded from trials of HIV vaccines because of concerns about harm to the fetus. However, the efficacy of vaccines to prevent transmission of HIV from an infected mother to her fetus can only be demonstrated in pregnant women. Three clinical trials of vaccines to prevent maternal-fetal HIV transmission have now enrolled infected pregnant women.

Certain populations targeted for vaccine trials may be considered vulnerable, not because they are unable to provide consent, but because they may be at greater risk of social harms as a result of their trial participation. Persons involved in illegal behaviors (such as injection drug user, prostitution, and, in certain jurisdictions, male-to-male sex) may increase their risk of detection as a consequence of trial participation. At the same time, it is important to include members of these groups in HIV vaccine trials, given the higher incidence of HIV infection in these groups, and given that members of these groups would be candidates for a vaccine once it is approved. Measures to protect their confidentiality are important to ensure their participation.

Members of racial minority groups are more highly represented among populations at increased risk of HIV infection, so they are more likely to participate in HIV vaccine trials. Members of racial minority groups may be less trustful of investigators, given the history of abuses of minorities in research, such as in the Tuskegee syphilis study. Community boards should be established to ensure that minority group participants' needs are addressed and that investigators are sensitive to cultural concerns.

Informed Consent

Rooted in the principle of respect for autonomy is the ethical obligation on the part of investigators to obtain informed consent from prospective research subjects. Federal law requires that all federally funded research be approved by external review boards, which have the responsibility to ensure that investigators have obtained informed consent. Virtually all academic institutions require that all research involving human subjects (not just that which is federally funded) secure such approval.

The process of informed consent requires the following: 1) prospective subjects must be provided with information relevant to their decision about participation; 2) they must understand that information; 3) they must provide consent voluntarily; 4) their consent must be documented. Prospective research subjects should be given the following information: a statement that explains that they are being asked to participate in research, not clinical care; the purpose of the research; the reason why they were selected; all procedures that are required, including the location, duration, and frequency of study visits; a description of foreseeable risks; the alternatives to the experimental intervention; a description about how confidentiality will be maintained; whether there will be compensation for injuries resulting from trial participation; information about who to contact for questions or problems; and a declaration that the subjects have both the right not to participate and to cease their participation at any time.

In addition to these general requirements, there are a number of special requirements for informed consent in HIV vaccine trials. If potential subjects are to be screened for HIV infection, they must provide informed consent for this screening. This is in addition to the informed consent that they must provide for participation in the trial. The informed consent process for HIV testing of potential research subjects should include the pre- and post-test counseling, as is required for HIV testing in other contexts, and referrals should be made available for those who test positive for HIV.

Potential subjects of HIV vaccine trials need to be informed of the following:

- The experimental vaccine has not been demonstrated to be effective, and it is unlikely that any HIV vaccine will be completely effective. In addition, the subject may be randomly assigned to a placebo vaccine. Compensation will not be provided for failure of the experimental vaccine to protect research subjects from HIV infection.
- Receipt of the experimental vaccine may complicate the diagnosis of HIV, because vaccinees may falsely test positive on conventional HIV screening tests. The investigators will make sure that more sophisticated tests are available to distinguish vaccine-induced positivity from true HIV infection.
- Trial participants should not be tested for HIV outside of the study, since knowledge of their

assignment could bias the study's results. They should also be told that investigators have made arrangements to provide trial participants with HIV testing, should they wish to be tested.

- Social harms may result from testing positive on an HIV screening test, such as problems with health or life insurance, employment, military service, and travel. All subjects will be provided with documentation of their trial participation.
- Anyone who participates in an HIV vaccine trial risks being socially stigmatized. Investigators also have the ethical obligation throughout the trial to provide subjects with any other information that might influence the subjects' continued willingness to participate in the trial.

Vaccine Trials in Developing Countries

Vaccine trials need to also be conducted in developing countries because AIDS is a devastating problem in these countries, and because the circulating HIV strains differ in each part of the world, so that findings from vaccine trials in developed countries may not be generalizable to developing countries. Local representative should be consulted at all stages of vaccine trials in developing countries.

Questions have been raised about whether it is ethically acceptable to recruit persons who have little control over their ability to avoid exposure to HIV, such as women whose male partners refuse to wear condoms. Such persons, however, may be targeted for vaccination, once an HIV vaccine is approved.

In developing countries, both local and Western requirements for informed consent should be met. In some societies, permission for trial participation is granted by some individual other than the potential research subject, such as a community leader or the female subject's husband. This does not abrogate the responsibility of the investigator to obtain consent from the potential subject as well.

Potential subjects should have an adequate understanding of the study and its risks in order to provide informed consent. If the potential subject is illiterate, investigators must provide information orally, using the local language or dialect.

In some societies, broad understandings about disease causation are completely different than Western understandings. Potential subjects and investigators need not have a completely shared understanding of disease causation, so long as no harmful consequences are likely to ensue.

In developing countries, there may not be available the more sophisticated tests that are necessary to distinguish vaccine-induced positivity from true HIV infection. In that case, investigators have the responsibility to make these sophisticated tests available to trial participants, should they need them.

Investigators also have the ethical obligation to ensure that the trial does not interfere with other health care or public health efforts. Finally, investigators and vaccine sponsors have an ethical obligation to make vaccine available to the communities where the trial was conducted; to ensure that vaccine is available to members of poor communities, they may have to provide it either at cost or free of charge.

Compensation for Adverse Reactions

There is general agreement that, although vaccine sponsors and investigators have no legal obligation to provide compensation to subjects for injuries incurred as a result of participation, there is an ethical obligation to do so. If compensation will not be provided, this should be explained to subjects as part of informed consent.

Incorporating an HIV Vaccine into Clinical Practice

In considering whether to incorporate a partially effective HIV vaccine into clinical practice, one should consider whether the benefits of a partially effective vaccine are outweighed by the harmful increase in risk behaviors that may result in reliance on the vaccine.

Less rigorous standards of informed consent are applied to clinical practice, even though the consequences of vaccination are just as important. There is no requirement for signed written consent, except for certain types of medical interventions, typically surgery and uncommon procedures. For public health interventions, the requirements for informed consent have been limited (although the requirements for informed consent for HIV screening is an exception). The risk that confidentiality will be breached in the clinical setting is greater, because insurance companies and other outside parties have access to patients' medical information.

LIABILITY AND COMPENSATION FOR ADVERSE REACTIONS

Responsibility for Injury and Compensation

With every injury, the question arises whether its financial losses should be shifted to someone else, and if so, to whom. Although the injured person inevitably bears the physical and emotional consequences of injury, financial losses may be either: 1) left where they lie, with the injured person, or 2) transferred, in whole or in part, to someone else by requiring that party to compensate the injured person. There are no other options; the losses do not disappear. The threshold question, therefore, is whether it is necessary or desirable to compensate people who incur particular injuries.

Reasons for Compensating Injuries

Arguments for and against compensating people who are injured have been based on economic, ethical, and social policy grounds. Economic arguments tend to focus on total social costs of injuries and do not necessarily justify compensation for all injuries. Whether society believes it has a moral obligation to ensure that injured persons are compensated may depend upon how society perceives the injured person. In different circumstances, compensation can be: 1) morally required, because not providing it is unjust; 2) morally desirable, but not morally required; or 3) not morally required and possibly unjust. Compensation has also been viewed as a pragmatic means to provide for people in need.

Tort liability for adverse reactions to vaccines has been justified as a reasonable method of compensating people who are injured from specific causes, but more commonly as providing a deterrent to creating products that pose unreasonable risks of injury to others. Compensation and liability for injury appear to be linked in policy discussions of vaccine-related injury because of a general sense that injured vaccine recipients deserve compensation, but that vaccine producers should not be responsible for paying compensation for all the injuries that occur.

Social Goals of Allocating Responsibility for Injury

If injury compensation is desirable or morally required, responsibility for providing compensation may be allocated to the vaccine manufacturer, the person who prescribed or administered the vaccine, the government, or some other party, depending upon the goals to be achieved. Any of the following might serve as goals for allocating responsibility for adverse reactions to a future HIV vaccine to different parties:

1. The development of an effective vaccine to prevent HIV infection or AIDS.
2. The marketing and distribution of an HIV vaccine.
3. The marketing and distribution of an HIV vaccine at a reasonable cost to users.
4. The use of HIV vaccine to prevent HIV infection or progression to AIDS.
5. Compensating persons injured as a result of vaccination with an HIV vaccine.
6. Minimizing the total social cost of HIV vaccine development, marketing, and injury compensation.
7. Minimizing the total costs of HIV infection, including prevention and transaction costs.

None of these goals can be achieved solely by assigning responsibility (or liability) for injuries. Rather, by assigning responsibility to different parties, society may encourage or discourage progress toward specific goals. The choice of system depends upon the goals to be achieved by liability and compensation and how alternative systems affect the achievement of other important goals, such as prevention of disease, deterrence of injury-producing products and activities, and the just distribution of resources.

Systems that satisfy one goal may undermine another. For example, a system that minimized the costs of compensation to vaccine makers might encourage vaccine development, but also reduce incentives to limit potential safety risks. A system that required vaccine makers to provide generous financial assistance might achieve the goal of equitable compensation, but might be too expensive for many companies that society, for other reasons, wishes to attract to vaccine development. If government were to assume responsibility for compensation, the cost to government might conflict with other societal goals to minimize government expenditures or to fund other important programs. Any system that limits compensation to injuries from one specific cause, like an HIV vaccine, raises questions of fairness to people with similar injuries from a different cause. A compensation system limited to persons with adverse reactions to an HIV vaccine invites the question why people living with HIV infection or AIDS or other serious illnesses or injuries should not be compensated as well.

Potential Deterrents to HIV Vaccine Development

Companies in private industry necessarily make choices about what products to make. Because new biologic products require a substantial investment of both time and money, choices may have long-term consequences for a company's product line. Thus, the decision whether or not to invest in the production facilities and equipment, as well as human expertise, necessary to produce an HIV vaccine is a complicated business decision in which companies must weigh the financial risks against the financial rewards.

Scientific Obstacles

The major obstacles to developing an HIV vaccine are scientific. Unfortunately, too little is known about how to produce an immune response in human beings that would protect against infection or development of disease to be assured than an effective vaccine can be produced in the foreseeable future. The National Institute of Allergy and Infectious Disease's decision in June 1994 not to proceed with large Phase III field trials of the leading candidates, for lack of adequate promise of effectiveness, is indicative of the difficulty of surmounting scientific and technical obstacles.

Potential Market for HIV Vaccines

If scientific obstacles can be overcome and an HIV vaccine appears technically feasible, the major factor influencing vaccine development is its expected return on investment or profitability. Profitability depends on the size of the market for an HIV vaccine and the price at which it can be sold. Although the worldwide population at risk for HIV infection numbers in the millions, the relevant market for HIV vaccine sales consists of paying purchasers: individuals who can pay for vaccination either out-of-pocket or with insurance and government agencies that purchase vaccine for distribution to individuals.

Not everyone in the potential market may be willing to buy an HIV vaccine, either because they do not wish to be vaccinated or because they cannot afford the market price. The United States may be the most profitable market for HIV vaccines. The prices at which vaccines can be sold are limited in many foreign countries, either by government regulation or competition from foreign vaccine makers who may receive government subsidies. Many developing countries have severely limited budgets for vaccine purchases and are unable to pay in the hard currency demanded for most transnational sales. A disproportionate number of people at risk for HIV infection are unable to pay for vaccination and are not likely to obtain vaccines without government assistance. Government purchasers, however, may demand substantial discounts from market prices, as the U.S. federal government does for pediatric vaccines, which limits the potential revenues from vaccine sales.

Potential Liability

An HIV vaccine would have considerable appeal to companies that believe that market demand will be strong, the price will not be regulated, and users would pay the price. HIV vaccine development may appear unattractive to companies that perceive any of these factors to be absent. Liability for vaccine-related injuries may affect the profitability of vaccines. If the financial costs of defending and paying expected liability claims are predicted to be too large a proportion of expected revenues, then companies are likely to pursue more profitable lines of product development. Thus, liability may influence decisions about whether to develop a specific product, but it is weighed with other factors. If scientific and financial factors argue against pursuing HIV vaccine development, it is unlikely that changes in liability can outweigh them.

The evidence that liability may deter some companies from developing an HIV vaccine comes from anecdotal reports that several companies interrupted HIV vaccine research or testing and sought immunity from liability before they would consider proceeding. Other factors, however, including scientific problems with the candidate vaccine, inadequate financing, poor market predictions, patent problems, and internal corporate restructuring, may have influenced their decisions about whether to pursue testing. One company later developed a new candidate HIV vaccine. Another proceeded with testing after all. A third attempted to test its preventive vaccine candidate in a single location but enrolled only two subjects before the trial was closed after about a year. The same company actively pursued tests of a therapeutic vaccine. At the same time, other companies developed and tested their candidate vaccines without raising liability concerns. Almost 30 candidate vaccines have been in clinical trials.

In summary, decisions about whether to develop an HIV vaccine, or any other product, entail predictions about its scientific, technical, and financial feasibility and profitability compared with alternative investments. However, the number of companies engaged in HIV vaccine development and testing is encouraging. More companies are engaged in HIV vaccine research than in research for any other type of vaccine. Potential liability may have concerned a few companies, but it is not likely to stop HIV vaccine development.

Tort Liability for Adverse Reactions to Vaccines

Principles of Strict Liability and Negligence

Like manufacturers of all products, vaccine makers are responsible under state law for personal injuries caused by their own negligence or by a defect in their products. Negligence is conduct by the manufacturer that deviates from standards of acceptable conduct adhered to by the ordinary manufacturer of similar products and that causes harm to the product user. Strict liability holds the seller (including a manufacturer) responsible for physical harm caused by a product that is in a defective condition unreasonably dangerous to the user. As a practical matter, most people claiming vaccine-related injury assert several causes of action to avoid losing their claim because of a technical characterization. Thus, the distinction primarily determines the success of a specific cause of action, rather than whether a claim is brought at all.

Product defects

Traditionally, product defects have been divided into three categories: 1) manufacturing defects, 2) design defects, and 3) errors or omissions in warnings accompanying the product. Concern about liability for vaccine-related injuries tends to focus more on strict liability for design defects and inadequate warnings, and less, if at all, on liability for negligence or strict liability for manufacturing errors. Critics of the former two causes of action argue that drug and vaccine makers should be exempt from liability because their products confer significant benefits and their designs and labeling are approved by the FDA. Supporters of liability argue that no exemption should be granted because not all drugs provide significant social benefits, and that manufacturers should be held to at least the same standards as manufacturers of ordinary consumer goods because consumers are vulnerable to undetectable risks in pharmaceutical and biological products. Courts have upheld both positions.

Design defects

An increasing number of states have held that makers of FDA-approved prescription drugs or vaccines are entirely exempt from strict liability for design defects, regardless of the product in question, largely for reasons of public policy. Other states have refused to grant a blanket exemption from liability for all drugs and vaccines. Instead they would exempt only those drugs and vaccines that are shown to be unavoidably unsafe, on a case-by-case basis.

Warnings of risks

In view of the impossibility of creating a risk-free vaccine, manufacturers have an obligation to provide a warning of the vaccine's inherent risks. The history of the legal doctrine and its application in litigated cases parallels that of the doctrine of informed consent to medical care.

A vaccine manufacturer's duty to warn differs from a physician's duty to obtain informed consent for medical care in one respect, however: who is entitled to receive the warning. The doctrine of informed consent to medical care requires a physician to tell his or her patient about the risks and benefits of taking a drug or vaccine, as well as any alternatives. Although the general rule is that all manufacturers have a duty to warn those who use their products of dangers that are not readily apparent, an exception, known as the "learned intermediary rule," permits the maker of prescription drugs or vaccines to warn only the prescribing physician, and not the patient who receives the product. This is because it is the physician—acting as a "learned intermediary" between the manufacturer and the patient—who ordinarily makes the medical judgment that a vaccine is appropriate to recommend for an individual patient.

Thus, vaccine manufacturers do not ordinarily have a duty to provide a warning directly to a vaccine recipient. Similarly, the National Childhood Vaccine Injury Act of 1986 barred any cause of action for a manufacturer's failure to warn a recipient (or a recipient's parent or guardian) about the risks of a childhood vaccine covered by the compensation program. It also created a rebuttable presumption that warnings approved by the FDA are adequate.

Under the learned intermediary rule, a warning is generally not considered inadequate unless the missing information would have caused a physician not to give the vaccine to the patient. A few reported cases have found specific warnings inadequate because they did not mention known risks of a vaccine. In most cases, warnings have been found adequate because they disclosed all reasonably known risks, or manufacturers have not been held liable because the warning would not alter the physician's decision to recommend the vaccine. Physicians have an independent obligation to obtain their patients' informed consent to immunization. This means that physicians are more likely than vaccine manufacturers to be the target of complaints that patients were not informed of vaccine risks.

Types or Uses of HIV Vaccines

The above principles of liability apply to manufacturers of all vaccines, regardless of whether they are preventive (intended to prevent) or therapeutic (intended to treat or cure infection or disease), and regardless of whether the vaccines are experimental (investigational) or approved and licensed. The likelihood of adverse reactions and liability claims occurring may differ, however, depending upon the way in which a vaccine is used.

Investigational Vaccines

The potential liability for adverse reactions to investigational preventive vaccines is less than that for marketed vaccines. Although the legal basis for liability is the same in both cases, both the likelihood of claims and the probability that any such claims would succeed in practice is far lower with respect to investigational vaccines than with marketed vaccines. Historically, there have been no reported product liability cases involving vaccine research, probably because there has been a very low incidence of injury among research subjects in general. Claims of defective design are also minimized, if not precluded entirely, by the fact that the research is being conducted to find out whether the vaccine works and whether it has dangerous side effects.

Therapeutic Vaccines

Therapeutic HIV vaccines, which are used to treat people who are already infected with HIV, are more comparable to drugs than to preventive vaccines. Patients who take therapeutic vaccines may be willing to accept accompanying risks in order to receive any benefit the therapeutic vaccine might afford. Adverse reactions may be difficult to distinguish from other symptoms arising from existing illness. The potential for damages is also limited because of the perceived limited life expectancy of people with AIDS. Perhaps for these reasons, there has been little concern about liability for adverse reactions to therapeutic vaccines.

Potential Adverse Reactions to HIV Vaccines

In the absence of any approved HIV vaccine, predictions about adverse reactions are based on somewhat limited experience with the candidate vaccines in clinical trials, laboratory research, and theoretical hypotheses. The following are the most commonly mentioned hypotheses.

Low Levels of Effectiveness

There has been speculation among researchers that some candidate HIV vaccines now in clinical trials may ultimately prove effective in only a small percentage of the vaccinated population. If the vaccinated population is at risk for HIV infection, as anticipated, then some proportion may become infected after taking a vaccine of limited efficacy, even if the vaccine is not defective. Claims based on low levels (or lack) of effectiveness have not been brought against existing vaccines. The likelihood of success of a claim of lack of effectiveness of an HIV vaccine is speculative, but probably small as long as those who take the vaccine are warned of its limited efficacy and advised to take precautions against exposure to HIV infection.

Enhanced Susceptibility to Infection or Disease Progression

Researchers have theorized that candidate vaccines might have the potential to increase one's susceptibility to infection with HIV or other organisms, or to increase the rate of disease progression in people who become infected with HIV in spite of vaccination. Both hypotheses raise the possibility of a claim for defective design if they are not investigated, or a claim for inadequate warning if they are not disclosed. The likelihood of a successful claim would depend upon whether the manufacturer knew or should have known that the vaccine was capable of causing the reaction, and whether the plaintiff could prove that the vaccine did cause the reaction in his or her case.

Development of Cancer

There has been speculation that, because HIV is a retrovirus, an HIV vaccine might cause cancer many years after vaccination. Although a manufacturer is not liable for injuries caused by unforeseeable dangers in its products, there may be some question as to whether a manufacturer adequately investigated a suggested risk. Given the need for an HIV vaccine, it appears unlikely that a manufacturer would be held responsible for distributing a vaccine with a risk that could not be verified at the time it was released.

Vaccine-Induced HIV Infection

Non-recombinant vaccines that use killed, inactivated, or attenuated virus raise the possibility that the manufacturing process might inadvertently fail to remove or render harmless part of the virus that could actively infect a person. Although claims of vaccine manufacturing errors have been rare in the past, the consequences of a batch of vaccine accidentally escaping inactivation are sufficiently serious to make this type vaccine unappealing to many vaccine makers. However, companies may not wish to pursue a type of vaccine that might produce HIV infection, regardless of exposure to liability, especially if they believe that they cannot eliminate the risk of manufacturing error.

Social Harms

HIV vaccination may pose risks of social harm that are not adverse reactions to the vaccine itself. People who receive HIV vaccines may be especially vulnerable to denials of health or life insurance or permission to travel abroad, loss of employment or housing, segregation in institutions, or rejection by family and friends. Most such harms result from lawful conduct for which the vaccine recipient would have no legal recourse. Manufacturers are not ordinarily responsible for the bigotry of others. Physicians who administer HIV vaccines may be the more likely target for any claim that a vaccine recipient was not adequately warned about possible discrimination.

Susceptibility of HIV Vaccines to Liability Claims

Preventive vaccines may be more susceptible to claims of liability than most drugs and biologics, primarily because they are used in large numbers of healthy people. As with drugs, the majority of claims have affected only a few vaccines, and the number of reported cases that impose liability on the vaccine maker is very small. Thus, although the probability of *claims* of liability may be higher than that for drugs, the probability of actual *liability* is quite low.

Plaintiffs rarely succeed on a claim of design defect, probably because of the difficulty of proving that a safer, equally effective vaccine could have replaced a vaccine that was approved by the FDA. Although most states still permit claims that a vaccine was defectively designed, only one vaccine (Quadrigen) has been found to have a defective design (in a warranty, not product liability, action). No reported court decision after 1969 has held a vaccine maker liable for a design defect.

Few courts have found a vaccine maker liable for an inadequate warning of risks. More extensive and sophisticated warning statements may have increased manufacturers' protection against such liability. In addition, vaccine makers are largely exempt from any duty to warn vaccine recipients themselves of vaccine risks. Instead, manufacturers have a duty to warn the prescribing physician, who bears the responsibility for disclosing vaccine risks to patients. Thus, physicians may now be more vulnerable to claims (of lack of informed consent) than vaccine makers.

Fear of liability for adverse reactions to vaccines may have been based on a perception in the 1970s and early 1980s that courts were expanding the grounds for product liability. That expansion appears to have halted, although it cannot be assumed that it would never recur. Since liability itself is so rarely imposed, the fear of liability may be more accurately described as fear of having to litigate at all. This is understandable, given the time and expense of pursuing and defending claims. Complaints about the litigation process, however, are not limited to cases involving HIV vaccines (there have been none). Concerns about the efficiency and fairness of tort litigation as a means of resolving disputes are generic. This does not mean that an alternative means of allocating responsibility for injury and compensation is not warranted for other reasons. It does mean that any alternative that is intended to remedy tort litigation's inefficiencies would have application beyond HIV vaccines.

Alternative Compensation Options

The following outlines several major options for allocating responsibility for compensating adverse reactions to HIV vaccines.

Tort Liability Reform

Tort liability imposes legal responsibility for compensating injuries. Tort reform proposals seek to change the substantive grounds for liability, the procedures or evidence used in litigation, or the amount of compensation payable. Any single reform can only be unidirectional: it either increases or decreases the opportunity for a plaintiff to bring or succeed on a claim.

Currently, most tort reform proposals seek to limit the liability of potential defendants. By themselves, limitations on liability are cost control measures, not compensation mechanisms. Such limitations are best suited to circumstances in which the primary goal is to save potential defendants money and where providing compensation to those who would not qualify under the reform is not relevant or desirable.

Reforms expanding plaintiffs' opportunities to recover compensation would further a goal of increased compensation, but are likely to increase total costs. Reforms such as scheduling compensation are intended to make compensation more consistent across different claimants with similar injuries, without necessarily altering the grounds for recovery.

Other reforms are intended to reduce the time and expense of litigation and the possibility of inconsistent results, without changing the bases for liability. Similar proposals to reform the law of medical malpractice and product liability have been the subject of considerable debate. If considered for HIV vaccines, they may have to be considered for other types of injuries.

Voluntary Contractual Arrangements

Private companies and individuals are free to reduce the time and expense of resolving claims by voluntarily agreeing to provide compensation without the necessity of litigation or legislation. The voluntary contract model, exemplified by the Moore-Gephardt bill introduced in Congress (99th Congress, 1st Session, 1985) but never passed, would permit a vaccine maker or administering physician to agree, at the time of vaccination, to pay the vaccine recipient compensation for out-of-pocket expenses promptly if an adverse reaction occurred. Such contracts may encourage compensation even in cases in which the vaccine recipient would have no recourse in tort law. They may work reasonably well in circumstances in which the payor and payee know each other and where the cause of injury is relatively easy to establish. Neither circumstance is likely to apply to new HIV vaccines. The process of deciding how much, if any, compensation to offer resembles the process of settling a claim in litigation, and may be equally difficult in many cases.

Government-Funded Insurance Arrangements

Government-funded excess insurance

Government-financed insurance programs can fund compensation for injuries. Government might purchase private excess insurance or reinsurance or use its own revenues to finance compensation awards that exceed a predetermined amount. This would limit the amount of financial exposure private companies face from liability payments, and lower premiums for basic liability insurance. The primary disadvantage of government-funded excess insurance is the difficulty of estimating the amount of excess insurance needed for a new vaccine, and the amount of liability expenditures that should be considered excessive for manufacturers. Reinsurance systems do not alter the legal bases for liability and would not remedy concerns about inefficiencies of tort litigation and inconsistent awards. In addition, an excess insurance program might set a precedent for government reinsurance of liability expenses for other tort claims, from medical malpractice to automobile accidents.

Government-funded disability insurance

Vaccine-related injuries could be compensated through government disability insurance programs. For example, the Social Security program could be amended to specifically include coverage of injuries resulting from HIV vaccines. A more general expansion of disability insurance to cover injuries regardless of cause would be more in keeping with the general function of Social Security, which already covers AIDS-related disability. A general disability insurance program avoids hard questions of horizontal justice about why injuries resulting from one cause should be compensated while others are not. The cost of such a program may require new government revenues, but, because the costs of disability for the entire national population are relatively consistent over time, they are more predictable than the costs of compensating injuries caused by new HIV vaccines.

If the health care system is reformed to ensure universal coverage, a significant expense of injury would be covered outside the disability insurance program. In the absence of universal insurance coverage, continued pressure for financial assistance to pay for medical care may be expected.

Public No-Fault Compensation Systems

Federal and state governments have created several publicly administered injury compensation programs, such as state workers compensation programs, the Federal Black Lung Benefits Act, the Radiation Exposure Compensation Act, Virginia and Florida's Birth-Related Neurological Injury Compensation acts, and the National Vaccine Injury Compensation Program.

Most such programs provide compensation on a no-fault basis for specific injuries from specific causes. As long as the injury is demonstrated to result from the specified cause, compensation is granted without the need to prove negligence or legal responsibility for the injury. Parties that might be liable for the injury typically need not participate in the claims determination process. Administrative costs can be less than those of litigation. Compensation can be funded from different sources to achieve different goals.

No-fault compensation programs have the disadvantage of treating one group of people differently from others with similar injuries or needs. Those who do not qualify for compensation may object to such special treatment or demand equivalent treatment themselves as a matter of horizontal justice. The more programs that exist for specific causes, the more difficult it becomes to defend excluding the remaining injuries from a no-fault system.

No-fault systems that are limited to injuries from a specific cause, like adverse reactions to vaccines, require proving that an injury resulted from that specific cause. Determining causation is often difficult, time-consuming, and expensive, especially where the scientific evidence is uncertain or conflicting. Yet no-fault systems are often recommended in order to provide desired compensation in circumstances where causation is unclear or controversial. Thus, many of the complexities that make litigation frustrating and expensive are often necessarily part of cause-based, no-fault compensation proceedings.

No-fault compensation systems may sometimes generate more, rather than less, cost, depending upon the level of compensation to be awarded and the scope of eligibility for compensation. No-fault systems typically compensate more people than would recover compensation (or even file a claim) in tort law. In the absence of reliable estimates of the number and type of compensable injuries, it may be difficult to predict system costs.

The National Vaccine Injury Compensation Program may provide a model for compensating adverse reactions to HIV vaccines. A no-fault system funded by federal revenues (for administration) and surtaxes on vaccines (for compensation), it provides compensation for adverse reactions that are caused by specific vaccines. Although the program was originally intended to cover only vaccines required by state law for children before they enter school or day care, it has been amended to permit coverage of vaccines that are recommended for children. Adding HIV vaccines to the program would expand its scope beyond children's vaccines, but it would also avoid the need for creating a new administrative structure to provide compensation.

Table 1-1 lists the basic elements of a no-fault compensation program and key questions that must be answered in constructing a suitable system.

Alternative Incentives for HIV Vaccine Development

By themselves, compensation programs cannot guarantee that any vaccine is developed. If HIV vaccines are not sufficiently attractive to private industry for reasons of the difficulty and expense of research compared with the expected financial

TABLE 1-1: ELEMENTS OF A COMPENSATION PROGRAM

Eligibility
Who should be eligible for compensation?
U.S. citizens, U.S. residents, nonresidents?
What, if any, time period should be the limit for bringing claims?

Covered vaccines
Should the program cover all or only some vaccines? Investigational vaccines?

Compensable injuries
Should all injuries be covered, or only injuries at a minimum level of severity (in either physical or financial terms)?
Should injuries include HIV infection? Social harms?

Causation
How is causation to be determined?
Is causation understood well enough to permit a list of compensable injuries?
Who has the burden of proving causation?
What kind of evidence should be required to prove causation?

Compensation benefits
Is compensation to be calculated on the basis of actual losses, a fixed schedule of injuries, a fixed amount per person or injury, or some other basis?
Which, if any, actual expenses will be compensated?

Payment mechanisms
Should payment of compensation be made in a lump sum, periodic payments, by an annuity providing periodic income, or a health insurance policy providing coverage for medical expenses?

Decisionmaking athority and procedures
What entity is authorized to make decisions about eligibility and compensation?
Should any third party be required or permitted to participate in the decisionmaking process?
What, if any, type of review or appeal should be available?

Relationship to tort law
Should the compensation system be an optional alternative to the tort system or the exclusive source of compensation for claimants?
Should people who have filed claims in court be eligible for compensation?
If the program ceases operation or is repealed, what, if any, rights should the claimants have?

Financing
What should be the source of funding for the compensation and administration? Government revenues? Taxes on products or manufacturers? Private insurance?

Period of operation
Should the program's continuance be contingent upon future events, such as the development of a vaccine, the sale of a vaccine at a specified price, the disposition of a maximum number of claims, adequate funding or some other event?

SOURCE: Office of Technology Assessment, 1995.

return, then other initiatives will be necessary to encourage vaccine development. Among the types of initiatives that might foster increased attention to HIV vaccine development are:

- Tax incentives for investment in vaccine development.
- Mechanisms for increased collaboration and in- formation-sharing among vaccine researchers to increase productivity and expedite research.
- Simplification of collaborative arrangements between government and industry researchers.
- Expanded access to preclinical nonhuman animal models for testing investigational vaccines.
- Expedited review by the FDA of applications for vaccine licensing.

- International harmonization of national vaccine licensing standards.
- Guaranteed purchase of vaccine supplies by government.
- Expanded patent protection for approved vaccines.
- National coordination of vaccine research and distribution policies.
- Creation of a National Vaccine Authority to foster research and product development by providing grants, facilities, and consultation, as well as arranging procurement contracts.

Social goals for HIV vaccines go beyond mere development and marketing of a vaccine. The vaccines developed should be reasonably safe and effective to prevent the continued expansion of a devastating epidemic. FDA regulation is one mechanism to assess the safety and effectiveness of vaccines. One of tort law's objectives is to provide additional incentives to produce safe and effective products. Whatever one's view of the FDA or tort law's effectiveness in this respect, some mechanism to ensure adequate quality in vaccines is necessary. In addition, effective mechanisms for distributing and encouraging the use of vaccines, especially by those unable to buy them, will be required if the benefit of HIV vaccines is to be realized.

Potential for Adverse Reactions from HIV Vaccines 2

The potential safety problems in the development and introduction of a vaccine for the prevention of HIV, type 1 (HIV-1) infection are addressed in this chapter.[1] Ethical, social science, and legal issues are presented more fully in chapters 3 and 4.

This chapter begins with a brief review of the biological basis for development of a vaccine to prevent AIDS. Next, principles underlying the preparation of a protective vaccine are reviewed, including observations on the unprecedented hurdles posed by HIV infection compared with successful vaccines developed in the past. This chapter also discusses the biological basis for safety concerns and why the nature, frequency, and severity of adverse reactions with HIV vaccines cannot be predicted at this point. In addition to adverse events that may be associated with *biological* mechanisms of injury, important adverse *social* consequences, termed "social harms," are addressed here and in chapters 3 and 4.

This chapter has been written for a diverse target audience, including legislators, policymakers, lawyers, ethicists, social scientists, and the AIDS community, in addition to biological scientists. Experts in the several disciplines will recognize the abbreviated and simplified approach in some areas. A more

by
David T. Karzon
Vanderbilt University Medical Center
Nashville, TN

[1] In this background paper, reference to HIV will refer to human immunodeficiency virus, type 1 (HIV-1), unless otherwise noted. HIV-1 has been found throughout the world. Human immunodeficiency virus, type 2 (HIV-2) is found in West Africa and is in the same retrovirus family as HIV-1. Infection with either HIV-1 or HIV-2 can lead to the development of AIDS.

technical discussion of the theory and proposed mechanisms of HIV vaccine risks are presented in appendix A.[2]

ROLE OF VACCINES IN THE CONTROL OF INFECTIOUS DISEASE

Options for the Control of Infectious Diseases

There are three major options for controlling HIV infection: 1) halt transfer of virus from person to person through education and behavioral changes; 2) treat HIV-infected individuals with therapeutic drugs after infection is recognized; 3) prevent disease through introduction of "prophylactic" HIV vaccines[3] that prevent the establishment of infection. The possible uses of an HIV vaccine are described in box 2-1. The magnitude of the medical, social, and political impact of the AIDS epidemic will, for the foreseeable future, require continued intensive efforts using all three options.

Measures to control HIV infection have met formidable difficulties, and infection is spreading uncontrollably around the globe. Prevention of viral transfer by limiting risk behavior and the extensive research directed at development of drug treatments have had limited success (2). Treatment of infected pregnant women with the antiviral drug zidovudine (AZT) has decreased transmission of HIV infection to newborns, a significant achievement.

Vaccines capable of preventing infectious diseases are generally regarded as the most successful instrument of cost-effective, humane health care. Vaccines are credited with the global elimination of smallpox and, more recently, elimination of poliomyelitis from the Americas (26)—(105). In addition, the childhood vaccines, measles, mumps, and rubella (MMR), Haemophilus influenza type B (HIB), and diphtheria, tetanus, and pertussis (DTP)—have markedly reduced the number of cases and deaths from infectious diseases. More widespread use of influenza, pneumococcus, and hepatitis B virus (HBV) vaccines, in addition to the availability of hepatitis A virus (HAV) and varicella (chickenpox) vaccines, will add significantly to reduction of morbidity and mortality from infectious diseases. The historical success of conventional vaccines in preventing and even eradicating disease has stimulated an extensive quest for a safe and effective preventive HIV vaccine. This chapter will review the progress toward development of an HIV vaccine through 1994.

How a Vaccine Works

HIV is the most intensively studied virus of all time. Details of its molecular structure, replication strategies,[4] host-cell interactions,[5] and pathology are known. Despite a decade of research and advances in biotechnology, a successful HIV vaccine lies at least several years ahead. Most currently licensed vaccines for infectious diseases were developed when much less was known about the target microbe and its infection. The reasons an HIV vaccine has been so difficult to prepare, the unique features of the virus that elude vaccine control, and the implications for possible safety problems from an HIV vaccine will are discussed below.

Stated in its simplest form, a viral vaccine consists of a microorganism (such as a virus or-

---

[2] Selected review articles are noted in the references. However, references are also cited in the text insofar as they may be linked to design and outcome of clinical trials of HIV vaccines.

[3] This background paper will focus on prophylactic HIV vaccines, and not on therapeutic HIV vaccines. Prophylactic vaccines prevent infection or disease in uninfected individuals (so-called classic prophylaxis) or reduce their infectivity should the vaccinated individual subsequently become infected. Therapeutic vaccines prevent or reduce disease progression in infected individuals, or reduce disease transmission to persons who come in contact with infected individuals.

[4] The viral genome is reproduced in a process called *replication*.

[5] In microbiology, the *host* refers to the organism or cells that are being infected by the microorganism.

BOX 2-1: The Spectrum of Possible Strategies for Use of HIV Vaccines

HIV vaccines have been proposed for prevention of HIV infection (classic prophylaxis) and for therapy of HIV infection (as a form of post-infection immunotherapy). HIV vaccines have also been advocated as a tool to reduce the infectivity of HIV-infected individuals (i.e., to reduce the risk of transmission of HIV from infected vaccinees to their contacts or offspring). These approaches have been reviewed previously (9, 13, 29, 80) and are briefly outlined below.

1. *Classic Prophylaxis.* The classic prophylactic vaccination strategy requires a high rate of vaccination in the general population at childhood or adolescence, yielding individual immunity as well as "herd immunity" (inhibited spread of infection through the population) if a sufficient percentage of the general population is immunized. Examples of successful classic prophylactic vaccination strategies include the worldwide smallpox vaccination program and, in the Unites States, the mandatory childhood vaccination program.

2. *Targeted prophylactic vaccination.* Another well-established strategy is to prevent infection by targeting "at-risk" populations for vaccination. An example of this prophylactic vaccination strategy is the targeting of tropical disease vaccines, such as yellow fever, to travelers.

3. *Immediate post-exposure vaccination.* Falling between prophylaxis and treatment is the concept of vaccination immediately after exposure to an infectious pathogen to prevent establishment of permanent infection. Rabies vaccine, in which anti-rabies immunoglobulins are administered immediately following exposure to rabies virus, is a model for this vaccination strategy.

An immediate post-exposure HIV vaccine would be most useful in cases of accidental exposures to HIV, such as following a needle-stick injury. A clinical trial of such a vaccine, however, would be unlikely to yield significant results due to the low rate of HIV infection following needle sticks or other accidental exposures (72).

4. *Therapeutic vaccination.* Therapeutic vaccination to prevent disease progression in an infected individual has been proposed for several pathogens and has a long history as a concept (13). However, there are few examples of the successful application of this vaccination strategy for any infectious disease, with a recent report of decreased genital herpes lesions following vaccination with herpes glycoprotein a noteworthy exception (93).

Until recently, there has been little evidence that envelope-based HIV vaccines (77) or whole inactivated HIV vaccines (81) have had therapeutic benefits in HIV-infected individuals. However, recent results from a Phase II trial of a whole inactivated envelope depleted virus vaccine in HIV-infected individuals suggests the possibility of an antiviral effect from the vaccine (94).

Likewise, there are no examples of a vaccine that can prevent disease transmission from infected vaccinees to susceptible contacts. But passive transfer of antibodies to infected pregnant women has been discussed as a potential means for reducing maternal-fetal transmission of several infectious agents, including HIV.

There has been discussion of development of a therapeutic vaccine for HIV-infected women of childbearing age to prevent infection of their offspring, since there is a 15 to 50 percent probability of transmission of HIV infection from untreated infected mothers to their newborns. Recently, however, a clinical trial showed that the antiviral drug AZT (zidovudine), when given to infected mothers during pregnancy, was able to reduce the rate of maternal-fetal HIV transmission from 24 to 8 percent (Pediatric ACTG Protocol 076). Thus, the efficacy of AZT in reducing maternal-fetal HIV transmission is the standard against which the efficacy of any vaccine to reduce maternal-fetal transmission will be compared.

(continued)

BOX 2-1: The Spectrum of Possible Strategies for Use of HIV Vaccines (Cont'd.)

5. *Vaccines to reduce infectivity.* Another strategy involves the vaccination of uninfected members of high risk groups to reduce their infectivity in the event of subsequent infection; in this case, the vaccine is not expected to actually prevent chronic infection in subsequently exposed individuals, but to decrease their infectivity by reducing the rate of viral replication. Presumably, the reduction in the rate of viral replication would probably be accompanied by a decreased rate of disease progression, and so this vaccination strategy represents a variant of the classic prophylactic vaccination strategy. There are no examples of human vaccines that follow this strategy, but an analogous situation occurs naturally in some diseases (e.g., tuberculosis, Hepatitis B infection), where persistently infected individuals that mount a strong immune responses have been shown to have decreased infectivity. This decreased infectivity has also been shown to occur in vaccinated monkeys that are infected with SIV (85, 86). HIV vaccines that do not clear all virus (achieve "sterilizing immunity") may also reduce infectivity, although this has not been demonstrated.

This vaccination strategy has not yet received much attention from experts in the field of HIV vaccine research. Investigators would have difficulty demonstrating the efficacy of a vaccine to reduce infectivity because it would require a clinical trial that followed not only a large number of high-risk vaccine and placebo recipients, but the recipients' contacts as well.[1] In addition, conclusions about the effect of the vaccine on the transmissibility of infection could only be drawn from observation of incidence of HIV infection among those persons whose only risk for HIV infection is from contact with a vaccine trial participant (e.g., the vaccinee's offspring or monogamous sexual partners). Nevertheless, this may be the vaccination strategy that has the greatest chance of success in controlling the AIDS epidemic in the foreseeable future. Therefore, designing the necessary studies to test the efficacy of vaccines to reduce infectivity is important.

The efficacy of a vaccine to reduce infectivity could be tested, for example, in a clinical trial involving intercity truckers in India. These truckers are at high risk for HIV infection due to their frequent contact with female sex workers. The wives of these truckers, however, tend to be monogamous. Such a trial would require investigators to monitor incidence of HIV infection not only in the truckers participating in the trial, but in their wives as well. Another way to test this strategy would be to vaccinate uninfected women of child-bearing age who are at high risk of acquiring HIV, and then monitor HIV infection incidence in these women and their offspring.

The efficacy of this vaccine in reducing the infectivity of subsequently infected individuals may also be approximated by testing the vaccine in individuals that are already infected with HIV. Such a trial would require enrollment of far fewer participants. To demonstrate the efficacy of such a vaccine in reducing infectivity, however, one would still need to follow up the vaccinees' monogamous sexual contacts. Furthermore, a vaccine may not be nearly as effective in reducing infectivity when given after infection as it is when given before infection.

SOURCE: David Schwartz, "Analysis of 'Worst Case Scenarios' for Theoretical Risks Associated with Experimental HIV Vaccines," unpublished contractor report prepared for the Office of Technology Assessment, U.S. Congress, Washington, DC, July 7, 1994.

---

[1] For example, assuming a 5-percent annual incidence of HIV infection in the high-risk target population, and 5-percent annual transmission from this population to their monogamous sexual partners, there would be a 0.25 percent annual incidence of HIV infection among the sexual partners. More than 40,000 participants from the high-risk target population would be required for a Phase III efficacy trial of a vaccine using this strategy.

TABLE 2-1: Immune Response Elements		
Type of Immune response	**Elements**	**Function of elements**
Humoral immunity	Antibody produced by B lymphocytes	Inactivates free virus
Cellular immunity	T lymphocytes CD4+ CD8+	Helper cells Cytotoxic lymphocytes
	Macrophages	Immune intermediary cells
Mucosal immunity	Antibody plus immune cells	Blocks mucosal invasion

SOURCE: Office of Technology Assessment, 1995.

bacteria) or its components, in a safe form, designed to protect against future disease. Administration of a vaccine stimulates the body's immune system to generate protective defenses specifically directed against the microorganism. This vaccine-induced protective immune response is rapidly restimulated when a vaccinated individual is subsequently exposed to the microorganism. Thus, the vaccine "primes" the immune system to respond to a microorganism, so that upon exposure to that microorganism, spread of the microorganism through the body is dampened before it can cause disease (51). This is the mechanism by which traditional vaccines protect against establishment of infection.

Immune Response Elements

Selection of starting material for a vaccine begins with identification of the important sites on the microorganism that stimulate the immune system. These sites are known as *antigens*, which are usually composed of proteins, which are long chains of amino acids.[6] The term *epitope* describes the specific amino acid sequence and configuration of the antigenic protein. Epitopes are the functional sites that are recognized by the body's immune defense system, and that induce the body to produce an immune response. These epitopes are incorporated in various forms into the vaccine.

Knowledge of the nature of the elements of the immune system and how each element functions is important in understanding how a new vaccine is designed. The immune system can be thought of as having three major response elements: 1) *humoral immunity*, the immune response to foreign substances from antibody[7] circulating in the blood; 2) *cellular immunity*,[8] immune response from a network of immune white cells in the blood and tissues, and 3) *mucosal immunity*, a specialized system of antibody and immune cells located at the smooth, moist mucous membranes (mucosa) that cover-inner body surfaces, including the routes of sexual transmission of HIV: the vagina, anus, and penile urethra (table 1-1).

Each of the three immune response elements plays a unique role and each may be stimulated differentially by altering the design of the vaccine or its method of administration (1, 62, 63). One type of immune white cell, the B lymphocyte, produces antibody. Each antibody is antigen-specif-

[6] Proteins are composed of long chains of amino acids. A protein's shape, properties, and biological functions are determined in part by the specific sequence of its constituent amino acids. *Peptides* are short amino acids.

[7] Antibodies are blood proteins produced in B lymphocytes, a type of white blood cell, in response to the introduction of a specific antigen (e.g., an invading virus, incompatible red blood cells, inhaled pollen grains, or foreign tissue grafts). Once produced, the antibody has the ability to combine with the specific antigen that stimulated antibody production, and thereby render the antigen harmless, a process called neutralization.

[8] Cellular immunity is also called *cell-mediated* immunity.

TABLE 2-2: Design of Contemporary Viral Vaccines

Preparation	Vaccine
Live attenuated virus	Adenovirus Measles Mumps Polio Rubella Smallpox (vaccinia)[b] Varicella[a] Yellow Fever
Inactivated whole virus	Hepatitis A[a] Japanese Encephalitis Polio Rabies
Protein subunit (recombinant)	Hepatitis B
Protein subunit (purified)	Influenza

[a] Under review for licensure.
[b] No longer recommended; smallpox globally eradicated.

SOURCE: Office of Technology Assessment, 1995.

ic and can bind and inactivate ("neutralize") virus particles that are free in the circulation but cannot inactivate virus located inside of infected cells. Another type of white cell, the T lymphocyte, participates in cellular immunity. Subtypes of T lymphocytes include CD4+ (helper T) lymphocytes and CD8+ (cytotoxic T) lymphocytes. Cytotoxic T lymphocytes can kill cells undergoing active viral infection. CD4+ (T helper) lymphocytes are necessary for the development of mature functional lymphocytes. A third type of immune white cell, the macrophage, is an important intermediary in the development of the immune response.

Historically Successful Vaccines

Review of the design of contemporary viral vaccines provides background for understanding the strategies available for the design of an HIV vaccine. Contemporary viral vaccines, in fact, follow only a few basic designs (table 2-2). Eight are live attenuated (weakened) vaccines, four are inactivated (killed) whole virus vaccines, and two are protein subunit vaccines. Hepatitis B is the sole vaccine prepared using recombinant biotechnology (gene splicing) techniques. Both attenuated and inactivated poliovirus vaccines are available. Most successful viral vaccines are live attenuated and, less frequently, inactivated whole-virus products.

A common feature of vaccines currently in use is their ability to induce durable circulating antibody, usually persisting for many years. A low level of antibody directed against the virus may be sufficient for protection against establishment of viral infection. For some viruses, such as measles virus, the rapid immune recall due to vaccine priming may be sufficient to protect against infection; for protection against other viruses, such as influenza virus, a preexisting threshold level of virus-specific antibody is necessary. For other vaccines, a vaccine-induced cytotoxic T lymphocyte response may also participate in protection (e.g., varicella).

Currently used vaccines are capable of preventing the initial viral infection from becoming established and progressing to *disease*; they are not capable of preventing the initial viral *infection*. This distinction is important to understanding the requirements for an effective HIV vaccine. Live attenuated vaccines, composed of live virus that has been altered to make it incapable of producing disease, most closely reproduce the immune state seen after natural infection. Attenuated vaccines may induce, in addition to circulating antibody, a

TABLE 2-3: HIV Structural Elements and Their Function

Structure	Viral Function	Immune Significance
Envelope proteins	Cell attachment and penetration	Induce antibody
gp160	Precursor of gp120, gp41	
gp120	External protein	
gp41	Membrane anchor	
Internal proteins		Important CTL sites
gag	Structural, viral assembly	
pol	Facilitates replication	
Auxiliary proteins (6) e.g., *nef*	Regulate level of virus activity	Selective deletion produces attenuated virus vaccine
RNA genome	Genetic code for all viral proteins (virus has a latent DNA stage in host chromosome)	Use of infectious DNA as vaccine

KEY: CTL = Cytotxic T lymphocytes.

SOURCE: Office of Technology Assessment, 1995.

cytotoxic T lymphocyte response and mucosal immunity. Further, unlike nonreplicating vaccines, live attenuated vaccines generally do not require multiple primary and booster doses. In practice, before the era of modern biotechnology, inactivated whole virus and live attenuated viruses were usually tried empirically, and live attenuated vaccines were preferred as a more reliable source of long-term protection.

Historically Unsuccessful Vaccines

The number of infectious agents for which we have failed to develop a satisfactory vaccine, even those targeted as high priority (49), is far greater than the number for which we have been successful. Examples of viruses for which we have failed to develop a vaccine include the viruses herpes simplex, infectious mononucleosis, cytomegalovirus, respiratory syncytial virus, and rotavirus; vaccines against many sexually transmitted disease agents, such as syphilis and gonorrhea; vaccines against parasitic diseases, such as malaria and schistosomiases; and vaccines against numerous bacterial infections, including tuberculosis. Individually, these infections are characterized by such features as chronic persistence of the organism, restriction of the organism to mucosal sites, genetic variability of the organisms, and lack of spontaneous recovery from the disease that they cause. Vaccines that have been successful are more likely to be directed against acute, self-limiting systemic[9] infections, where immune responses can readily clear residual organisms.

HIV IS A UNIQUE VIRUS

HIV Structure: Starting Point for Vaccine Design

A brief description of HIV structural elements and their function will facilitate later discussion. The virus is bounded by a membrane with the gp160 protein projecting through the membrane surface or envelope (see table 2-3 and Figure 2-1). The envelope gp160 protein is composed of, and is precursor to, the gp120 and gp41 envelope proteins.[10] The envelope protein gp120 bears the V3

[9] Systemic infections involve the whole body, in contrast to localized infections, which may involve one specific organ or body part.

[10] The "gp" refers to its composition of glycoproteins (proteins bound with sugars), and the numbers 160, 120, and 41 refer to a measure of each glycoprotein's weight.

THE POPULATION COUNCIL

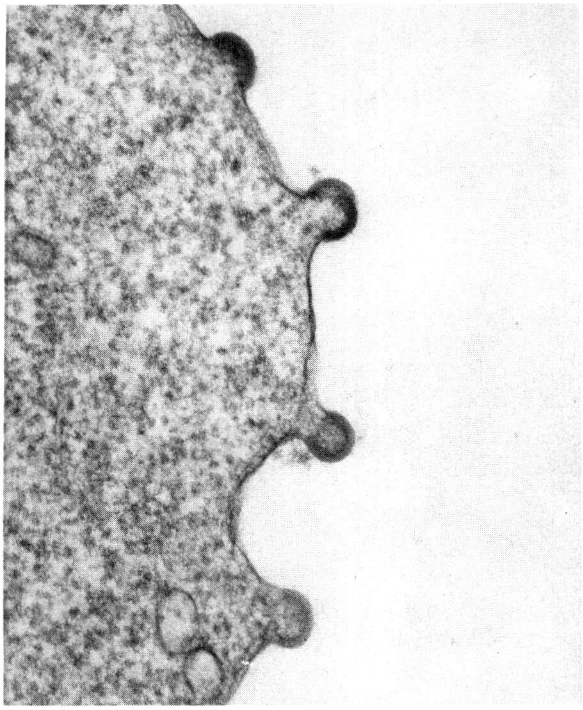

Electron micrograph of HIV virions budding from an infected cell.

THE POPULATION COUNCIL

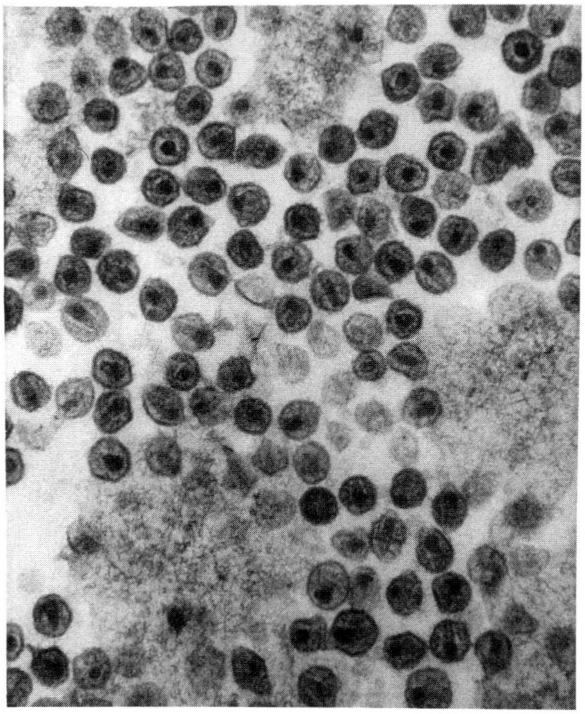

Electron micrograph of free HIV virions.

loop, which is the site of attachment of the human immunodeficiency virus to its receptor on the surface of the CD4+ lymphocyte. The V3 loop of the gp120 protein is also the site for induction of neutralizing antibody (antibody that specifically binds to, or "neutralizes," the antigen); antibody to gp120 can block HIV from entering and propagating in cells.

The viral membrane encloses two major internal components, the *gag* and *pol* proteins, and several small auxiliary proteins that control the rate of virus replication[11] (see figure 2-1). The genetic information, or genome, of HIV is composed of ribonucleic acid (RNA); by contrast, the human genome (and that of most other species) is composed of deoxyribonucleic acid (DNA). The RNA genome of HIV is associated with the internal proteins. Epitopes on the gp120 and *gag* proteins, as well as those on other internal proteins, can induce cytotoxic T lymphocyte responses necessary for cellular immunity (4).

Properties of HIV That Handicap Vaccine Development

Because of several unique features of HIV, the model for an effective HIV vaccine is much more complicated than the model for contemporary vaccines. HIV is endowed with an unusual set of capacities that enable it to evade or manipulate normal immune defenses (table 2-4). These capacities are listed below:

1. HIV is capable of evading immune surveillance by integrating its genome into the genome of infected cells. During replication, the human immunodeficiency virus undergoes a stage where its RNA genome is transcribed into DNA by a process called "reverse transcription." As a necessary part of its life cycle inside

[11] These small auxiliary proteins are called *regulatory* or *accessory* proteins.

FIGURE 2-1: Morphology of HIV-1 and Diagram of the Structural Relation of Major Viral Proteins

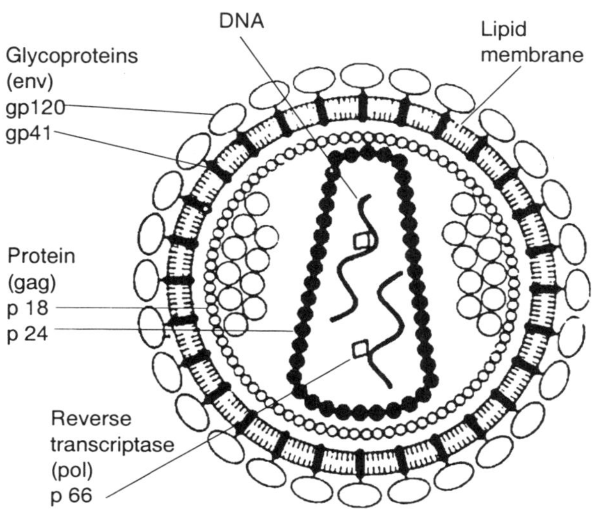

SOURCE: G.C. Schild, and P.D. Minor, "Human Immunodeficiency Virus and AIDS: Challenges and Progress," *Lancet* 335:1081-1084, 1990.

TABLE 2-4: Mechanisms by Which HIV Evades Immune Control

- Latency in chromosomal DNA
- Extensive genetic diversity
- Virus infects and destroys critical immune cells
- Spread by macrophage and direct cell fusion
- Silent transmission during prolonged latent infection
- Transmitted by three routes, as free- or cell-associated virus
- Recovery from infection not known, providing no clues to protective mechanisms
- Primate models offer no clear guidance to protective mechanisms

SOURCE: Office of Technology Assessment, 1995.

the cell, HIV DNA must integrate into the DNA of the human chromosome in the cell nucleus. While the HIV genome is integrated into the human genome, it is hidden from immune surveillance and cannot be recognized and eliminated. While it is integrated, the HIV genome is latent and not replicating. HIV may persist in this sanctuary, later to reactivate, replicate, and shed new virus from the cell.

2. The virus can undergo genetic change through a process of rapid genetic mutation and selection of viral mutants resistant to preexisting antibody. Viral mutations can occur at epitopes, the key sites normally recognized and attacked by antibody and immune cells. These mutations may render the epitopes unrecognizable, allowing the virus to avoid immune elimination. During the lengthy course of infection in a single individual, new genetic variants of HIV emerge.

Globally, at least six major subtypes (clades) of HIV have been identified based upon genetic analysis (70). Subtype B has been isolated in the Americas, Western Europe, and in parts of Southeast Asia. Substantial genetic variation is found even within each subtype of HIV (73). A significant consequence of the genetic diversity of HIV is that the immune response directed to one HIV strain may not necessarily protect an individual from other subtypes of HIV or from different strains within the same subtype of HIV. Therefore, there is consensus that HIV strains used to prepare vaccines must match HIV specimens that are freshly isolated from infected individuals in the region where the vaccine is to be used (so called "fresh primary field isolates") (103).

3. Virus spreads through the body soon after initial contact with the surface mucus membranes (the mucosa) of the vagina, anus, and penile urethra, the sites of sexual transmission. The virus selectively invades and can injure the very cells that play central roles in immune defense, the CD4+ (T helper) lymphocytes and the macrophages.
4. Virus that infects and is sheltered by macrophages may spread to other sites, such as the central nervous system, a body compartment

where access of immune cells and antibody is poor.[12] Virus can also spread by direct cell-to-cell contact through a process of direct fusion, again avoiding immune inactivation.

5. HIV infection is chronic, with a variable number of years of apparent clinical wellness preceding the onset of HIV-related illnesses. Despite the presence of vigorous, sustained antibody and cytotoxic T lymphocyte responses to HIV, the virus continues to multiply to high concentrations (titers) in immune cells in lymphoid tissues of the body. The virus remains silently transmissible. When a sufficient number of CD4+ lymphocytes are injured and lost, the acquired immunodeficiency syndrome, AIDS, becomes clinically apparent, with eventual death. The progression of HIV-related immune dysfunction is classically monitored by measuring the fall in concentration of circulating CD4+ lymphocytes.
6. HIV can be transmitted by three different routes, which, in itself, can complicate the task of developing a vaccine that can induce an effective immune blockade. HIV is acquired by sexual contact with mucosa of the vagina, rectum, or penis; by direct inoculation into the blood stream; or by transfer from mother to fetus or infant through the uterus, at birth, or through breast milk. Protecting the mucosa against infection presents special challenges because of the difficulty in inducing mucosal immunity through vaccination. Virus may be transmitted as free virus or as virus carried inside cells (see photos 2-1 and 2-2). It is more difficult to block the transmission of virus in infected cells; different immune mechanisms are required.
7. Unlike other viral infections that are self-limited, there are few, if any, instances of recovery from HIV infection to offer clues for understanding the key immune response elements that are necessary for protection from the virus.
8. Animal models of human HIV infection, using monkeys and other primates, have not yet yielded definitive guidance to the immune elements necessary for protection.

ANIMAL MODELS

What Has Been Learned from Animal Models?

Animal models of infection historically have contributed to the development of vaccines in two general ways: 1) use of animal models has helped to define interactions between the virus and the infected organism or *host*, particularly in understanding the immune responses necessary for control of infection; and 2) animal models have provided a system to predict the behavior of a candidate vaccine in man. The primate model can be used to provide an initial assessment of vaccine concepts, test a vaccine's immune potential, provide evidence of protection against challenge virus, and screen the vaccine for safety. Scientific opinion varies concerning the significance and validity of primate studies as a guide to HIV vaccine development and as a criterion for judging the eligibility of a vaccine for participation in efficacy trials (83). However, as our understanding expands, patterns of primate infection are emerging that should permit more focused studies.

Primate Systems

The chimpanzee is the only animal in which HIV will replicate. However, chimpanzees have severe limitations as animal models. Chimpanzees are expensive and their supply is limited; a typical study may involve two chimpanzees given experimental vaccine and one chimpanzee receiving placebo vaccine for comparison. In the chimpanzee, the virus causes a minimal persistent infection, waning over time, with no disease manifesta-

[12] The central nervous system includes the brain and spinal cord, and is separated from the other body compartments by the "blood-brain" barrier. Certain immune response components, including certain white cells and antibody, are limited in their ability to traverse this brain barrier.

tions. Some fresh human HIV isolates may actually fail to infect chimpanzees.

Macaque monkey infection with simian immunodeficiency virus (SIV) provides an important parallel to HIV infection in humans. SIV, a retrovirus that is in the same virus family as HIV, is highly virulent in macaques, with induction of high concentrations (titers) of antibodies and persistent infection leading to an AIDS-like syndrome within 6 to 24 months of the infection. The rapidity of disease progression varies with the level of virulence[13] of the SIV strain used. Unlike chimpanzees, the macaque is readily available.

Human immunodeficiency virus, type 2 (HIV-2) causes human AIDS restricted to West Africa. HIV-2 is more closely related to SIV than HIV-1, grows poorly in monkeys, and does not grow at all in chimpanzees.

Protection Under Optimal Conditions

There are examples of vaccine protection or partial protection in primates, largely under optimal circumstances, for example where vaccinated primates were exposed to virus immediately following the final dose of vaccine (which corresponds to the height of the immune response elicited by the vaccine), where vaccinated primates were "challenged" with virus that was homologous to (i.e., of the same strain as) the virus used in the preparation of vaccine, and where small doses of cell-free virus were inoculated directly into the blood stream by the intravenous route (8, 30, 47, 83, 101). Also, large doses of antibody administered to the chimpanzee have been shown to provide passive protection from infection with HIV for several hours, but no longer (24).

Studies using the SIV/macaque model have shown that it may not be necessary for a vaccine to attain sterilizing immunity (to clear all virus) to protect against disease (44). If this is also true of HIV in humans, it may lower the requirements for an effective HIV vaccine. Importantly, vaccine protection against SIV infection of the vaginal mucous membranes of macaques has been accomplished recently using microspheres, which permit slow release of antigen (58).

Live attenuated vaccines show a high level of protection against SIV infection in macaques. The promise of live attenuated vaccines and their safety concerns are discussed later in this chapter (19, 20, 21).

Inconsistent Results in Primate Studies

Primate studies conducted over the past decade have been subject to inconsistent results that are sometimes difficult to duplicate. It is now appreciated that the outcome of a vaccine challenge experiment can vary depending on the relative virulence of viral infection in different primates, the choice of virus strain, the dose of virus, the route of viral inoculation, the history of the virus, and other specific conditions of viral challenge (10, 83). Understanding these variables allows investigators to select primate systems that pose higher or lower hurdles for vaccine protection. For example, protection against HIV infection in the chimpanzee (the HIV/chimpanzee model) appears to be more readily accomplished than protection against the more lethal SIV infection in the macaque (the SIV/macaque model). Success in the less virulent HIV/chimpanzee model frequently cannot be duplicated in the more virulent SIV/macaque model. Both models are helpful in understanding HIV in humans. The HIV/chimpanzee system models silent persistent HIV infection of humans; the SIV/macaque model parallels HIV disease progression in humans.

IMMUNE CORRELATES OF PROTECTION

Knowledge of the specific elements of an immune response required to protect against HIV infection (the immune correlates of protection) would help guide the design of an effective HIV vaccine. Two approaches to understanding such correlates are available: 1) experiments using experimental vaccines in primates, and 2) observations that may

[13] The *virulence* of a microorganism refers to its capacity to produce disease.

suggest the development of a protective immune response in human HIV infection. While primate studies have shown examples of protection under limited circumstances, as yet the immune responses required for a successful HIV vaccine remain undefined. Levels of antibody induced in primates by vaccines are, in themselves, not well correlated with protection against HIV infection.

What is the evidence for natural immunity to HIV infection in man? Studies of the natural history of long-term survivors of HIV infection have helped us know what are the clinical indicators of sustained favorable prognosis in HIV infection. But these studies have been less useful in helping us understand the requirements for a protective immune blockade to HIV infection (57). Studies of individuals who have remained seronegative[14] despite intense exposure to HIV, such as infants of seropositive mothers (78) and multiply-exposed men (17) have shown that some of these individuals have developed protective patterns of immune response, suggesting that "natural immunization" to HIV infection may occur.

DEVELOPMENT AND CLINICAL EVALUATION OF HIV VACCINES

U.S. Program of HIV Vaccine Development

The U.S. Public Health Service established a program of discovery, development, and clinical trials directed toward making available a safe and effective preventive HIV vaccine. The effort is centered at the National Institutes of Health (NIH) with the National Institute of Allergy and Infectious Diseases (NIAID) as the lead institute. Fundamental and applied studies of HIV molecular biology, pathogenesis, and immunopathology and of HIV vaccine development have been fostered by a variety of funding strategies, enabling interactive research among scientists in the U.S. and abroad.

The NIAID Division of AIDS (DAIDS) created a network of primate centers to study HIV infection in the chimpanzee and SIV infection in lower primates. The DAIDS AIDS Vaccine Clinical Trial Network (AVCTN) has several components. The AIDS Vaccine Evaluation Group (AVEG) includes six AIDS Vaccine Evaluation Unit (AVEU) trial sites at university research centers. Each unit has an associated Community Advisory Board. Other AVCTN elements include a Central Immunology Laboratory, which develops standards and performs most of the immunological assays, a Mucosal Immunology Laboratory, and a Data Coordinating and Analysis Center. A Data and Safety Monitoring Board exercises independent oversight of HIV vaccine trials.

The process of testing a candidate vaccine in clinical trials is initiated by a sponsor, which presents preclinical data to the Food and Drug Administration's (FDA's) Center for Biologicals Evaluation and Research (CBER) for review. FDA assesses data from laboratory studies of the vaccine, data from animal studies, and other "preclinical data" for evidence of the vaccine's safety, potency, and potential for efficacy. The FDA is also responsible for approval and oversight of experimental protocols as vaccines progress through clinical trials.

Vaccine sponsors may present data from preclinical studies of their vaccines to the AIDS Vaccine Selection Group; the group will consider this material in determining which vaccines will be entered into federally funded AVEG trials. A unified approach to trial design, clinical assessment, laboratory assays, and data analysis permits direct comparisons among multiple vaccine strategies and products.

Other major participants in HIV vaccine development include the National Cancer Institute, the

[14] An individual that is *seronegative* for HIV infection has a negative result on a test for HIV infection, and a *seropositive* individual has a positive test. The enzyme-linked immunosorbant assay (ELISA) is the most commonly used screening test for HIV infection. The ELISA indirectly determines whether one is HIV infected by testing for the presence of antibodies to HIV. Because antibodies to HIV may not appear for two or more weeks after initial HIV infection, some "seronegative" individuals may actually be infected with HIV.

Centers for Disease Control and Prevention (CDC), vaccine manufacturers, universities, the World Health Organization (WHO), and the Department of Defense. These participants contribute capacities for research, product development, and conduct of clinical trials in the United States and other developed countries, as well as in the developing world.

Design of Clinical Trials (Phases I and II)

Promising candidate vaccines are selected for initial assessment of immune responses and safety in carefully monitored, prospectively randomized, double-blind, placebo-controlled clinical trials.[15] Phase I and II are described below, and Phase III (large controlled clinical trials of a vaccine's efficacy) are described in a later section. The FDA approval process involves three phases.

Phase I focuses on an assessment of vaccine safety and the immune responses to the vaccine. Phase I study protocols involve 25 to 100 individuals who are randomly assigned to either a placebo control group or one or more experimental groups. Recruitment for Phase I studies involves selection of healthy noninfected individuals who are prescreened and undergo a full physical and laboratory examination. Volunteers are selected to be at low risk for HIV infection to minimize their potential for acquiring confounding HIV infection during the trial. Trial participants receive detailed individual counseling and education on the experimental nature of the vaccine, the design of the trial, and possible adverse consequences of the vaccine. Informed consent for trial participation is obtained from each volunteer. The effects of varying the vaccine's dose of antigen, schedule of administration, and ratios of adjuvant to antigen are determined in Phase I studies.

If the immune responses to the vaccine and the safety profile of the vaccine warrant further studies, it may undergo Phase II trials, which involve up to a few hundred individuals. These studies refine and enlarge the database, may directly compare products or sequences, or may include individuals at higher risk of acquiring infection.

Role of Industry

The role of U.S. industry, traditionally a world leader in vaccine development and marketing, deserves special comment. There is a long list of candidate vaccines in trials or in development (tables 2-5, 2-6, 2-7). Not all vaccines in development will be eligible for Phase I trials. HIV vaccine sponsors, to a large extent, are small biotechnology companies, private research institutions, and universities (98). Some of the large pharmaceutical manufacturers in the Unites States are not sponsoring an HIV vaccine. There may be different market forces affecting large companies and small companies that affect their decisions to become involved in HIV vaccine development. Some have argued that the compelling global progression of the AIDS epidemic warrants exploration of special incentives to attract increased participation of both small and large companies.

Corporate decisions to invest in the development of an HIV vaccine are based on several considerations, including the opportunity costs of vaccine development relative to drug development, the potential market for an HIV vaccine,

---

[15] A prospective, randomized, double-blind, placebo-controlled study design minimizes threats to the validity of the study. Prospective studies are ones where the investigator observes the participants from the beginning of the study on; in retrospective studies, observations are made after the study is completed. A randomized trial refers to one in which participants are randomly assigned to experimental and control groups; random assignment helps ensure that each of the groups are equivalent. A double-blind trial is one in which both the clinician and the subject are unaware of the group to which the subject has been assigned; this minimizes the risk of bias that may be introduced when either the clinician or subject is aware of the subject's assignment. A *controlled trial* is one in which one group of participants (the control group) is assigned to a receive a either a placebo or a standard comparison treatment. A *placebo* is an inert substance which, in the context of a controlled trial, is made to appear identical to the active experimental treatment. Comparison of one or more *experimental* groups with the control group allows the investigators to determine the impact of the experimental treatment.

TABLE 2-5: Current U.S. and Foreign Phase I/II Clinical Trials[a] of HIV Vaccine Candidates in Noninfected Adults

Vaccine	Developer	Trial sites or sponsor
Envelope proteins		
rgp160-LAI[b] (insect)[c]	MicroGeneSys	AVEG[d]/LIR
rgp160-LAI (mammalian)	Immuno AG	AVEG
rgp160-MN (mammalian)	Immuno AG	AVEG
rgp120-LAI (mammalian)	Genentech	AVEG
rgp120-MN (mammalian)	Genentech (Phase II)	AVEG
rgp120-SF2 (yeast)	Biocine	AVEG
rgp120-SF2 (mammalian)	Biocine (Phase II)	AVEG, SFGH
Virus-like particles		
Ty.p24.VLP	British Biotechnology, Ltd.	London, UK
Peptides		
V3-MAPS	United Biomedical, Inc.	AVEG, SFGH, China, Australia
V3-MAPS (15 component)	United Biomedical, Inc.	AVEG
V3 peptide PPD conjugated	SSVI	SSVI
V3 peptides PPD conjugated	SSVI	Israel
V3 peptides conjugated to *Pseudomonas aeruginosa* toxin A	SSVI	Switzerland
HGP-30 (p17 peptide)	Viral Technologies, Inc.	SFGH/United Kingdom
Vectors		
Vaccinia-gp160-LAI	Bristol-Myers Squibb	AVEG/University of Washington
Canarypox-gp160	Pasteur-Merieux-Connaught	AVEG
Combinations of Vaccines		
Vaccinia-gp160 plus rgp160	Bristol-Myers Squibb, MicroGeneSys	AVEG, University of Washington
Vaccinia-gp160 plus rgp120 (yeast) or rgp120 (mammalian cell produced)	Bristol-Myers Squibb, Biocine	AVEG
Vaccinia-gp160 plus rgp160 plus 3 envelope peptides	G. Beaud, Institut Jacques Monod; A. Burney, Universite Libre de Bruxelles	Paris, France
Vaccinia-gp160 plus rgp160 or rgp12 (MN, LA1 or SF2)	Bristol-Myers Squibb; Immuno AG; Genentech; Biocine	AVEG
Canarypox-gp160 plus rgp160	Pasteur-Merieux-Connaught (Virogenetics, Transgene)	PMSV/ANRS
Vaccinia - *env, gag, pol*	Therion	AVEG
rgp160 plus V3 peptide	Pasteur-Merieux-Connaught (Transgene)	PMSV/ANRS
rgp120 (LA1)) plus rgp120 (MN) (sequentially or simultaneously)	Genentech	AVEG

[a] All vaccines listed are in Phase I trials, unless otherwise indicated .

[b] HIV-strains represent a group of clade B isolates from the United States and Europe, which includes LAI, IIIB, MN, and SF2.

[c] Cell substrate for recombinant subunit protein.

[d] The AIDS Vaccine Evaluation Group is a component of the AIDS Vaccine Clinical Trials Network. The network includes Johns Hopkins University, Baltimore, MD; St. Louis University, St. Louis, MO;University of Rochester, Rochester, NY; University of Washington, Seattle, WA; Vanderbilt University, Nashville, TN. Former members were Baylor University, Houston, TX and University of Maryland, Baltimore.

KEY: AVEG = AIDS Vaccine Evaluation Group of AIDS Vaccine Clinical Trials Network; LIR = Laboratory of Immunoregulation; SFGH = San Francisco General Hospital, CA.

SOURCE: Adapted from M.C. Walker and P.E. Fast, *Clinical Trials of Candidate AIDS Vaccines* (in press).

TABLE 2-6: Current Clinical Trials of HIV Vaccine Candidates in Noninfected Adults that Compare Adjuvant Formulations.

Vaccine	Developer	Adjuvants Compared	Adjuvant Source	Trial Site
rgp120-MN	Biocine	Alum	Superfos/AS	AVEG
		MPL	Ribi ImmunoChem Res.	
		Liposome-encapsulated MPL with alum	C. Alving/WRAIR	
		MF59	Biocine	
		MF59 + MTP-PE	Biocine	
		SAF/2	Syntex/Biocine	
		SAF/2 + MDP	Syntex/Biocine	
rgp120-MN	Genentech	Alum	Reheis	AVEG
		QS21	Cambridge Biotech	
		Alum + QS21	Reheis/Cambridge Biotech	

KEY: alum = Aluminum hydroxide; AVEG = AIDS Vaccine Evaluation Group of AIDS Vaccine Clinical Trials Network; MDP = Muramyl dipeptide; MF59 = Microfluidized oil-in-water emulsion; MPL = Monophosphoryl lipid A; MTP-PE = Muramyl tripeptide-phosphatidylethanolamine; QS21 = Purified saponin adjuvant; SAF = Syntex adjuvant formulation; WRAIR = Walter Reed Army Institute of Research

SOURCE: Adapted from M.C. Walker, and P.E. Fast, *Clinical Trials of Candidate AIDS Vaccines*, in press.

whether the development of an effective HIV vaccine is scientifically feasible, and potential liability for unforeseen adverse reactions to HIV vaccines. Of the disincentives to HIV vaccine development, scientific feasibility is a primary concern. The development of an HIV vaccine is hampered by a lack of clear scientific objectives, a consequence of the undefined protective immune requirements for an HIV vaccine.

Concerns surrounding the safety of an effective vaccine may also play a role in corporate decisions. Notably, manufacturers have pursued the development of HIV vaccines composed of envelope subunit proteins, which have inherently more limited immune capability than HIV vaccines composed of whole inactivated virus or live attenuated virus. Manufacturers have not, however, pursued the development of inactivated virus vaccines or live attenuated virus vaccines because of the greater inherent potential for safety problems from these vaccines. This is despite the fact that HIV vaccines based on these more classical vaccine designs are far more promising. Recognizing this, research on attenuated virus vaccines for HIV has been supported by the DAIDS program. (Recently, some manufacturers have expressed interest in developing an inactivated virus vaccine.)

There appears to be no unanimity on the relative importance of concerns about potential liability in corporate decisions to invest in the development of an HIV vaccine. Some cite potential for liability as a part of the "cost of doing business," to be considered along with scientific feasibility, marketing potential, and other business considerations. Industry may need further encouragement through special incentives to undertake unusual risks.

ADVERSE REACTIONS

Safety Lessons Learned from Experience with Traditional Vaccines

Safety Standards for Prophylactic Vaccines

The standard of safety applied to prophylactic vaccines is higher than that applied to other tools in the medical armamentarium. Historically, vaccines, especially those designed for universal use in children, have been held to extremely high safety standards. A vaccine is given to uninfected, healthy individuals to prevent potential disease for which the vaccinee may or may not be at risk at a future time. In this setting, any significant injury, even occurring in one in a thousand or million recipients, may be considered unacceptable.

TABLE 2-7: Vaccine Strategies and HIV Vaccine Candidates in Preclinical Development

Candidate	Expression system/ production method	Adjuvant or delivery system	Developer
Strategy: Targeting of immune response to specific HIV neutralization (B cell) epitopes and/or cytotoxic T lymphocyte (CTL) epitopes.			
rgp160	Mammalian	Oil/water, 3-deacyl monophosphoryl Lipid A	SmithKline Beecham
rgp120	Insect	Oil/water, 3-deacyl monophosphoryl Lipid A	SmithKline Beecham
V3-MAPS[a]	Synthetic	Alum (slow release for mulation)	United Biomedical, Inc.
Ty.V3.VLP	Yeast	Alum/none	British Bio-tech., Ltd.
T1-SPIO(A)	Synthetic	IFA	B. Haynes, Duke University
V3-T helper epitope peptides (PCLUS 3-18, PCLUS 6-18)	Synthetic	IFA, QS21	National Cancer Institute,
CLTB-34, CLTB-36, p24E-V3MN	Synthetic chimeric V3-p24 gag peptides	Alum, QS21	Connaught
V3 and gag peptides[a] coupled to lysine copolymers	Synthetic	Alum	Yokohama City University, Japan
V3-BCG	Recombinant mycobacteria	—	Nagasaki and Osaka Universities, Japan
V3-BCG[a]	Recombinant mycobacteria	—	NIH, Japan
V3 peptide coupled to Mycobacterium protein	Synthetic	10K mycobacterium protein	SSVI
env peptides coupled to beta-gal	E. coli	IFA	WRAIR-Univax
CD4 binding domain peptomer	Synthetic, conformationally constrained	Alum	F.A. Robey, NIDR
HBcAg-v3 particles	E. coli	—	Max V. Pettenkofer-Institut, FRG
Recombinant rhinovirus - HIV V3 peptides	Recombinant human rhinovirus (HRV14)	—	Rutgers University
Recombinant mengovirus - HIV, V3, V4 peptides	Recombinant murine mengovirus (attenuated)	—	Institut Pasteur

(continued)

TABLE 2-7: Vaccine Strategies and HIV Vaccine Candidates in Preclinical Development (Cont'd.)

Candidate	Expression system/ production method	Adjuvant or delivery system	Developer
Strategy: Mimicry of attenuated or inactivated HIV			
Whole inactivated HIV	Inactivated with betapropiolactone, BEI, formaldehyde	Digitonin	Retroscreen, Ltd./ISI
HIV *env*, *gag*, *pol* pseudovirions[b]	Mammalian/vaccinia	Alum	Therion Biologics
HIV *env*, *gag*, *pol* pseudovirions[b]	Mammalian (Vero)	—	Connaught
Gag-V3 virus-like particles	Insect cells/baculovirus	—	Universität Regensburg, FRG
p55gag/V3 chimeric vaccinia	Recombinant vaccinia	—	Universität Regensburg, FRG
TBC-3B, (vaccinia-HIV *env*, *gag*, *pol*)[b]	Recombinant vaccinia	—	Therion Biologics
Vaccinia-HIV *env*, *gag*, *pol*[b]	Attenuated recombinant vaccinia (NYVAC)	—	Pasteur-Merieux-Connaught (Virogenetics)
Canarypox-HIV *env*, *gag*, *pol*[b]	Recombinant canarypox (ALVAC)	—	Pasteur-Merieux-Connaught (Virogenetics)
HIV expression vector coated with 1.0 micron gold particles	DNA	particle acceleration device	Agracetus
pM160, (HIV envelope gp160 DNA construct)	DNA	—	University of Pennsylvania School of Medicine
Strategy: Induction of mucosal immune responses in gastrointestinal and genitourinary tracts.			
Adenovirus-Hiv env or gag	Recombinant adenovirus (Ad4, Ad5, Ad7 vaccine strains)	—	Wyeth-Ayerst
Poliovirus-HIV	Recombinant poliovirus	—	—
Poliovirus-HIV envelope peptides	Recombinant dicistronic poliovirus	—	SUNY, Stony Brook
Poliovirus-HIV nef, gag, env	Recombinant poliovirus (Mahoney type 1, Sabin types 1 and 2)	—	Gladstone Institute, UCSF
Encapsidated recombinant poliovirus HIV env, gag, or pol minireplicons	Encapsidate recombinant poliovirus	—	UAB

(continued)

TABLE 2-7: Vaccine Strategies and HIV Vaccine Candidates in Preclinical Development (Cont'd.)

Candidate	Expression system/ production method	Adjuvant or delivery system	Developer
Strategy: Induction of mucosal immune responses in gastrointestinal and genitourinary tracts. (Cont'd.)			
Mengovirus-HIV nef	Recombinant mengovirus (attenuated M16 Murine strain)	—	Gladstone Institute UCSF
Shigella-V3 peptide	Recombinant Shigella flexneri (attenuated strain SC602)	—	Institute Pasteur, France
Salmonella-HIV gp120, p24, nef	Recombinant Salmonella typhi (CVD 908 vaccine strain)	—	University of Maryland
BCG-HIV env peptides	Recombinant BCG	—	Medimmune, Inc.
BCG-HIV	Recombinant BCG	—	—
Recombinant Lactococcus-V3 peptide	Fusion of V3 peptide to TT fragment C in Lactococcus lactis	—	University of Cambridge, UK
Env-PND-gag-HGP-30 conjugate	Synthethic peptide	Cholera toxin B	Viral Technologies, Inc.; Alpha-1 Biomedicals
rgp 120	Recombinant protein	Liposome/Cholera toxin	UAB/Connaught
V3-MAPS[a]	Synthetic	Microparticles	United Biomedical, Inc.
Tetravalent MAP-gp120 sequence coupled to a ipophilic moiety	Recombinant protein	Syntheitic lopophilic moiety	Vanderbilt University
Strategy: Development of HIV-2 vaccines			
Whole inactivated HIV-2	Triton or formalin inactivation	IFA, alum, RIBI adjuvant, ISCOMS	National Bacteriological Laboratory, Sweden
gp125	Purified native glycoprotein	ISCOMS, RIBI adjuvant	National Bacteriological Laboratory, Sweden
gp130	Purified native glycoprotein	IFA, alum	National Bacteriological Laboratory, Sweden
rgp160	Baculovirus	—	German Primate Center, FRG
Vaccinia-HIV-2 env, gag, pol	Attenuated recombinant vaccinia (NYVAC)	—	Virogenetics
Canarypox-HIV-2 env, gag, pol	Recombinant canarypox (ALVAC)	—	Virogenetics
Vaccinia HIV-2 env	Recombinant vaccinia	—	German Primate Center, FRG
Salmonella-HIV-2 env, gag	Recombinant Salmonella typhimurium	—	National Cancer Institute

[a]Contains non-clade B strains.

[b]Multiple genetic deletions introduced for safety.

KEY: BCG = Bacille-Calmette Guerin; bovine tuberculosis; IFA = incomplete Freund's adjuvant; LAI = group of closely related HIV isolates that includes LAV, IIIB, BRU, etc.; MAP = multiple antigent peptide; MAPS = multiple antigen peptide; MAPS = multiple antigen presentation system; NIDR = National Institute of Dental Research, National Institutes of Health, SSVI = Swiss Serum and Vaccine Institute, Berne, Switzerland; SUNY = State University of New York; TT = tetanus toxin; UAB = University of Alabama at Birmingham; UCD = University of California, Davis; UCSF = University of California, San Francisco; WRAIR = Walter Reed Army Institute of Research.

SOURCE: Adapted from Walker, MC., Fast, PE., *Clinical Trials* of Candidate AIDS Vaccines, in press.

By contrast, there is greater tolerance for adverse reactions accompanying the administration of a therapeutic drug given as treatment for an existing disease. Further, this tolerance is proportionate to the severity and unfavorable prognosis of the illness treated. For example, severe side effects may be considered acceptable in cancer chemotherapy.

The concept of an "acceptable" risk has not been applied to vaccines. Good public health practice at the population level may at times be in conflict with the goal of near-zero risk to the individual. Attenuated polio vaccine has eradicated poliomyelitis from the Americas, yet each of the few vaccine-associated paralytic cases annually has given rise to a compensation claim.

Types of Adverse Events Seen with Traditional Vaccines

Vaccines are prepared from biologically active starting materials with inherent potential for harmful effects. Early adverse reactions, occurring within hours or days after vaccination, may be local (e.g., sore arm) or systemic (e.g., fever, malaise), and typically are minor, transient, and without residual effects. Severe reactions have occurred very rarely to vaccines currently in use; these include anaphylaxis (a severe allergic hypersensitivity reaction) (e.g., tetanus toxoid) and neurologic disease (e.g., pertussis vaccine).

Causal relationships with illnesses occurring long after vaccination may be particularly difficult to document and to distinguish from the occurrence of unrelated diseases. Relationships may be perceived between illnesses and vaccination that are not, in fact, causally related. The difficulty in assigning cause is exhaustively reviewed in two reports by the Institute of Medicine (IOM) of the National Academy of Sciences (48, 49).[16] The IOM reports are based on accumulated experience with millions of doses of licensed vaccines used worldwide, many in use for decades. The findings provide the basis for compensable awards by the Vaccine Injury Compensation Program (Statutory Basis for the National Vaccine Plan: Title XXI of the Public Health Service Act, Public Law 99-660). The IOM reports point to need for: 1) research on mechanisms of induction of adverse events; and 2) prospective, long-term, post-marketing surveillance. Both undertakings are expensive and technically difficult.

Despite the inherent potential for injury from vaccines, licensed vaccines in the United States have a record of remarkable safety and have provided a highly cost-effective method of disease control.

Safety Experience in Phase I and II Trials

Trial Design Using Envelope-Based Vaccines

Initial approaches to HIV vaccine have concentrated on envelope proteins gp160 or gp120. Purified proteins have been produced in three different cell types by recombinant techniques. These envelope proteins may be combined with carrier mole-

---

[16] In a retrospective analysis of worldwide published studies, the weight of evidence for or against causality of possible adverse events was examined for each of the childhood vaccines. There often was difficulty in assigning cause, but difficulty also in proving lack of cause. Four types of primary evidence were considered: a) biological plausibility; b) case reports, case series and uncontrolled observational studies; c) controlled observational studies; and d) controlled clinical trials. Based on these categories of evidence, the presumed adverse events were classified into five levels of certainty: a) no evidence bearing on a causal relation; b) evidence inadequate to accept or reject a causal relation; c) evidence favors rejection of a causal relation; d) evidence favors acceptance of a causal relation; and e) evidence establishes a causal relationship.

These analyses are then reviewed in the context of the compensable injuries covered by the Vaccine Injury Compensation Program established by Congress in 1986. The childhood vaccines have been in widespread use for many years, and millions of doses have been administered. Despite this historical experience, the data was difficult to interpret. The vast majority of adverse events came from uncontrolled studies and individual case reports. The pathologic conditions under consideration often were uncommon or rare in the population. Because comparative age-specific incidence rates and relative risk estimates of the condition in the general population are rarely available, it was not possible to calculate a statistical rate of excess vaccine-related cases, if any. Controlled epidemiological studies are lacking (48, 49).

cules and injected into the individual to produce an immune response. A second method of immunization with envelope protein uses live vaccinia virus as a "delivery vector" (vaccinia/gp 160 vector); the vaccinia virus genome has been genetically altered to incorporate the HIV envelope gp160 gene. Replication of vaccinia virus in the dermal layer of the skin results in expression of gp160 protein, which in turn induces the immune response. From the initiation of the AVEG program in 1988, more than 1,400 volunteers have participated in trials of envelope-based HIV vaccines (tables 2-5 and 2-6). Twelve envelope-based vaccine products or combinations, formulations, and adjuvants[17] were used, prepared by five manufacturers using three subtype B virus strains. Additional independent trials of envelope-based vaccines have been conducted by U.S. and foreign sponsors.

Immune Responses

The immune responses provide an initial measure of the potential value of envelope vaccines and must be considered in context of adverse reactions accompanying the use of these vaccines (5, 4, 38, 53, 60, 61). Envelope-based vaccines have induced antibodies directed against the strains of virus used to prepare the envelope proteins (homologous strains). The titers (concentrations) of antibody induced by envelope-based vaccines were 5- to 10-fold lower than the titers of antibody found in HIV-infected individuals. Antibody titers are not sustained, falling rapidly after each dose of vaccine. Other subgroup B strains (heterologous strains) were neutralized less well, and freshly isolated strains were entirely resistant.

The evasion of neutralization by freshly isolated strains is of concern and remains under intensive study to determine its significance.

Envelope vaccines, with or without adjuvants, produced no consistent cytotoxic T lymphocyte responses. Priming with vaccinia/gp160 vector vaccine followed by a booster dose of envelope-based vaccine resulted in modest cytotoxic T lymphocyte responses in a few recipients. Envelope-based vaccines that were combined with new adjuvants to enhance vaccine immunogenicity produced modest increases in titers of neutralizing antibody; this enhanced immunogenecity occurred at the expense of an increased rate of local or systemic reactions in some of these vaccines.

Thus, envelope-based vaccines preferentially generated antibody responses and were disappointing in that they failed to generate substantial cytotoxic T lymphocyte responses. The antibody responses elicited by envelope-based vaccines have been judged by many scientists to be marginal with respect to their magnitude, duration, and cross-reactivity with other strains.

Safety Overview

Adverse reactions following vaccination with envelope-based products have been minimally greater than adverse reactions following placebo vaccination. (Eighteen percent of participants in trials of envelope-based vaccines received a placebo vaccination.) In general, the experience with envelope-based HIV vaccines suggests that they have a benign adverse reaction profile, similar to currently licensed vaccines. Sequential measures of biochemical, hematological, and immunological status and kidney and liver function tests showed no significant vaccine-related abnormal findings. Importantly, there has been no evidence of adverse effects on immune function, including CD4+ and CD8+ lymphocyte counts.

Early Self-Limited Adverse Reactions

Envelope-based vaccines with alum adjuvant were associated with local reactions at the injection site, consisting of mild pain, tenderness, redness, and swelling for one to two days. The incidence and type of systemic complaints, such as fever and malaise, were similar to those of placebo

[17] In immunology, an adjuvant is a substance, such as alum, that is added to a vaccine to non-specifically enhance the vaccine's immunogenicity (the vaccine's ability to produce an immune response).

recipients. Addition of some of the new adjuvants, Genentech QS21 and Chiron/Biocine SAF/2, induced transient moderate to severe local reactions and febrile flu-like illnesses for one to three days in a number of recipients (53). None of the vaccinees dropped out of the trials, missed school or work, or had residual consequences. No further studies were undertaken with these adjuvants.

Ten vaccinees developed a rash to several products, and one also developed painful joints (arthralgias). A positive antinuclear antibody (ANA) test (which may at times be associated with autoimmune disease, such as rheumatoid arthritis) was found in a few individuals. However, further testing ruled out any vaccine-related disease. Despite careful screening and counseling, 14 pregnancies occurred. There was no evidence of vaccine-related adverse effects.

Level of Attenuation of the Vaccinia Vector

The trials permitted comparison of the side effects of vaccinia/gp160 vector with the commercial vaccinia strain used to prevent smallpox, from which it had been derived. Smallpox vaccine virus, injected into the dermal layer of the skin, can spread and cause severe or fatal disease in rare instances, especially in individuals with compromised immune systems. The vaccinia vector has been attenuated (rendered incapable of producing disease) as measured in laboratory tests. Reactions to the vaccine resembled those seen following classical smallpox vaccination in individuals who had not been vaccinated previously (36). There were no differences in rates of pustule development at the inoculation site, regional lymph node swelling, or systemic symptoms. The vaccinia virus did not appear to be attenuated and, thus, could carry the risk of vaccinia complications known to occur with classical vaccination (75). Under the controlled conditions of the trial, occlusive dressings were used over the inoculation site, and no secondary spread to other individuals was observed. With broad use of an HIV vaccine, substitution of a more attenuated poxvirus vector, such as canarypox virus, is preferable.

Neoplasms

As of May 1994, 10 neoplasms (tumors) were observed in 9 different protocols (52). One of the neoplasms was benign. At the time of review, more than 1,300 volunteers were in AVEG trials, 18 percent of whom were assigned to a placebo control group. Those neoplasms that were malignant tended to occur in older groups. Analysis by the Data and Safety Monitoring Board and an ad hoc expert committee found no evidence that these neoplasms were linked to any vaccine. The wide variety of tumor types seen in these vaccinees was judged to be biologically incompatible with the hypothesis that there was a causal relationship between these neoplasms and vaccine. The occurrence of such coincidental events exemplifies the need for placebo-controlled trials of HIV vaccines, with careful long-term followup and independent review.

HIV Infections Among Trial Volunteers

A Phase II trial of envelope-based vaccine was conducted in 300 noninfected individuals from groups at high risk for HIV infection. These included men who have sex with men, injection drug users, sexual partners of infected individuals, and teenagers engaged in high-risk sexual behavior. A control group of individuals at low risk for HIV infection was also included for comparison. The trial has provided experience with recruitment, counseling, cohort retention, and compliance. It has also provided information about the acceptability of the vaccine and the effect of vaccine trial participation on risk behaviors. The trial was not designed to determine the efficacy of the vaccine because inadequate numbers of individuals were included. Despite counseling, HIV infections have occurred among vaccinees. "Breakthrough cases" of HIV infection in all protocols have been entered into a special study.

To date, 12 of the 1,400 individuals in AVEG trials since 1988 have become infected with HIV (37). Of the 12 breakthrough cases, three received placebo vaccine, eight an envelope-based vaccine, and one received a vaccinia/gp160 vector vaccine boosted with rgp160 vaccine. Five breakthrough cases received one to two doses of vaccine, and only four breakthrough cases received an adequate series of three to four vaccine doses. Notably, five of nine breakthrough cases occurred among volunteers enrolled in vaccine trials involving low-risk groups. Three additional infections occurred among individuals enrolled in an intramural NIAID trial, and two others occurred among individuals enrolled in non-NIAID vaccine trials, so that a total of 17 volunteers have become infected in envelope-based vaccine trials. Envelope-based vaccines of all participating manufacturers were involved (Genentech, Chiron/Biocene, Bristol-Myers Squibb/Oncogen and MicroGeneSys) (95).

Breakthrough infections among vaccine trial participants were to be expected because: 1) some volunteers received placebo; 2) the protective efficacy of the vaccine, if any, is not known; 3) maximum protection is afforded only after a full vaccine dosage schedule (involving 3 or more doses); and 4) antibody-dependent enhancement of infectivity must be considered as a possible reason for breakthrough infections.

Despite intensive counseling, on retrospective review, all HIV infections among vacinees accompanied high-risk behavior (5). Intensive study of recipient and donor viruses and of immune titers may provide clues to mechanisms of protection or failure.

Antibody-Dependent Enhancement

Some experts have questioned whether priming with an HIV vaccine can potentiate subsequently acquired natural HIV infection (12). The historical prototype giving rise to this concern is dengue virus, a tropical viral disease. The presence of serum antibodies induced by a first attack of mild dengue can facilitate the development of severe disease on subsequent infection with a related dengue virus (40). This "antibody-dependent enhancement" (ADE) of infection can be demonstrated in the laboratory by an increase in growth of virus in cell culture in the presence of antibodies from the serum of exposed individuals.

Recipients of envelope vaccines have been shown to develop small amounts of enhancing antibodies (66). The clinical significance of HIV vaccine-induced ADE is unclear. No direct evidence exists at this time that ADE has any clinical significance. Many scientists consider it to be an unrelated laboratory phenomenon only. Enhancement of disease has not been duplicated with HIV-1 or SIV in primate experiments, although it has been recommended that studies in primate models should continue (59, 67).

Other Mechanisms of Enhanced Disease

Historically, two other vaccines have been associated with an accompanying subsequent natural infection that is atypically severe: an experimental respiratory synitial virus (RSV) vaccine and a licensed measles virus vaccine (27, 54). Both were vaccines composed of whole virus inactivated by formalin. While the mechanisms of disease enhancement remain unclear, they both appear to occur by mechanisms unrelated to ADE of the dengue fever type. The enhanced disease experiences with these vaccines were wholly unexpected and have had a significant effect on further vaccine development. For measles, a live attenuated vaccine has supplanted the inactivated vaccine, and currently there is no licensed RSV vaccine. It has been suggested recently that inactivated RSV vaccine may induce inappropriate cytokines, or cell-to-cell communication substances, that are responsible for enhancement (35).

These experiences with vaccine-related enhancement of disease severity have only theoretical implications for HIV vaccines, such as inactivated whole-virus vaccines.

Induction of Autoimmunity

HIV vaccines may have potential for causing an immune reaction against the body's own tissues. Such "anti-self" antibodies could, in theory, be the basis for autoimmune injury (56, 84). Concern arises because HIV shares several envelope protein sequences that are identical (homologous) to sequences on human tissues, a phenomenon known as molecular mimicry. One example is the similarity of an HIV envelope protein region to a normal human blood type protein (32). Immunization with such viral structures can induce immune responses to the cells of vaccinated individuals. Adverse effects of the autoimmune type have not been observed among HIV vaccine recipients to date, although, in theory, autoimmune phenomena could appear months to years after vaccination.

NEW GENERATION VACCINES: IMPLICATIONS FOR SAFETY

Immune Goals Drive Vaccine Design and Enlarge Potential for Risk

As has been discussed, the immune determinants of protection against HIV infection remain undefined. The unique ability of HIV to evade immune controls in natural disease and in experimental systems suggests that all avenues of immune containment should remain on the research agenda. Based on classical theory, three elements may be required to prevent infection: 1) neutralization of free virus would be more effective with a more vigorous, broadly strain-reactive, sustained antibody response; 2) destruction of infected cells requires induction of cytotoxic T lymphocytes that recognize multiple HIV epitopes; and 3) protection against sexual transmission of HIV requires an antibody and cellular response at genital and rectal mucosal surfaces.

New vaccine strategies may be needed to fulfill these immune requirements (14). Some of the new-generation concepts are novel, never before applied to vaccines used in humans. Each vaccine formulation or variation on a formulation is regarded as a new product by the FDA, and separate evaluations of each are required. New approaches may carry special risks, some unique to that system. The potential for minimizing known, suspected, or theoretical risks is limited. Tests of vaccine *in vitro* laboratory studies and in animal models can be poor predictors, particularly of infrequent or late events. The major types of experimental vaccines in development are addressed below, along with implications for their safety (table 2-8).

Synthetic Peptides

Defined epitopes on viral proteins are simply and cheaply duplicated by artificial synthesis of short amino acid chains (41, 99). Specific B and T lymphocyte epitopes selected to stimulate antibody and cytotoxic T lymphocytes may be combined. Vaccines directed at multiple epitopes (multivalent vaccines) have been prepared containing subtypes of HIV that are endemic in diverse regions of the globe. Immune responses have been improved by arranging peptides into complex structural forms, as well as by adding new adjuvants or carrier molecules. Peptide-based vaccines have induced cytotoxic T lymphocyte responses in the SIV/macaque model. Clinical reactions to peptide products have been benign in initial clinical trials.

Live Vectors Carrying Genes Coding for Immunizing Antigens

A *vector* is a living virus or bacterium used as a carrier to express one or more "foreign" genes encoding desired antigens. Vectors under study include canarypox virus (a relative of vaccinia virus), adenovirus (a cause of respiratory disease), BCG (an attenuated bovine tuberculosis organism), Salmonella or Shigella (typhoid-like bacteria), and attenuated poliovirus. Canarypox can be altered to express HIV antigens, but canarypox does not itself multiply in the human. Canarypox therefore serves as a safe substitute for vaccinia as a vector (3, 15, 16, 69, 74, 91).

Live vectors have important advantages in inducing protective responses. First, protein antigen synthesized in a vector can induce cytotoxic T lymphocyte responses not expected with antigen administered as inert protein. Second, vectors carrying multiple *env*, *gag*, and *pol* genes but not RNA or other sequences essential for viral replication can assemble into a viral configuration, or *pseudovirion* (55). The nonreplicating structure of the pseudovirion is designed to duplicate advantages of a whole inactivated vaccine but eliminate its risks. Vaccines using *virus-like particles* (VLP) have also been produced without use of live vectors (102). Third, vectors that grow on body surfaces, such as adenovirus or Salmonella, can induce HIV local mucosal immune responses.

Live vectors also carry inherent safety concerns. The vector must be: 1) stably attenuated and unable to produce the natural human disease caused by the vector, 2) safe from unwanted spread to contacts and community at large, and 3) safe for individuals with impaired immunity. The safety problems that have occurred in licensed smallpox (vaccinia virus) vaccines allow us to predict potential safety problems with vaccines using live vaccinia virus vectors. These may include severe skin and mucous membrane infections, invasive and neurological diseases, and even death in susceptible immunosuppressed individuals (75).

Infectious DNA

The development of vaccines composed of pure viral genetic material, infectious or "naked" DNA, is a novel departure from traditional vaccines. Viral DNA coding for a single or multiple genes, injected directly into the muscle or skin, provides the genetic code for synthesizing new protein, which in turn behaves as a potent antigen. Persistent antibody and cytotoxic T lymphocyte responses have been induced in laboratory animals (42, 100). Mechanisms leading to the potent immune responses are not understood. Safety questions, which are highly theoretical at this time, involve possible tumor formation, production of autoimmune disease, or even the possibility of DNA transmission to the fetus.

Inactivated Whole Virus Vaccine

Development of inactivated as well as live attenuated HIV vaccines, using classical approaches, were seriously considered in early deliberations. Historically, the empiric use of either of these two pathways was generally successful with other viruses. These strategies have not been applied to HIV by vaccine manufacturers because each may carry significant risk.

TABLE 2-8: Vaccine Concepts and Their Stages of Development

Stage of development	Vaccine design
Phase I/II Trials	Envelope proteins (gp160, gp120) Vaccinia vector/gp160
Currently entering trials	Synthetic peptides Live vectors/multiple proteins Virus-like particles Pseudovirions Immune modulators/delivery systems
Preclinical research	Infectious DNA Inactivated whole virus Live attenuated virus

SOURCE: Office of Technology Assessment, 1995.

Preparation of a safe inactivated whole-virus vaccine, exemplified by the Salk-type of inactivated polio vaccine, requires inactivation of a high-titered preparation of live virus using gentle physical-chemical means to preserve full immunogenicity, yet ensuring inactivation of all live viruses. The process must guarantee absence of even a single infectious dose in large volumes (hundreds of thousands of patient units) of vaccine. There is a narrow margin between surviving virus and the destruction of viral immunogenicity; this was highlighted early in the use of licensed polio vaccine when a number of vaccinated individuals developed paralytic poliomyelitis from vaccine lots containing residual live virus (71). The safety problem was resolved by simple refinements in the inactivation process. By contrast, assuring inactivation of all HIV particles could prove difficult. In particular, concern exists as to whether cell cultures or animal models are sufficiently sensitive to detect the minimal residual live virus capable of infecting humans. There has also been theoretical concern regarding residual reactive viral DNA in the product.

In addition, the safety of the "lymphoblastoid" cell lines used to prepare the virus is unknown. "Adventitious agents," that is, unwanted agents growing silently in the cell cultures used to prepare vaccine stock, have posed safety problems in the past. As an example, SV_{40}, a monkey tumor virus, contaminated early lots of inactivated polio vaccine prepared in monkey cells (68).

The safety of an inactivated whole-virus vaccine for HIV was reviewed at a workshop in 1990. It was the consensus that a safe product is technically feasible but that product development should proceed with caution (82).

Live Attenuated Vaccine

Vaccines using live attenuated virus, exemplified by polio or measles vaccines, are capable of producing immune responses that closely mimic the solid, long-term protective immune response afforded by natural viral infection. In addition to a more vigorous and broader antibody response, attenuated virus vaccines may more effectively induce cytotoxic T lymphocytes and mucosal immunity compared with vaccines composed of inert antigens, such as envelope protein vaccines.

Using the SIV/monkey model, attenuated live virus vaccines have been constructed using selective deletions of nonessential auxiliary genes that are required for SIV replication (21). The attenuated virus is stable, not reverting to a virulent form of virus (i.e., a form of virus capable of producing disease) over an observation period of several years. Monkeys vaccinated with an SIV *nef* gene deletion show protection against challenge with large doses of virulent virus. By contrast, the control vaccinated monkeys acquired an AIDS-like disease and died in two years.

Safety Concerns Associated with Attenuated Virus

There are four primary safety concerns about attenuated viral vaccines that have been recognized (11, 22, 104).

1. *Level of attenuation.* Inadequate attenuation (reduction of virulence) of virus may result in a vaccine that induces the disease that it was designed to prevent; over-attenuated virus may fail to induce protective immune responses. However, even an appropriately attenuated virus may show virulent behavior when not constrained by a competent immune system, such as in vaccine recipients with immune systems compromised by cancers, immunosuppressant drugs, and other non-AIDS causes. The highly infectious nature of SIV administered orally to monkeys at birth, before the monkey's immune system has fully developed, has raised new questions about safety of vaccines in immunocompromised individuals (79).
2. *Stability of attenuation.* The vaccine strain could undergo genetic reversion to a more virulent form during the lengthy course of replication in the vaccinee. This risk is of particular concern with vaccines using attenuated strains of HIV, as the human immunodeficiency virus is characterized by rapid and frequent genetic mutations.
3. *Possibility of secondary spread.* Spread of attenuated virus to contacts of vaccinees (secondary spread) may provide the virus with further opportunity to revert to virulence (e.g., vaccine-induced poliomyelitis in contacts of vaccinees). However, if it can be assured that the level of attenuation of the virus remains stable, secondary spread of the virus may be beneficial, because the attenuated virus could induce protective immunity in contacts. Sufficient spread of the attenuated virus would result in the induction of herd immunity (as had occurred with poliovirus vaccine).
4. *Possibility of induction of tumors.* Other members of the retrovirus family regularly produce tumors (e.g., mouse tumors and a form of human leukemia). Theoretically, the prolonged residence of a live attenuated HIV vaccine strain in vaccinees could allow the retrovirus to produce tumors. Recent evidence for a direct role for HIV infection in the etiology of some T-cell lymphomas suggests a need to proceed cautiously while continuing to investigate the long-term potential of these vaccinees to produce tumors (92, 104).

The gene deletion approach to attenuation holds special promise. Deletion of one or more auxiliary genes essential for viral replication should make the risk of reversion to virulence unlikely. Because of safety concerns, viral mutants with multiple gene deletions are being explored for level of stability and attenuation, duration of protection, and long-term safety. It is hoped that these attenuated viral vaccines will prevent subsequent superinfection with a second, virulent but genetically different HIV strain.

The protective mechanism of attenuated SIV vaccine is unclear. It is not correlated with antibody or cytotoxic T lymphocyte responses, and mucosal immunity is not involved. This observation raises the question of whether another means of blocking virus exists. Attenuated vaccines in the SIV/monkey model offer interesting opportunities to explore immune determinants of protection.

New Approaches to Improve Vaccine Performance

Mucosal Immunity

No vaccine has yet provided an immune barrier at the mucosal membranes of the rectum, vagina, and urethra—the sites of sexual transmission of HIV (62, 63, 64). The mucosal administration of vaccine vectors that grow on mucosal surfaces may provide a critical tool for the prevention of HIV transmission by sexual routes. Antigen uptake from mucosal surfaces is poor compared with injection. New strategies to improve the uptake of antigens from mucosal surfaces involve use of biodegradable microspheres, cholera toxin B, liposomes (phospholipid droplets), and immunostimulating complexes (iscoms) to enhance passage of antigen through cell membranes for more efficient processing (58).

New Adjuvants and Delivery Vehicles

Adjuvants are nonviral materials incorporated into vaccine formulations to augment the magnitude or spectrum of immune responses to vaccines (31). Since the 1940s, however, alum compounds have been the only adjuvants accepted for vaccine products licensed by the FDA. Adjuvants have been discovered largely empirically, and are commonly derivatives of bacteria or plants. They may be combined with chemical surfactants (emulsifiers), forming complexes with specific HIV proteins or individual peptides. The introduction of new adjuvants into clinical practice has been slowed by concerns about the adjuvant's toxicity. Significant transient toxicity was shown in comparative trials of experimental adjuvants (table 2-6).

Exploration of adjuvants is currently undergoing a renaissance in an effort to selectively enhance HIV antibody, cytotoxic T lymphocyte, or mucosal immune responses. The hope is to move from an empiric to a rational approach to attaining specific immune response goals.

The microsphere is a new delivery vehicle that can add flexibility to the antigen's disposition (23, 58, 65). Antigen is coated with an inert plastic polymer, which becomes soluble in body tissues. The microsphere particle size and polymer composition can be altered to target a single dose of antigen to specific tissue sites such as mucous membranes, and to release the antigen in pulses, obviating the need for a multiple dose vaccination schedule.

Cytokines

Cytokines comprise a family of soluble substances (e.g., 1L-2, 1L-4, interferons, etc.) that mediate functions of immune cells. Cytokines can play a significant role in providing protective immune responses following vaccination (18). Specific cytokines may be included in a vaccine, or may be induced in the body by altering the form in which vaccine antigens are presented.

Any of the above approaches to improve vaccine performance may have unexpected side effects. So far, several new adjuvants have caused early transient difficulties and have been withdrawn from use.

SOCIAL HARMS AS ADVERSE EVENTS

Adverse consequences or harms may be expected, not attributable to the biological properties of the vaccine, but rather falling into the realm of "social injury" (2, 90). Vaccines may cause a "false-positive" screening tests for HIV infection. This vaccine-induced seropositivity can result in discrimination against false-positive individuals, such as in eligibility for military service, employment, health or life insurance, or restriction of travel.

Seropositivity following inoculation with envelope vaccines can usually be distinguished from HIV infection by the Western blot test which is used to confirm the results HIV of enzyme-linked immunosorbant assay (ELISA) tests used in HIV screening. Volunteers in NIAID-sponsored trials have received identification documents certifying their participation in these trails, although AVEG personnel have had to intervene to provide validation of confounding Western blot confirmatory tests (5).

The problem may become more acute in the future as new generation vaccines that include many more types of antigenic proteins than are currently used may render the Western blot test unable to distinguish vaccine-induced seropositivity from true HIV infection. Reliance must then be placed on time-consuming and expensive polymerase chain reaction (PCR) tests which detect the presence of virus directly, and on viral cultures. Simpler methods of distinguishing vaccine-induced immune responses from immune responses induced by natural infection are being actively pursued.

Participation in an HIV trial, in itself, may engender social harms. Others may perceive a volunteer's participation in the trial as implying that the volunteer is in a group at special risk of acquiring HIV infection, and this may result in personal stigmatization of the volunteer. Further, volunteers who are immunized with one candidate vaccine may be precluded from participating in clinical trials of subsequent, possibly more effective, vaccine products. Also, trial participants may assume that they are protected from HIV infection, and as a consequence may increase their risk-taking behaviors. This increased risk-taking behavior may occur despite intensive counseling on the possibility of assignment to placebo vaccine and the unknown efficacy of the trial vaccine.

HIV vaccines will fall short of protecting all recipients. None of the currently licensed vaccines in public health use, even the most effective, vaccines protects all recipients; estimates of protection range from 50 to 70 percent for influenza vaccine, to 95 percent for measles and polio vaccines. Failure of vaccine to protect is expected in clinical trials. These failures may be perceived as vaccine-induced enhancement of infection, manifest as an increased susceptibility or a more aggressive course of infection. Lastly, questions of responsibility and legal liability for vaccine injury, provision of health care, or other services to trial participants remain unresolved (2). The concept of social harms is developed further in the discussion of efficacy trials below. These issues are also discussed in further detail in chapters 3 and 4.

CLINICAL TRIALS IN HIV-INFECTED INDIVIDUALS

Infected Pregnant Women

Prevention of newborn HIV infection by vaccination of the infected mother deserves special note. HIV-infected pregnant women transmit infection to 15 to 40 percent of their progeny. In this complicated situation, vaccination can potentially prevent infection of the fetus or newborn and treat the infection of the mother. The goal of a vaccine in this setting is to favorably alter the immune status of the mother during pregnancy, thereby lowering the risk of transmission of the virus from mother to fetus (vertical transmission) (98).[18]. Possible risks to the mother, fetus, and newborn have not been formally tested in clinical trials of HIV vaccines. Previously, pregnancy has been cause for exclusion in all Phase I and II trials. Despite counseling designed to exclude pregnancy, overall 16 pregnancies have occurred in AVEG trials conducted in uninfected subjects with no adverse events attributable to vaccine.

[18] The use of vaccines to prevent vertical transmission is reviewed by M. Walker and P. Fast, 1995(98).

TABLE 2-9: Current Cinical Trials in HIV-Infected Pregnant Women

Vaccine	Developer	Trial site
In HIV infected pregnant women		
rgp160-LAI	MicroGeneSys	AVEG, ACTG
rgp120-MN	Genentech	AVEG, ACTG
rgp120-SF2	Biocine	ACTG
In infants born to HIV-infected women		
rgp120-MN	Genentech	ACTG
rgp120-SF2	Biocine	ACTG

KEY: ACTG = NIAID AIDS Clinical Trial Group; AVEG = AIDS Vaccine Evaluation Group of AIDS Vaccine Clinical Trials Network.

SOURCE: Adapted from M.C. Walker, and P.E. Fast, *Clinical Trials of Candidate AIDS Vaccines,* in press.

While there is no a priori reason to expect adverse events, such as injury to the developing fetus or newborn, from HIV vaccine, the outcomes of these pregnancies will be carefully monitored. Injuries to the newborn that are causally related to the vaccine must be distinguished from the recognized high background rate, approximately 3 percent, of naturally occurring birth defects or developmental problems in newborns. Phase I clinical trials of HIV vaccine in 23 infected pregnant women, using three rgp120 vaccine products, are in progress (table 2-9) (106). The vaccine products were pre-screened for fetal toxicity in rodents. No significant vaccine-related adverse events occurred in mothers or in the 20 infants that have been delivered to date.

In regions of the developing world where there is a high incidence of HIV infection and where effective chemotherapy (Zidovudine) is not widely available, trials of vaccines to prevent vertical HIV transmission remain appropriate. These trials should be a high priority, because HIV-infected infants usually progress rapidly to severe disease.

Trials of Therapeutic Vaccine for Treatment of Established Infection

Use of an HIV vaccine as an agent to treat individuals with established HIV infection (therapeutic vaccination) is based upon concepts that are different from vaccine used as a preventive agent (prophylactic vaccination). In established infection, a vaccine is used for its potential to favorably modulate the immune system. The objective of therapeutic vaccination is to selectively enhance the immune processes that reduce viral replication and increase viral suppression. This, in turn, may control or eliminate persistent virus and delay or prevent disease progression.

However, there has never been a vaccine that has been able to slow progression of an infectious process once the infection has been established. Post-exposure immunization in some viral infections, such as rabies, is only effective if the vaccine is administered early in the incubation period of the virus, before infection is established in the target organ. Approximately 35 Phase I and II trials of therapeutic HIV vaccines are active in the United States and abroad, using envelope and core proteins, novel vectors, inactivated virus, and other products (98).

Several things can be learned from trials of therapeutic HIV vaccines that bear on the development of a preventive HIV vaccine. First, the more favorable risk/benefit ratio in a treatment setting versus a preventive setting, permits more widespread study of novel products. Second, trials of therapeutic vaccines permit the assessment of the safety and specificity of immune responses to the vaccines (77). Third, there has been no clear evidence that therapeutic vaccines benefit the course of HIV infection, although more definitive randomized, controlled Phase II clinical trials are in progress. Finally, there is no evidence that HIV infection has been accelerated or enhanced in recipients of therapeutic HIV vaccines. One study of HIV vaccines in chimpanzees reported a

TABLE 2-10: HIV Vaccine Efficacy Trials

	Total sample size[a]			
	Annual rate HIV infection			
Length of Trial	1%	2%	3%	4%
2 years	28,896	14,540	9,690	7,290
2.5 years	22,266	11,224	7,496	5,650
3 years	18,294	9,238	6,180	4,668

[a] Two-arm study, 90% power to detect a 30% reduction in the risk of infection; 10% annual loss to followup.

SOURCE: Wasima N. Rida, Division of AIDS, NIAID, Bethesda, MD, June 1995.

transient rise in HIV-infected cells after vaccination; this transient increase in HIV-infected cells was of unknown significance (28).

PHASE III EFFICACY TRIALS

General Concepts of Efficacy Trial Design

The capability of a vaccine to protect against infection is determined in Phase III efficacy trials (96) (97). The quality and quantity of vaccine-induced immune responses measured in Phase I and II trials may predict, but do not demonstrate, efficacy of the vaccine. The second major function of the Phase III efficacy trial is to provide a more definitive assessment of vaccine safety.

Efficacy trials of HIV vaccines will be large, complex, lengthy, and expensive. The design requires a prospectively randomized, double-blind, placebo-controlled study, which will involve several thousand subjects assigned to one or more vaccines or to placebo. The trial site must be prepared with competence in epidemiology capabilities in behavioral, clinical and laboratory roles, and data management skills. The number of subjects, duration of recruitment, and followup are determined by several key variables. These include the number of arms (i.e., vaccine and placebo groups) in the study, seroincidence (annual rate of new infection), length of recruitment period, rate of retention, assumptions about level of efficacy of the experimental vaccines, and the definition of infection or disease endpoint(s) or outcomes that are measured. An example is provided in table 2-10.

Persistent infection accompanied by delay or prevention of clinical disease or reduced transmission of virus requires many years or lifetime followup.

Possible endpoints, including "intermediate endpoints" in vaccine trials, are described in table 2-11. Documentation of the validity of intermediate endpoints as predictors of vaccine protection will require intensive laboratory studies. Multiple efficacy trials will be needed; the initial vaccine formulations may well be less than optimal.

Preparing for Efficacy Trials in the United States

Successive vaccine candidates with potential for improved efficacy and safety will be compared in randomized, double-blind, controlled clinical trials with prior vaccines serving as benchmarks. HIV efficacy trials in the U.S. will be unique in the history of vaccinology. While the underlying epidemiological and statistical principles of trial design are the same as those used in trials of classical vaccines, the groups that are targeted for HIV vaccination and their community settings have special characteristics. This, together with the special biological and social implications of HIV infection, has a great impact on the conduct and outcome of the trial (43, 45, 96, 97).

Populations with high rates of seroconversion (incidence of HIV infection) are required, such as intravenous drug users and men who have sex with men. Such communities may feel disenfranchised and socially stigmatized, have concerns regarding access to health care and other services, and harbor distrust of the government and of

TABLE 2-11: Possible Outcomes of HIV Vaccine Efficacy Trials and Levels of Protection

Possible outcomes of trial	Interpretation
Sterilizing immunity	Vaccine has prevented infection.
Minimal infection without antibody	Vaccine has induced immune memory only.
Abortive infection	Early transient viremia and/or antibody response; vaccine has prevented establishment of infection.
Modified infection	Vaccine has decreased viral load, delayed disease, or reduced transmission.
Unmodified infection and disease	Vaccine has failed.
Rapid progression or increased incidence	Immune enhancement of infection as a result of vaccination.

SOURCE: Office of Technology Assessment, 1995.

scientific experimentation (90). These underlying ethical, social, legal, and political issues will require sensitive attention.

In anticipation of conducting large-scale efficacy trials, preparatory studies have been initiated (89, 96). Several thousand injection drug users and homosexual and bisexual gay men with a high HIV seroincidence are under study in the HIV Evaluation Network (HIVNET), sponsored by the NIAID, CDC, and the National Institute of Drug Abuse. The goals are multiple: 1) to study sociocultural factors affecting recruitment and retention; 2) to measure the frequency of risk behaviors, to assess the effect of trial participation, counseling, and unblinding on risk behaviors, and to develop strategies to reduce the frequency of risk behaviors (undocumented changes in personal risk behavior can have confounding effects on the apparent efficacy of a vaccine) (87); 3) to determine the basis for attitudes toward vaccine acceptance; 4) to develop educational strategies and consent forms appropriate to the subject groups; and 5) to study the dynamics of trial acceptance and feasibility. Information derived from such studies will enhance the feasibility and readiness to undertake full-scale HIV vaccine efficacy trials in the U.S. Continued research into the measurement of socio-behavioral variables is critical to planning, trial design and data analysis.

Criteria for Selection of a Vaccine for Efficacy Trials

The criteria for selecting an HIV vaccine candidate that merits study in a Phase III efficacy trial has been extensively discussed over the past few years. Because we do not know what specific type of immune response is required to provide protection from HIV infection, the criteria to be used to select vaccine candidates are not sharply defined. Discussions have involved consideration of the following elements: 1) evidence of safety and immunogenicity of the vaccine in Phase I and II trials; 2) the vaccines ability to induce high-titered, broadly reactive, and sustained levels of antibody capable of neutralizing primary field HIV isolates; 3) the vaccines ability to induce cytotoxic T lymphocyte responses, and 4) evidence of vaccine protection in a primate model. However, in the face of scientific uncertainty and a rapidly evolving knowledge base, the relative emphasis and stringency given to each of these criteria have varied in successive recommendations. More clearly defined criteria for selection of vaccine candidates for entry into Phase III efficacy trials would be of obvious value.

Envelope Proteins as Candidates for Efficacy Trials

Two candidate vaccines, Biocine SF2 with MF59 and Genentech MN with alum adjuvant have completed Phase II trials. A Phase III clinical trial of envelope vaccine would test the following hypothesis: can neutralizing antibody, with certain limitations in its magnitude, cross-reactivity, durability, and mucosal localization, protect a high-risk population with a measurable level of efficacy?

In June 1994, the NIAID AIDS Subcommittee and AIDS Research Advisory Committee (ARAC)

TABLE 2-12: Factors Considered in Determining Whether to Proceed With Efficacy Trials

Biological factors	Factors favoring efficacy trials	Factors weighing against efficacy trials
Safety	▪ Only minimal transient local and systemic reactions have occurred.	▪ Breakthrough infections; Possibility of immune enhancement.
Immune response	▪ Neutralizing antibody has been induced by envelope vaccines. ▪ CTL may not be essential.	▪ Need increased titer, duration, and cross-reactivity of antibody in response to envelope protein, as well as neutralization of primary isolates ▪ CTL may be important to protection.
Primate model	▪ Envelope vaccine protects chimpanzees against mild HIV infection under limited conditions.	▪ Envelope vaccine offered; poor protection in more stringent SIV/monkey disease model.
Social, political, ethical factors	▪ Vaccine need is a public health imperative.	▪ An inconclusive trial may result, with loss of public confidence.
	▪ Infrastructure for trials is ready.	▪ A better behavioral database is needed.
	▪ Modest protection valuable.	▪ Trial may involve large investment of funds and human resources for questionable gains. False security may increase risk-taking.
	▪ Scientific gains may result, e.g., immune determinants of protection.	▪ Trial lacks sensitivity to detect immune determinants of infection.
	▪ Product is ready.	▪ Setback for industry if trials fail.

KEY: CTL = cytotoxic T lymphocytes.

SOURCE: Adapted from A. Hause, "Report on the April HIV Vaccine Working Group Meeting,' paper presented at the NIAID AIDS Research Advisory Committee (ARAC) meeting, June 17, 1994.

recommended that Phase III clinical efficacy trials with the envelope vaccines should not proceed in the United States at that time (25). Factors contributing to the decision included scientific, political, and ethical issues (39) (table 2-12). There was a significant level of scientific uncertainty regarding the wisdom of immediate efficacy trials, with advocates on both sides of the question. Two trial designs were discussed (46). A definitive three-armed trial with a sample size of 9,000 high-risk individuals would permit detection of statistically significant protection from a vaccine with only 30 percent efficacy. Alternatively, a smaller trial, involving 4,500 individuals, would allow detection of significant protection from a vaccine with 60 percent efficacy, but have little chance of detecting the protection from a vaccine with 30 percent efficacy.[19]

Phase I and II clinical trials of HIV vaccines continue. New generation products recently entered into Phase I trials or in the preclinical pipeline are designed to expand the quality and quantity of the protective immune response to the vaccine. These products should be available for consideration for Phase III efficacy trails within two to three years.

Monitoring Adverse Events in Efficacy Trials

The long-term followup of large numbers of vaccinees and controls allows for surveillance of events that are infrequent or occur after an interval of years. The prospectively defined populations that participated in vaccine efficacy trials constitute unique epidemiologic cohorts, not easily du-

[19] Larger trials are able to defect smaller degrees of vaccine efficacy.

plicated after controlled efficacy trials are completed. "Vaccinated cohorts" from efficacy trials could be compared to the unvaccinated cohorts that are currently under epidemiologic and virologic surveillance.

Provision for long-term followup should be an integral part of the design of efficacy trials, allowing surveillance of safety issues, such as enhanced infection, autoimmune disease, tumors, or reversion to virulence. Rigorous assessment will be required before acceptance of a causal relationship between a vaccine and adverse events. Despite difficulties and expense, decades of experience with childhood vaccines emphasize the singular need for maintaining followup capability.

Efficacy Trials in the Developing World

While the current document addresses domestic issues, it is clear that HIV-1 efficacy trials at international sites will be an important and integral part of the process of developing and evaluating AIDS vaccine candidates. Such sites provide opportunities to study diverse population groups in highly endemic areas, including heterosexual and maternal-infant transmission of HIV, a variety of cultural and health settings, and vaccines targeting a multiplicity of HIV subtypes. In addition, it affords the possibility of direct benefit to the participating population in a tangible way. Vaccine affordability, ease of administration (given in a few doses or orally), and stability of protection will be critical to widespread use of vaccine. The NIAID and U.S. Department of Defense (DOD) are developing sites in concert with national governments in the Americas, Africa, and Asia. A multivalent peptide vaccine is currently the only approach in advanced stage of development that addresses the diversity of global subtypes. Opportunities for assessing subtype B strains are available in the Americas and Western Europe, as well as in a locus in Thailand.

The June 1994 decision to defer Phase III clinical efficacy trials in the U.S. does not preclude clinical efficacy trials of envelope-based vaccines in the developing world. Applying standards of safety and efficacy to populations with a rapid and uncontrollable rise in HIV infection alters the risk to benefit ratio of the vaccines. While ethical principles of such decisions remain universal, it is recognized that biological circumstances can validly affect the decision process. The attendant risks of adverse reactions or social harms in a developing world setting engender a separate level of issues, involving U.S. industry, institutions, and investigators, as well as the host foreign nationals. Issues surrounding vaccine trials in developing countries are discussed in chapters 3 and 4.

CHAPTER 2 REFERENCES

1. Ada, G.L., "Modern Vaccines: The Immunological Principles of Vaccination," *Lancet* 335:423-526, 1990.
2. AIDS Action Foundation, *HIV Preventive Vaccines: Social, Ethical, and Political Considerations for Domestic Efficacy Trials* Report of a Working Group Convened by the AIDS Action Foundation, July, 1994.
3. Aldovini, A., and Young, R.A., "Humoral and Cell-Mediated Immune Responses to Live Recombinant BCG-HIV Vaccines," *Nature* 351:479-482, 1991.
4. Autran, B., and Letvin, N.L., "HIV Epitopes Recognized by Cytotoxic T-lymphocytes," *AIDS* 5:S145-S150, 1991.
5. Belshe, R.B., et al., "HIV Infection in Vaccinated Volunteers," *Journal of the American Medical Association* 272(6):431, 1994.
6. Belshe, R.B., et al., "Neutralizing Antibodies to HIV-1 in Seronegative Volunteers Immunized with Recombinant gp120 from the MN Strain of HIV-1," *Journal of the American Medical Association* 272(6):475-48, 1994.
7. Belshe, R.B., Clements, M.L., and Keefer, M.C., "Interpretation of Serodiagnostic Tests for HIV in the 1990s: Social Risks of HIV Vaccine Studies in Uninfected Volunteers," *Annals of Internal Medicine,* in press.
8. Herman, P.W., et al., "Protection of Chimpanzees from Infection of HIV-1 After Vaccination with Recombinant Glycoprotein

gp120 but not gp160," *Nature* 345:622-625, 1990.
9. Berzofsky, J.A., "Approaches and Issues in the Development of Vaccines Against HIV," *Acquired Immune Deficiency Syndrome* 4:451-459,1991.
10. Bolognesi, D.P., "Prospects for an HIV Vaccine," *Scientific American Science & Medicine* March/April:44-53, 1994.
11. Bolognesi, D.P., "A Live-Virus AIDS Vaccine?," *Journal of NIH Research* 6:59-62, 1994.
12. Burke, D.S., "Human HIV Vaccine Trials: Does Antibody-Dependent Enhancement Pose a Genuine Risk?," *Perspectives in Biology and Medicine* 35(4): 511-530, 1992.
13. Burke, D.S. "Vaccine Therapy for HIV: A Historical Review of the Treatment of Infectious Diseases by Active Specific Immunization with Microbe-Derived Antigens," *Vaccine* 11:883-891, 1993.
14. Cease, K.B., and Berzofsky, J.A., "Toward a Vaccine for AIDS: The Emergence of Immunogiology-Based Vaccine Development," *Annual Review of Immunology* 12:923-928, 1994.
15. Chatfield, S., Strugnell, R., and Dougan, G., "Live *Salmonella* as Vaccines and Carriers of Foreign Antigenic Determinants," *Vaccine* 7:495-498, 1989.
16. Cheng, S-M., et al., "Robust Expression of the SIV Envelope Protein by a Recombinant Human Adenovirus Host-range Mutant," *Vaccines 91* (Cold Spring Harbor, NY: Cold Spring Harbor Laboratory Press, 1991).
17. Clerici, M. et al., "Cell-Mediated Immune Response to Human Immunodeficiency Virus (HIV) Type 1 in Seronegative Homosexual Men with Recent Sexual Exposure to HIV-1," *Journal of Infectious Diseases* 165:1012-1019, 1992.
18. Clerici, M., and Shearer, G.M., "A T_H1 T_H2 Switch is a Critical Step in the Etiology of HIV Infection," *Immunology Today* 14:107-111, 1993.
19. Daniel, M.D., et al., "Protective Effects of a Live Attenuated SIV Vaccine with a Deletion in the *nef* Gene," *Science* 258:1938-1941, 1992.
20. Desrosiers, R.C., et al., "Vaccine Protection Against Simian Immunodeficiency Virus Infection," *Proceedings of the National Academy of Science USA* 86:6353-6357, 1989.
21. Desrosiers, R.C., "HIV with Multiple Gene Deletions as a Live Attenuated Vaccine for AIDS," *AIDS Research and Human Retroviruses* 8:411-421, 1992.
22. Desrosiers, R.C., "*Yes*, It Is Time To Consider Use of a Live-Attenuated Virus Vaccine Against HIV-1," *Journal of NIH Research* 6:54-59, 1994.
23. Eldridge, J.H., et al., "Biodegradable Microspheres as a Vaccine Delivery System," *Molecular Immunology* 28:287-294, 1991.
24. Emini, E.A., et al., "Prevention of HIV-1 Infection in Chimpanzees by gp120 V3 Domain-specific Monoclonal Antibody," *Nature* 355:728-730, 1992.
25. Fauci, R., "The Dilemma of Developing and Testing AIDS Vaccines," paper presented at the *International Conference on AIDS,* Tokyo, Japan, July 1994.
26. Fenner, F., et al., "Smallpox and Its Eradication," (Geneva, Switzerland: World Health Organization, 1988).
27. Fulginiti, V.A., et al., "Altered Reactivity to Measles Virus. Atypical Measles in Children Previously Immunized With Inactivated Measles Virus Vaccines," *Journal of the American Medical Association* 202:1075-1080, 1967.
28. Fultz, P.N., et al., "Transient Increases in Numbers of Infectious Cells in an HIV-infected Chimpanzee Following Immune Stimulation," *AIDS Research and Human Retroviruses* 8:313-317, 1992.
29. Garrison, L., and Clements, M.L., "Development of New Vaccines for AIDS," *Comprehensive Therapy* 15(7):47-55,1989.

30. Girard, M., et al., "Immunization of Chimpanzees Confers Protection Against Challenge with Human Immunodeficiency Virus," *Proceedings of the National Academy of Science USA* 88:542-546, 1991.
31. Goldenthal, et al., "Safety Evaluation of Vaccine Adjuvants: National Cooperative Vaccine Development Meeting Working Group," *AIDS Research and Human Retroviruses* 9(suppl 1):S47-S51, 1993.
32. Golding, H., et al., "Identification of Homologous Regions in Human Immunodeficiency Virus I gp 41 and Human MHC Class II ß 1 Domain," *Journal of Experimental Medicine* 167:914-923, 1988.
33. Golding, H., et al., "Common Epitope in Human Immunodeficiency Virus (HIV) 1-gp41 and HLA Class II Elicits Immunosuppressive Autoantibodies Capable of Contributing to Immune Dysfunction in HIV-1 Infected Individuals," *Journal of Clinical Investigation* 83:1430-1435, 1989.
34. Gorse, G.J., et al., "Vaccine-induced Antibodies to Native and Recombinant HIV-1 Envelope Glycoproteins," *Vaccine* 12(10):912-918, 1994.
35. Graham, B.S., et al. "Priming Immunization Determines Cytokine MRNA Expression Patterns in Lungs of Mice Challenged with Respiratory Syncytial Virus," *Journal of Immunology* 151:2032-2040, 1993.
36. Graham, B.S., et al., "Augmentation of HIV-1 Neutralizing Antibody by Priming with gp160 Recombinant Vaccinia and Boosting with rgp160," *Journal of Infectious Diseases* 167:533-537, 1993b.
37. Graham, B.S., "Panel Discussion on Infected Vaccinees," paper presented at *The Seventh Annual Meeting of the National Cooperative Vaccine Development Groups for AIDS: Conference on Advances in AIDS Vaccine Development,* Reston, VA, November 6-10, 1994.
38. Graham, B.S., "Serologic Responses to Candidate AIDS Vaccines," *AIDS Research and Human Retroviruses,* in press.
39. Haase, A., "Report on the April HIV Vaccine Working Group Meeting," paper presented at the NIAID AIDS Research Advisory Committee meeting, June 17, 1994.
40. Halstead, S.A., "In Vivo Enhancement of Dengue Virus Infection in Rhesus Monkeys by Passively Transferred Antibody," *Journal of Infectious Diseases* 140:527-533, 1979.
41. Hart, M.K., et al., "Synthetic Peptides Containing T and B Cell Epitopes from Human Immunodeficiency Virus Envelope gp120 Induce Anti-HIV Proliferative Responses and High Titers of Neutralizing Antibodies in Rhesus Monkeys," *Journal of Immunology* 145:2677-2685, 1990.
42. Haynes, B.F., "Scientific and Social Issues of Human Immunodeficiency Virus Vaccine Development," *Science* 260:1279-1286, 1993.
43. Haynes, J.R., Fuller, D., and Eisenbraun, M., "In Vivo Delivery of HIV and SIV Antigen-encoding Vectors by Particle Bombardment as an Alternative to Live Recombinant Viruses for the Induction of Humoral and Cellular Immunity," *AIDS Research and Human Retroviruses* 9(Suppl 1):S75, 1993.
44. Hirsch, V.M., et al., "Prolonged Clinical Latency and Survival of Macaques Given a Whole Inactivated Simian Immunodeficiency Virus Vaccine," *Journal of Infectious Diseases* 170:51-59, 1994.
45. Hoff, R., et al., "Monitoring Immunogenicity and Infection in HIV Vaccine Efficacy Trials," *AIDS Research and Human Retroviruses* 9(supp 1):S71-S73, 1993.
46. Hoff, R., et al., "HIV Vaccine Trial Design," paper presented at the NIAID AIDS Research Advisory Committee meeting, June 17, 1994.
47. Hu, S.L., et al., "Protection of Macaques Against SIV Infection by Subunit Vaccines of SIV Envelope Glycoprotein gp160," *Science* 255:456-459, 1992.
48. Institute of Medicine, *Adverse Events Associated with Childhood Vaccines; Evidence Bearing on Causality* (Washington, DC: National Academy Press, 1994).

49. Institute of Medicine, *Research Strategies for Assessing Adverse Events Associated with Vaccines* (Washington, DC: National Academy Press, 1994).
50. Karzon, D.T., Bolognesi, D. P., and Koff, W.C., "Development of a Vaccine for the Prevention of AIDS, A Critical Appraisal," *Vaccine* 10:1039-1052, 1992.
51. Karzon, D.T., "Preventive Vaccines," *Textbook of AIDS Medicine*, S. Broder S, T. Merigan, and D. Bolognesi (eds.) (Baltimore, MD: Williams & Wilkins, 1994).
52. Keefer, M.C., et al., "Safety Profile of HIV Vaccination: First 1,000 Volunteers of AIDS Vaccine Evaluation Group," *AIDS Research and Human Retroviruses* 10(suppl 2):S139-S140, 1994.
53. Keefer, M.C., et al. "Studies of High Doses of an HIV-1 Recombinant gp160 Candidate Vaccine in HIV-1 Seronegative Humans," *AIDS Research and Human Retroviruses,* in press.
54. Kim, H.W., et al. "Safety and Antigenicity of Temperature-sensitive (Ts) Mutants Respiratory Syncytial (RS) Virus in Infants and Children," *Pediatrics* 52:56-63, 1973.
55. Klein, M.R., et al., "Persistent High gagCTLp Frequency and Low Viral Load in Long-term Asymptomatic HIV Infection," IXth International Conference on AIDS, Berlin, Germany, June 1993 [abstract WS-B03-3].
56. Levy, J.A., "Pathogenesis of Human Immunodeficiency Virus Infection," *Microbiological Reviews* 57(1):183-289, 1993.
57. Levy, J.A., "Long-term Survivors of HIV Infection," *Hospital Practice* pp.41-52, October 15, 1994.
58. Marx, P.A., et al., "Protection Against Vaginal SIV Transmission With Microencapsulated Vaccine," *Science* 260:1323-1327, 1993.
59. Mascola, J.R., et al. "Summary Report: Workshop on the Potential Risks of Antibody-Dependent Enhancement in Human HIV Vaccine Trials," *AIDS Research and Human Retroviruses* 9(12):1175-1184, 1993.
60. McElrath, et al., "Immune Responses Elicited by Recombinant Vaccinia—HIV Envelope and HIV Envelope Protein: Analysis of the Durability of Immune Responses and Effect of Repeated Boosting," *Journal of Infectious Diseases* 169:41-47, 1994.
61. McElrath, M.J., et al., "Evaluation of HIV-1-specific Cytotoxic T Lymphocyte Responses Utilizing B Lymphoblastoid Cell Lines Transduced with the CD4 Gene and Infected with HIV-1," *Journal of Virology* 68(8):5074-5083, 1994.
62. McGhee, J.R., et al., "The Mucosal Immune System: From Fundamental Concepts to Vaccine Development," *Vaccine* 10:75-88, 1992.
63. Mestecky, J., Kutteh, W.H., and Jackson, S., "Mucosal Immunity in the Female Genital Tract: Relevance to Vaccination Efforts Against the Human Immunodeficiency Virus," *AIDS Research and Human Retroviruses* 10(suppl.):S11-20, 1994.
64. Miller, C.J., McGhee, J.R., and Gardner, M.B., "Mucosal Immunity, HIV Transmission and AIDS," *Laboratory Investigation* 68:129-145, 1992.
65. Moldoveanu, Z., et al., "Oral Immunization with Influenza Virus in Biodegradable Microspheres," *Journal of Infectious Diseases* 167:84-90, 1993.
66. Montefiori, D.C., et al., "Absence of a Clinical Correlation for Complement-mediated, Infection-Enhancing Antibodies in Plasma or Sera from HIV-1-infected Individuals," *AIDS* 5:513-517, 1991.
67. Montefiori, D.C., "In Vivo Correlates of HIV and SIV Humoral Immunity and Infection-Enhancement," *AIDS Research Reviews*, W.C. Koff, F. Wong-Saal, and R.C. Kennedy (eds.) (New York, NY: Marcel Dekker, 1992).
68. Mortimer, E.A., et al. "Long-term Follow-up of Persons Inadvertently Inoculated with SV_{40} as Neonates," *New England Journal of Medicine* 305:1517- 1518, 1981.

69. Moss, B., "Vaccinia Virus: A Tool for Research and Vaccine Development," *Science* 252:1662-1667, 1991.
70. Myers, G., et al. (eds.), *Human Retroviruses and AIDS 1992* (Los Alamos, NM: Los Alamos National Laboratory, 1992).
71. Nathanson, N., and Langmuir, A.D., "The Cutter Incident: Poliomyelitis Following Formaldehyde-inactivated Poliovirus Vaccination in the United States During the Spring of 1955. I. Background," *American Journal of Hygiene* 78:16-28, 1963.
72. Nelsing, S., Nielsen, T.L., and Nielsen, J.O., "Occupational Exposure to Human Immunogenicity Virus Among Health Care Workers in a Danish Hospital," *Journal of Infectious Diseases* 169:478,1994.
73. Ou, C.Y., et al. "Molecular Epidemiology of HIV Transmission in a Dental Practice, *Science* 256:1165-1171, 1992.
74. Panicali, D., and Paoletti, E., "Construction of Poxviruses as Cloning Vectors: Insertion of the Thymidine Kinase Gene from Herpes Simplex Virus into the DNA of Infectious Vaccinia Virus," *Proceedings of the National Academy of Science USA* 79:4927-4931, 1982.
75. Redfield, R.R., et al., "Disseminated Vaccinia in a Military Recruit with Human Immunodeficiency Virus (HIV) Disease," *New England Journal of Medicine* 316:673-676, 1987.
76. Redfield, R., et al. "A Phase I Evaluation of the Safety and Immunogenicity of Vaccination With Recombinant gp160 in Patients with Early Human Immunodeficiency Virus Infection," *New England Journal of Medicine* 324:1677-1684, 1991.
77. Redfield R.R., et al., "Evaluation of the Safety and Immunogenicity of Vaccination with Recombinant gp160 in Patients with Early Immunodeficiency Virus Infection," *New England Journal of Medicine* 324:1678-1684, 1991.
78. Rowland-Jones, S.L., et al., "HIV-specific Cytotoxic T-cell Activity in an HIV-exposed but Uninfected Infant," *Lancet* 341:860-861, 1993.
79. Ruprecht, R., et al., "Vaccine Strategies to Prevent Congenital Infection," paper presented at *The Seventh Annual Meeting of the National Cooperative Vaccine Development Groups for AIDS: Conference on Advances in AIDS Vaccine Development*, Reston, VA, Nov. 6-10, 1994.
80. Sabin, A.B., "Improbability of Effective Vaccination Against Human Immuno deficiency Because of Its Intracellular Transmission and Rectal Portal of Entry," *Proceedings of the National Academy of Sciences* 89:8852-8855, 1992.
81. Salk, J., "Prospects for the Control of AIDS by Immunizing Seropositive Individuals," *Nature* 327:473-476, 1987.
82. Schultz, A.M., Koff, W.C., and Lawrence, D.N., "Workshop on HIV Inactivated Vaccines," *Vaccine* 8:516-517, 1990.
83. Schultz, A.M., Hu, S, "Primate Models for HIV Vaccines," *AIDS* 7:S161-S170, 1993.
84. Schwartz, D.H., "Potential Pitfalls on the Road to an Effective HIV Vaccine," *Immunology Today* 15(2):54-57, 1994.
85. Shafferman, A., et al., "Protection of Macaques with Simian Immunodeficiency Virus Envelope Peptide Vaccine Based on Conserved Human Immunodeficiency Virus Type 1 Sequences," *Proceedings of the National Academy of Sciences* 88:7126-7130, 1991.
86. Shafferman A., et al., "Prevention of Transmission of Simian Immunodeficiency Virus from Vaccinated Macaques that Developed Transient Virus Infection Following Challenge," *Vaccine* 11:848-852,1993.
87. Sheon, A.R., "Behavioral Aspects of HIV Vaccine Efficacy Trials," paper presented at *Second International Conference on Vaccines,* Alexandria, VA, March 22, 1994.
88. Sheon, A.R., "Vaccines: New Technologies and Applications," paper presented at *Second International Conference on Vaccines,* Alexandria, VA, Mar. 22, 1994.

89. Sheon, A.R., "NIAID Vaccine Preparedness Initiative: Overview," presentation to AIDS Action Foundation Steering Committee Meeting, Santa Monica, CA, Feb. 1-3, 1994.
90. Sheon, A.R., "HIV Vaccine Preparedness Initiative," *AIDS Research and Human Retroviruses*, in press.
91. Shibata, R., Adachi, A., "SIV/HIV Recombinants and Their Use in Studying Biological Properties," *AIDS Research and Human Retroviruses* 8:403-490, 1992.
92. Shiramizu, B., Herndier, B.G., and McGrath, M.S., "Identification of a Common Clonal Human Immunodeficiency Virus Integration Site in Human Immunodeficiency Virus-associated Lymphomas," *Cancer Research* 54:2069-2072, 1994.
93. Strauss, S.E., et al., "Placebo-Controlled Trial of Vaccination with Recombinant Glycoprotein D of Herpes Simplex Virus Type 2 for Immunotherapy of Genital Herpes," *Lancet* 343:1460-63,1994.
94. Trauger, R.J., et al., "Effect of Immunization with Inactivated gp120-Depleted Human Immunodeficiency Virus Type 1 (HIV-1) Immunogen on HIV-1 Immunity, Viral DNA, and Percentage of CD4 Cells," *Journal of Infectious Diseases* 169:1256-64,1994.
95. U.S. Department of Health and Human Services, Public Health Service, National Institutes of Health, National Institute of Allergy and Infectious Diseases, *HIV Infection in Vaccine Trial Volunteers*, (Bethesda, MD: National Institutes of Health, June 1994).
96. Vermund, S.H., "The Efficacy of HIV Vaccines: Methodological Issues in Preparing for Clinical Trials," *HIV Epidemiology: Models and Methods*, A. Nicolosi (ed.) (New York, NY: Raven Press, Ltd., 1994).
97. Vermund, S.H., Schultz, A.M., and Hoff, R., "Prevention of HIV/AIDS with Vaccines," *Current Opinion in Infectious Diseases* 7:82-94, 1994.
98. Walker, M.C., and Fast, P.E., "Clinical Trials of Candidate AIDS Vaccines," in press.
99. Wang, C.Y., et al., "Long-term High-titer Neutralizing Activity Induced by Octameric Synthetic HIV-1 Antigen," *Science* 254:285-288, 1991.
100. Wang, B., et al., "Gene Inoculation Generates Immune Responses Against Human Immunodeficiency Virus Type 1," *Proceedings of the National Academy of Science USA* 90:4156-4160, 1993.
101. Warren, J.T., and Dolatshahi, M. "Annual Updated Survey of Worldwide HIV, SIV, and SHIV Challenge Studies in Vaccinated Nonhuman Primates," *Journal of Medical Primatology* 23:184-225, 1994.
102. Weber, J., et al., "A Phase I Clinical Study of the Safety, Toxicity, and Immunogenicity of the Ty, p24, VLP in Healthy Volunteers-Interim Report," *AIDS Research and Human Retroviruses* 8:1311, 1992.
103. World Health Organization Global Programme on AIDS, *Report of a Technical Working Group on Establishment of a WHO Network for HIV Isolation and Characterization* (Potters Bar, United Kingdom: 1991).
104. World Health Organization Working Group, "Feasibility of Developing Live Attenuated HIV Vaccines: Conclusions and Recommendations," *AIDS Research and Human Retroviruses* 10:221-222, 1994.
105. Wright, P.F., et al., "Strategies for the Global Eradication of Poliomyelitis By the Year 2000," *New England Journal of Medicine* 325:1774-1779, 1991.
106. Wright, P.F., "Active Immunization of HIV-Positive Women During Pregnancy," paper presented at *The Seventh Annual Meeting of the National Cooperative Vaccine Development Groups for AIDS: Conference on Advances in AIDS Vaccine Development,* Reston, VA, Nov. 6-10, 1994.

Ethical Issues in the Design and Conduct of HIV Vaccine Trials | 3

by
Nancy E. Kass
Johns Hopkins University School of Hygiene and Public Health Baltimore, MD

Although of crucial importance, human trials of HIV vaccines should not go forward without appropriate attention to ethical considerations. This chapter provides an overview of the ethical considerations that arise in the design and conduct of clinical trials of preventive HIV vaccines.[1] The primary focus of this chapter is on Phase III (efficacy) trials; however, many ethical issues relevant to early stage (Phase I and II) clinical trials and to the marketing of HIV vaccines are also addressed.

This chapter begins with a review of some basic ethical principles and background information about clinical trials. The chapter then discusses ethical issues in clinical trial design, sample selection, informed consent, trial termination, and compensation for adverse reactions. The chapter concludes with a discussion of ethical issues relevant to clinical trials in developing countries, and issues arising from the incorporation of HIV vaccines into clinical practice.

BASIC ETHICAL PRINCIPLES

All biomedical research should be conducted in a manner that seeks not to violate three primary bioethical principles: 1) beneficence, 2) respect for autonomy, and 3) justice (3).[1] The principle

[1] This paper is concerned with *ethical* obligations, rather than *legal* ones. Ethical obligations tell us how we ought to act, in accordance with a series of morals, values, and principles. In certain contexts, including in the research context, organizations have put forward codes of behavior to guide ethical conduct. Typically, these codes are not binding legally, and at most, carry weight in determining the standard of care. Legal obligations tell us what we are required to do, in accordance with a government's legal system, as defined by regulations, legislation, and court decisions. Breach of legal obligations typically results in specified penalties.

of beneficence addresses one's obligations to ensure the well being of others. Included within the principle are both the obligation to do no harm (called nonmaleficence) and the obligation to do good. In the context of clinical trials, the principle of beneficence requires that the welfare of research participants be protected. Participants must not be exposed to undue or excessive risks. This obligation may not be waived merely by informing subjects of these risks.

Moreover, initial responsibility for ensuring that risks are not excessive lies with the investigator, the vaccine sponsor, and an external review board. This responsibility may not be delegated to the research participant, for two reasons. First, research volunteers are unlikely to understand the risks of research as well as do the investigators and research sponsors. Second, it is a central tenet of research ethics that, unless personal benefit can be gained from trial participation, there are certain risks that are just too great for anyone to consent to, regardless of one's level of understanding of those risks. In trials involving human research subjects, an external review board, in collaboration with the investigators, is charged with assessing whether a given level of risk is justified. External review boards are given this responsibility because of concern that investigators directly involved in the study have interests that may bias their assessment of research risks. Also, external review boards typically include lay persons and persons from disciplines other than that of the investigator, who provide balance in the assessment of the reasonableness of risks.[2]

There are further obligations arising out of beneficence. When persons are included in research who might be particularly vulnerable to being exploited (e.g., prisoners, children, persons with little formal education), beneficence requires us to provide special protections to ensure that these participants are not harmed by the research.

Respect for autonomy, or respect for persons, obligates investigators to recognize research subjects as individuals who have the right to make their own decisions, even when those decisions are based on values or world views that are different from those of the investigator. The doctrine of informed consent (described below) is derived from the principle of respect for autonomy.

Justice requires fairness in the distribution of both benefits and burdens. In research, this requires that no individuals or populations bear a disproportionate share of the risks of research without justification, and that all populations have access to the benefits of research participation.

Each of these three principles create independent obligations that may conflict. For example, decisions about what is the "reasonable" level of risk above which participants cannot be exposed (based on beneficence) may conflict with the right of potential participants to determine this level for themselves (based on respect for autonomy). Another example is the potential conflict among the obligation of external boards to protect certain groups or individuals from research risks (based on justice), the obligation to allow individuals to make that assessment for themselves (autonomy), and the obligation to obtain findings that will benefit society as a whole (beneficence). There are no clear rules for balancing these obligations. In actual practice, the investigators and an outside board first determine what harms are unreasonable. If the risks of trial participation are not unreasonable, potential research participants must provide "informed consent" to trial participation-research participants should be given information about the trial in question, including its risks, and allowed to decide whether they wish to participate, according to their own values and preferences.

CLINICAL TRIALS OF VACCINES

There are two main categories of vaccines being developed for HIV: prophylactic vaccines and therapeutic vaccines. Prophylactic HIV vaccines

[2] For further history of Institutional Review Boards, see R.J. Levine, 1988 (20).

have as their primary purpose the prevention of infection (although, in certain cases, the term is used for vaccines intended to prevent establishment of infection). Therapeutic HIV vaccines are given to persons who are already infected to slow, halt, or reverse the progression of disease. In this sense, therapeutic vaccines are similar to any other treatment.[3] This chapter discusses ethical issues surrounding clinical trials of prophylactic HIV vaccines.

While the three phases to the testing of vaccines in human populations were described in detail in chapter 2, the focus of this chapter is on ethical issues related to the conduct of clinical efficacy (Phase III) trials of HIV vaccines, although many of these issues are also relevant to the conduct of Phase I and Phase II trials. The final portion of this chapter discusses some ethical issues related to the use of an approved HIV vaccine in clinical practice.

ETHICAL ISSUES IN THE DESIGN OF CLINICAL TRIALS

These are a number of ethical considerations in the design of a clinical trial of a prophylactic HIV vaccine. Fundamentally, a trial that is not designed to yield valid, scientifically new, or confirmatory results is unethical and should not be conducted because no burden or risk on the part of research participants is justified if some benefit is not likely to result. Assuming that there is scientific justification to proceed with a clinical trial, specific questions related to design must be addressed.

Is Randomization Ethical?

Benjamin Freedman argued that it is only ethical to randomly assign trial participants to an experimental intervention where there is "clinical equipoise—"that is, where there is uncertainty in the medical or scientific community generally about whether the intervention is beneficial (10). This does not require, however, that the investigators themselves not have a "treatment preference."

Because HIV is such a serious condition and the consequences of erroneous vaccine research findings would be great, it may be less ethical to conduct a vaccine trial that does not randomly assign trial participants. Randomized clinical trials are not the only means of assessing effectiveness, but because they minimize the potential for bias, they are considered the "gold standard" for clinical research (30). Randomized trials of HIV vaccines are particularly important because factors that affect HIV transmission, such as risk behaviors or concurrent infection with other sexually transmitted diseases, have the potential to bias the results of an observational study of vaccine efficacy.

Once there is consensus that an HIV vaccine is protective, it would not be ethical to conduct a vaccine trial that randomly assigns research participants to a placebo vaccine.[4] It is ethical to conduct randomized clinical trials to test hypotheses, but not to provide confirmatory data.

Will Trial Participants Receive Counseling About Risk Behaviors?

Any clinical trial of an HIV vaccine should include behavioral counseling about risks for HIV transmission at every study visit. This is ethically required, not only because the vaccine is unlikely to be completely efficacious and some participants in a randomized trial will not receive the vaccine, but also because there is a responsibility to provide trial participants with some benefit if possible at not too great an expense. Moreover, the provision of behavioral counseling reinforces the message to trial participants that vaccines are but one part of an overall strategy to prevent HIV transmission, which also includes the avoidance of behaviors that increase one's risk of infection. This will also be an important message to convey

[3] The possible uses for an HIV vaccine are described in chapter 2, box 2-1, "The Spectrum of Possible Strategies for Uses of HIV Vaccines."

[4] After an HIV vaccine is approved, new generation experimental vaccines would be tested against the approved vaccine.

when HIV vaccines are incorporated into clinical practice.

Although the power of a study to detect differences between vaccine and placebo recipients will be reduced if the recipients' baseline rate of seroconversion falls, ethically the most effective behavioral counseling should be provided to participants.

Are Procedures Adequate for the Confidential Handling of Research Data?

In research, it is imperative that all aspects of data collection, including recordkeeping, data storage, and the sharing of information be performed in a manner that maintains participants' confidentiality. Persons known or even suspected of being HIV positive have experienced discrimination in housing, employment, and insurance, as well as social discrimination from peers (14). Because the HIV-related information gathered in HIV vaccine trials is particularly sensitive, the maintenance of confidentiality in these trials is especially important.

Procedures should be established to maintain the confidentiality of trial participants. A number of practical measures should be taken. For example, participants should be assigned unique identification numbers, and all interactions with participants should be conducted using those unique identifiers (or first names if trial participants prefer), rather than the trial participants' full names. A "master key" that links participants' full names to their unique identification numbers should be kept in a locked cabinet or other secure place, and accessible by only a limited number of investigators.

The participants' full names should not be revealed to those who interview the participant, draw his or her blood, provide behavioral counseling, administer the vaccine, or otherwise personally interact with the participant. All written information and specimens should be labeled with the participants' unique identifiers, and these should be kept in locked storage units or computer files with controlled access. Most important, staff at all levels should be trained in procedures for maintaining confidentiality.

Participants in clinical trials of HIV vaccines should be assured that they may have access to their files once the trial is completed. Participants should be provided with documentation of their participation in the HIV vaccine trial, as it may be needed later to demonstrate, for example, that vaccine is the source of a false-positive HIV screening test.

Some researchers have sought to bill participants' insurers for any trial-related procedures (e.g., laboratory analyses, screening tests, etc.). The primary legal reason why insurers rarely pay for these procedures is that insurance policies only provide reimbursement for "medically necessary" treatments. One's decision to participate in a clinical trial is completely discretionary and the efficacy of the preventive therapy or treatment is unproven, so the experimental therapy cannot be considered medically necessary. There is also an important ethical reason such claims should not be filed: the filing of claims would pose unjustifiable risk to trial participants' confidentiality. In HIV vaccine trials, the filing of a claim would require the disclosure of the participants' names and sensitive HIV-related information to individuals who have no relationship to the trial. The disclosure of sensitive HIV-related information may put the participants' access to future coverage at risk. Therefore, payment for trial-associated medical procedures should be the responsibility of the investigators and vaccine sponsors, and funds for these procedures should be included in the trial budget.

Is There Community Involvement in the Planning and Conduct of the Trial?

Although the importance of a community board is usually emphasized in discussions of clinical trials in developing countries, a community board is equally important for trials conducted in the United States or other developed countries. A community board often is comprised of approximately 10 persons, usually trial participants, who meet with the investigators periodically throughout the course of the trial, beginning with its developmental stage. Community boards often review and make recommendations about how the trial should be conducted. In some settings, new staff must be interviewed and approved by the board before they are hired. The community board benefits both the trial participants and the investigators. Participants can contact board members, who may seem more accessible than investigators, with questions and concerns. The members of the board are intended to be representative of trial participants, and will help ensure that participants' rights are protected. Researchers are likely to benefit from participants' greater involvement and, perhaps, "ownership" of the research, that is engendered by the community board; this could result in greater retention and better adherence by participants to study protocols.

SELECTION OF SAMPLE

There are a number of ethical considerations in recruitment and selection of trial participants. Generally, individuals suitable for clinical efficacy (Phase III) trials are from populations with a high incidence of HIV infection, and should be from communities with sufficient willingness and infrastructure to support a trial (31). A candidate vaccine should be tested in the populations in which it would be used in clinical practice because a study's findings may not be generalizable to populations other than those from which the study sample was chosen.

Special Populations

Historically, a major thrust of research ethics has been the protection of vulnerable populations from enrollment in human subject research without their (or their guardians') knowledge or consent (an autonomy-based concern) or without justification for their specific inclusion (a justice-based concern) (25, 33). More recently, concerns about not burdening any population disproportionately have been supplanted by concerns that there be fair access among populations to what may be the benefits of participation in research. In both cases, the key concern is one of justice: all populations have a right to the potential benefits of research, and no population, particularly those unable to provide voluntary consent, should bear the burdens of research unjustly.

"Vulnerable" populations, or those that may be unable to provide valid informed consent, can be divided into two general categories. First are those who have the mental capacity to consent, but, because of their situation, do not have the practical ability to provide consent *voluntarily.* Examples of this category of vulnerable populations include prisoners, women in certain societies, some desperately ill patients, or those in a dependent relationship with the investigator, such as medical students or patients. Second are those who are unable to consent by virtue of a characteristic or condition inherent to them. Examples include children and persons with mental illness or mental retardation who do not have the mental *capacity* to provide consent. The obligation to protect vulnerable participants, particularly in light of gross harms to which they have been submitted in the past,[5] remains paramount. At the same time, all of these populations also have a claim to what may be considered the benefits of participating in a trial.

In determining whether to include any vulnerable population in research, two questions should be answered. First is whether it is necessary to include the vulnerable population to obtain knowledge that cannot be gained from studying other, less vulnerable populations. For example, one can only determine the efficacy of a drug or vaccine for children by conducting clinical trials involving children. Second, do the members of the vulnerable population (or their guardians) consider the research to be of benefit to themselves.

---

[5] An initial expose of unethically conducted biomedical research was presented in a book by Beecher and colleagues in 1966 (4).

The question of whether to include pregnant women in clinical trials has been given particular attention in recent years (24). Until recently, pregnant women have largely been excluded from clinical trials because of concerns about risks to the fetus. However, the only way to study whether a vaccine prevents transmission of HIV from mother to fetus (vertical transmission) is to include infected pregnant women in clinical trials. As discussed in chapter 2, although pregnant women have been excluded from HIV vaccine trials in the past, there are now clinical trials of vaccines to interrupt vertical transmission that have enrolled infected pregnant women.

Certain populations at increased risk for HIV infection may be considered vulnerable, not because of a hampered ability to provide consent, but because they are at particular risk of social harms from trial participation. For example, some high-risk behaviors are illegal (e.g., injection drug use, prostitution, and, in certain jurisdictions, male-to-male sex). Members of these high-risk groups may increase the chance of detection as a result of trial participation. At the same time, such high-risk individuals are targeted for HIV vaccine clinical efficacy trials because they have high rates of seroconversion and because they offer an opportunity to study the interaction between the vaccine and specific risk behaviors. Investigators should assure these potential research participants that their confidentiality will be protected.[6]

Members of Racial and Ethnic Minority Groups

African American and Hispanic persons are likely to be recruited for HIV vaccine trials in greater proportion than their representation in the population, given that they are highly represented among groups at risk for HIV infection. There is reason to believe that African American and Hispanic persons are more likely to be suspicious of the intentions of investigators, given the history of abuses of members of racial minority groups in clinical research, most notably in the Tuskegee syphilis study (29). Involvement of community boards and "gatekeepers" is especially important from the outset of HIV vaccine trials to better ensure that trial participants' needs are addressed and that investigators are sensitive to cultural concerns.

It is also important to ensure that members of racial minority groups are recruited for participation in research trials given that the prevalence of infection is higher among these groups and that many members of these groups would be candidates for a vaccine once approved.

INFORMED CONSENT

Rooted in the principle of respect for autonomy is an ethical obligation on the part of investigators to engage potential research participants in the process of informed consent and to obtain adequate consent from all participants.[7] The U.S. Public

[6] Investigators may want to obtain a Federal certificate of confidentiality to better ensure protections for this category of participants. Public Health Service Act, § 301(d), 42 U.S.C. The Act states that special protection will be granted "sparingly" to research projects of a "sensitive nature where the protection is judged necessary to achieve the research objectives." 42 U.S.C. § 301(d). Examples of the types of research that may qualify are those that collect "information relating to sexual attitudes, preferences, or practices; alcohol, drugs, or other addictive products; illegal conduct; information that if released could reasonably be damaging to an individual's financial standing, employability, or reputation; information that would be recorded normally in a patient's medical record, and the disclosure of which could reasonably lead to social stigmatization or discrimination; information pertaining to an individual's psychological well-being or mental health." Researchers who have obtained a certificate of confidentiality "may not be compelled in any Federal, State, or other local civil, criminal, administrative, legislative or other proceedings to identify [research participants]."

[7] See Beauchamp and Childress, 1989 (3), for further discussion of ethical principles.

Health Service established a policy in 1966 (revised substantially in 1974)[8] that all federally funded research must be approved by external review boards that have as part of their responsibility ensuring that investigators obtain informed consent.[9] Essentially all academic institutions require that all research involving human subjects (not just that funded by the federal government) secure such approval. The need for this external oversight arose from the recognition that there may be conflicts of interest among clinical investigators.

The process of informed consent for a clinical trial involves: 1) providing the prospective participant with information relevant to his or her decision about participation in the trial, 2) ensuring that the participant understands that information, 3) ensuring that the participant is choosing to participate voluntarily, and 4) documenting the consent of the participant.[10]

The following information should be provided to potential participants: an explanation that they are being asked to participate in research, not clinical care; a statement of purpose of the research; an explanation of why they were selected; a description of all procedures that they may undergo, including duration, location, and frequency of study visits; a description of the "foreseeable" risks and benefits (both to the participant and others); the alternatives to trial participation (or to the experimental therapy or intervention); a description of how confidentiality will be protected; a description of whether there will be compensation for injuries resulting from participation; a list of those of who can be contacted for questions or problems; and a declaration that participants have the right both not to participate in the trial and to cease their participation at any time, and that by so doing, the receipt of medical care or other benefits will not be compromised.

In addition to these general requirements, there are considerations specifically for HIV vaccine trials. Any clinical efficacy trial examining HIV transmission will need to limit its sample to persons who are not HIV-infected. Therefore, all potential enrollees will first be screened for HIV infection. There needs to be an informed consent process for this testing that is distinct from the informed consent process for enrollment in the research trial. The usual procedures for pre- and post-test counseling must be adhered to. In addition, information should be provided to the potential enrollee that explains that a positive HIV test renders the potential subject ineligible for participation. Moreover, some means of referral for those found to be infected must be established.

Particular problems may arise from HIV testing, in that certain states require the names of all persons who test positive for HIV be reported to the state health department. If such name reporting is required in the state where the research is being conducted, this should be disclosed to potential trial participants and included in the consent form. If the investigators, however, have received an exemption from this requirement, then there is the concern that persons will volunteer for the trial just to receive a confidential HIV screening test,

---

[8] 45 Code of Federal Regulations, §§ 46.101-46.509.

[9] Institutional Review Boards (IRBs) are established by an institution conducting medical research to assess the legal, ethical, and scientific aspects of research on human subjects. IRB approval is required by the Department of Health and Human Services (DHHS) before proposals can receive federal funding. IRBs must review research protocols on a regular basis, but not less than once a year.

Federal regulations for human subjects research require both a generalized as well as specific informed consent for subjects to ensure that they understand the nature of the trial, the lack of any expected benefit, and the risks that are involved. 45 C.F.R. 46.101 (1993). Additional requirements apply to trials involving pregnant women and prisoners. The regulations are administered by the DHHS Office of Research Risks. Agencies and departments outside of DHHS are also required to adopt similar requirements. Although U.S. courts have not always relied on federal requirements to determine the standard for informed consent in clinical trials, failure to comply with these requirements could also give risk to a suit in tort.

[10] For a much more detailed discussion of informed consent see, e.g., Faden and Beauchamp, 1986 (8); and Appelbaum, et al., 1987 (2).

but with no intention of ultimately participating in the trial.

Once potential trial participants are selected from a pool of eligible persons, they should be provided with specific information as part of the disclosure component of the informed consent process, and investigators must ensure that each potential participant understands this information:

1. *The meaning of incomplete efficacy.* Potential trial participants should be informed that the investigators have no assurance that the particular vaccine being tested will actually be effective in preventing HIV infection, and, even if the candidate vaccine is effective, it is not likely that it would be completely effective in preventing HIV infection. Trials participants should therefore avoid high-risk behaviors, as they would had they never received the vaccine.
2. *The meaning of a placebo and the meaning of randomization.* Potential participants in a randomized clinical trial should be informed that there is a chance that they will not receive the experimental vaccine, and they should be informed of the likelihood of that chance. In some trials, investigators are choosing to provide the control arm of studies with an alternative vaccine, such as Hepatitis B vaccine, rather than a placebo vaccine. If so, this should be disclosed to potential trial participants.

   Various analogies have been used to explain the concept of random assignment, including the flipping of a coin or choosing marbles from a jar, depending on the number of experimental and control groups employed in the study. What is most important is that participants understand that they may not be assigned to the group(s) receiving the experimental vaccine, that this assignment is made by chance, that they will not be told if they have received the experimental vaccine until the study is completed, and that the persons administering the vaccine as well as most of the other research personnel will also not know to which group they have been assigned.
3. *The importance of not being tested outside of the study.* Potential participants should be informed that they must commit to not be tested for HIV outside of the trial since that could reveal whether they have received the experimental vaccine. Participants' knowledge of their assignment could bias the results of the trial by affecting the participants' risk behaviors, their reports of side effects, and so forth. Admittedly, many investigators have hesitated to warn potential participants to not obtain HIV testing outside of the study, fearing that this knowledge may increase the likelihood that participants would obtain such testing.

   At the same time, participants should be told that if they need to know whether they have become infected with HIV, they may obtain HIV tests from the investigators. Investigators would use the appropriate tests to diagnose HIV infection, and would inform participants if they have become infected with HIV.
4. *That vaccine recipients testing positive on commonly used HIV screening tests may suffer social harms as a result.* Potential trial participants should be made aware that certain social harms may occur as a result of trial participation. Vaccinees may test positive on the ELISA (enzyme-linked immunosorbant assay) screening test, and other commonly used screening tests, which may result in problems in obtaining health or life insurance, employment, military service, or in travel to other countries. Participants should also be told that they will receive a document that certifies their participation in the vaccine trial and explains that they may test positive for that reason. More specific tests may be used to determine whether they are infected with the virus; if requested, these tests would be conducted at the investigators' expense.

   Potential participants should be told that vaccination may increase the difficulty of diagnosing HIV infection. Standard ELISA screening tests cannot determine whether a vaccinee is HIV infected; more specific tests must be used.

5. *That other social or personal harms might result.* Others may assume that trial participants are members of groups at increased risk for HIV infection and social stigmatization could result. Some have suggested that social harms from trial participation be monitored, just as are biological adverse events. A board could be established to monitor and review social harms and decide if these harms to trial participants are sufficiently severe to warrant termination of the trial.
6. *That participation in this trial may make participants ineligible for other HIV vaccine trials.* Because multiple vaccinations may confound interpretation of results, trial participants that receive the experimental HIV vaccine may not be eligible for participation in trials of subsequent and trials of possibly more effective HIV vaccines.

Cause of the large amount of information that must be conveyed in the informed consent process, some investigators have chosen to give potential participants a written test of their understanding of this information. (Tests could also be administered orally to participants who cannot read.) This test would be completed upon enrollment and at each subsequent visit. A participant's continued participation in the trial could be made contingent on their successful completion of the test. Participants who do not "pass" the test would receive more education before the test is readministered.

Investigators and sponsors have an ethical obligation to ensure that there is an independent Data Safety and Monitoring Board (DSMB) to examine trial data at preestablished intervals for convincing evidence of either significant effectiveness or unacceptable harm from the experimental vaccine requiring termination of the trial.

Investigators also have the ethical obligation throughout the trial to provide participants with any other information that may reasonably be expected to influence their willingness to participate, and to evaluate whether continued participation in the trial is in the participants' best interests. The ethical obligation of investigators goes beyond providing information to the DSMB; it also could include information that becomes available through the vaccine research of others, HIV research in other realms, such as behavioral research, or relevant changes in public policy, if this can reasonably be expected to influence participants' willingness to participate.

RESEARCH IN DEVELOPING COUNTRIES[11]

It is not ethical for investigators or vaccine manufacturers to conduct trials in developing countries merely because it is less expensive or more convenient. To ignore the need for effective vaccines in developing countries, however, would be ethically unacceptable because HIV is an overwhelming problem in so many of these countries. Moreover, strains of HIV from different parts of the world vary, as do cofactors that influence transmission of infection and disease progression;[12] thus, findings from vaccine trials conducted in the United States or other developed countries, would not be generalizable to developing countries. For these reasons, it is appropriate to conduct HIV vaccine trials in developing countries that have a high incidence of HIV infection. Box 3-1 describes international guidelines for human subjects research.

[11] International guidelines for human subjects research developed by the World Health Organization (WHO) and the Council for International Organizations of Medical Science (CIOMS) are described in box 3-1. See also Lurie, et al., 1994 (23); Katongole-Mbidde, 1993 (16); and Lawrence, et al., 1993 (19).

[12] HIV is not a single, genetically homogenous virus, but exists in multiple strains, which differ among individuals from different regions, as well as among individuals from the same region (22). It has been estimated that isolates of HIV differ as much as forty percent in their envelope sequences (9), and that at least five major families or clades of HIV exist around the globe (12).

BOX 3-1: CIOMS Guidelines for Human Subjects Research

In 1993, the Council for International Organizations of Medical Sciences (CIOMS), in collaboration with the World Health Organization (WHO), approved a revised set of guidelines for human subjects research (6). *The International Ethical Guidelines for Biomedical Research Involving Human Subjects* begins with a statement of general ethical principles, and includes 16 guidelines.

The introduction to the guidelines notes that one of the reasons for the revision of the guidelines, initially promulgated in 1982, was the prospect of clinical trials of HIV vaccines and drugs for AIDS.

Guideline 8 provides that, in conducting human subjects research in developing countries, investigators must ensure the following: that persons in developing countries will not ordinarily be involved in research that may equally well be carried out in developed countries; that the research should be responsive to the health needs and priorities of the community in which the research is being conducted; that every effort should be made to secure the informed consent of individual research participants; and that proposals for the research should be reviewed and approved by an ethical review committee.

Guideline 15 states that the agency that is initiating the research should submit the research protocol to ethical and scientific review according to the standards of the initiating country, and the ethical standards applied should be equal to those applied to research conducted in the initiating country. The guideline also states that the appropriate authorities of the host country should assure themselves that the proposed research also meets the host country's own ethical requirements.

Although the guidelines do not address liability for adverse reactions, guideline 13 states that participants who suffer physical injury as a result of their participation are entitled to equitable compensation; the guideline does not define, however, what compensation is equitable. The sponsor of the research, whether it be a pharmaceutical company, a government, or an institution, should agree to provide compensation before the human subjects research is initiated, and research participants should be informed that such compensation is available. The guidelines also state that the ethical committee has the responsibility to determine what injuries are compensable and by whom.

SOURCE: R. E. Stein, Blicker & Stein, Washington, DC, "Selected Issues of AIDS Vaccine Liability," unpublished contractor report prepared for the Office of Technology Assessment, U.S. Congress, Washington, DC, Sept. 30, 1994.

Local representatives should be included in the preparation and conduct of the vaccine trial. Such involvement will enhance mutual respect, which is ethically linked to respect for autonomy. Moreover, from a practical perspective, inclusion of local representatives can help ensure the success of the trial. Local representatives can provide a conduit for information relevant to the logistical operations of the research, can enlist support for the research, and can provide outside investigators with a greater understanding of local customs and expectations. Involvement of a senior investigator from the local site is crucial, as is the involvement of other local scientists. To involve local scientists, outside investigators may need to provide them with further training.

Recruitment

Questions have been raised over whether it is ethically acceptable to recruit participants who have little control over their ability to contract HIV infection, such as women whose male partners refuse to wear condoms or are not forthcoming about their own HIV status. However, this is the context in which some vaccines would be administered if proven to be efficacious. For this reason, it is appropriate to include such populations, with a commitment to trying to encourage these persons to protect themselves. It has been argued that it would be unethical to recruit participants from a community that denies the existence of HIV infection (16, 23, 27). Recruitment of these participants would be ethically acceptable only if targeted education were provided as part of recruitment.

Informed Consent

The issue of how to obtain valid informed consent in developing countries is paramount.[13] Many of the issues that arise are the same as when obtaining consent in developed countries and many are not unique to HIV trials. Those that are special will be given attention here.

Ethics requires that both local and Western standards of informed consent be followed. Although there are debates about whether there exists "ethical universalism" (one set of principles that applies everywhere) or "ethical pluralism" (different principles in different contexts of cultures) (21), societies have different rules about who may grant permission for participation in research. In some societies, permission must be granted by a community leader or by someone other than the research participant (e.g., a woman's husband). Ethics requires that all local customs and requirements be met out of respect for both the community and the individuals involved; however, this does not abrogate the obligation of the investigator to seek and obtain consent from the potential trial participant as well. Although some may consider this latter obligation to be ethnocentric on the part of Westerners, this remains the ethical standard for international research (6).

Potential trial participants should have an adequate understanding of the study and its components in order for informed consent to be valid. If the potential trial participants are illiterate, this would alter the means by which informed consent is obtained. Information would need to be provided in the local language or dialect and read to potential participants rather than conveyed in written form. Visual aids or diagrams might be included among the materials given to the potential participants. Similarly, if some sort of a "test" of understanding is required, this would need to be conducted orally.

A more difficult situation occurs if the broad understanding of disease causation is completely different from Western understandings (1). For valid informed consent, it is not necessary for potential participants and investigators to have a completely shared understanding of disease causation. If the differences mean that, by virtue of participating, harmful consequences are likely to ensue, however, these persons cannot ethically be enrolled. Differences in beliefs must be evaluated on a case-by-case basis, and balanced with the need to ensure that any potential benefits of research participation not be denied to such populations.

Developing countries may not have the sophisticated tests necessary to detect HIV infection in vaccinees. Outside investigators should provide support, including these specific tests and necessary technical assistance. Investigators should also assist participants in securing documentation that they were enrolled in a vaccine trial. Although most vaccinees from developing countries would not have use for such documentation, it may be helpful in certain contexts, such as for immigration.

Other Responsibilities of Investigators

Investigators have the ethical obligation to not interfere with other prevention or public health efforts and not to draw the necessary number of local, trained health care personnel away from other important responsibilities. It also may be necessary to provide training to local personnel.

Once the vaccine is marketed, justice obligates the researchers and vaccine sponsors to make vaccine available to the community in which the trial was conducted. In developing countries, the obligation to ensure access to the benefits of vaccine

[13] See Council for International Organizations of Medical Sciences and World Health Organization, 1993 (6). See Box 3-1.

research would require the manufacturer to provide the vaccine for free or at cost.

COMPENSATION FOR ADVERSE REACTIONS

Although there may be no *legal* obligation to provide compensation for injuries incurred through research, it is generally agreed that there is an *ethical* obligation to do so (6, 18). Moreover, it need not be demonstrated that there was negligence on the part of researchers, but simply that harm resulted that would not have occurred had the person not participated in the trial. If compensation will not be provided, this should be explained in the informed consent process and included as part of the informed consent statement. Compensation need not be provided for harms that are not a direct result of research participation, such as for HIV infections not caused by the vaccine. Compensation decisions should be guided by the laws of the country in which the trial is occurring (17).

Potential trial participants should be informed that, even if investigators plan to provide compensation for harms resulting from trial participation, compensation will not be provided for harms resulting from the vaccine being less than completely effective in preventing HIV infection.

INCORPORATION INTO CLINICAL PRACTICE

A number of important ethical issues arise when a vaccine is approved and is used in clinical practice.

Efficacy

HIV vaccines are unlikely to be completely effective or efficacious. (The efficacy of licensed vaccines for other serious diseases ranges from 50 to 95 percent). Persons who believe that they are protected against infection because of the vaccine may be more likely to engage in high-risk behaviors. Further research is needed about the magnitude of this change in risk behaviors, and whether this outweighs the benefits of a partially effective vaccine. The public will need to be educated about the partial nature of protection from an HIV vaccine.

One model of HIV vaccine efficacy concluded that "earlier use of a 60 percent effective vaccine would prevent more new HIV infections than later use of a more efficacious vaccine" (7). Nonetheless, this model considered the theoretical efficacy of vaccines, rather than their effectiveness in actual populations whose risk-taking behaviors may increase in response to vaccination, affecting the incidence of infection.

Informed Consent in Clinical Practice

The informed consent process in clinical practice is less rigorous than that applied in research. Although the law requires that clinical trials be approved by external review boards and that research participants sign detailed written informed consent forms, there are no similar legal requirements for informed consent in clinical practice.

In clinical practice, written informed consent is only required for certain types of medical interventions, typically surgery and nonroutine medical procedures. Public health interventions in particular have an extremely limited tradition of informed consent (although one exception is the informed consent process for HIV testing). Generally, American common law requires that the patient be given sufficient information upon which to make "an intelligent and informed choice" (32). Case law does not provide clear guidance, however, about the requirement for an "intelligent and informed" choice. Some courts have concluded that all information must be provided to participants, and others have found that information that a "reasonable" person would consider to be relevant must be provided. Negligence typically is based on a breach of the standard of care, and a tradition of rigorous informed consent is not part of the standard of care in clinical practice.

This is not to say that most clinicians fail to ensure that each patient has an adequate level of understanding before consent to medical interventions is obtained. However, the lack of standardization and regulation of informed consent means that the extent to which this happens is unknown.

For HIV vaccines the consequences of an inadequate informed consent process may be severe. For consent to vaccination to be adequate, patients will need to understand that the vaccine is not completely effective and that they should continue to practice protective behaviors. Patients would also need to know the consequences of their testing positive on standard HIV screening tests. They also will need to be aware of the potential social harms from vaccination, particularly since vulnerable and "at risk" groups may be targeted for the first rounds of immunization. The risk of breach of confidentially is greater in clinical practice, because outside parties (such as insurance companies) have access to medical records. Lapses in confidentiality would increase the potential for social harms to vaccinees.

CONCLUSION

Scientific progress is occurring in the development of HIV vaccines and some vaccines have entered clinical trials. Clinical testing of vaccines should not move forward, however, without the incorporation of appropriate ethical standards. A lack of attention to ethical principles not only would be morally reprehensible, but would lead to less effective research and compromised clinical findings.

CHAPTER 3 REFERENCES

1. Ajayi, O.O., "Taboos and Clinical Research in West Africa," *Journal of Medical Ethics* 6:61-63, 1980.
2. Appelbaum, P.S., Lidz, C.W., and Meisel, A., *Informed Consent: Legal Theory and Clinical Practice* (New York, NY: Oxford University Press, 1987).
3. Beauchamp, T.L., and Childress, J.F., *Principles of Biomedical Ethics* (New York, NY: Oxford University Press, 1989).
4. Beecher, H.K., "Ethics and Clinical Research," *New England Journal of Medicine* 274:1354-1360, 1966.
5. "Can a Healthy Subject Volunteer To Be Injured in Research?" *Hastings Center Report* 31-33, August 1986.
6. Council for International Organizations of Medical Sciences (CIOMS) and World Health Organization (WHO), "International Ethical Guidelines for Biomedical Research Involving Human Subjects," *Proceedings of the XXVIth CIOMS Conference,* Geneva, Switzerland, 5-7 February 1992, published by CIOMS, 1993.
7. Dixon, D.O., et al., "HIV Vaccine Trials: Some Design Issues Including Sample Size Calculation," *Journal of Acquired Immune Deficiency Syndrome* 6:485-496, 1993.
8. Faden, R.R., and Beauchamp, T.L., *A History and Theory of Informed Consent* (New York, NY: Oxford University Press, 1986).
9. Federal Coordinating Council on Science, Engineering, and Technology, Committee on Life Sciences and Health *The Human Immunodeficiency Challenge: Issues in Development and International Trials* (Washington, DC: July 1993).
10. Freedman, B. "Equipoise and the Ethics of Clinical Research," *New England Journal of Medicine* 317:141-145, 1987.
11. Fultz, P.N., et al., "Vaccine Protection of Chimpanzees Against Challenge with HIV-1-Infected Peripheral Blood Mononuclear Cells," *Science* 256:1687-1690, 1992.
12. Gardner, M., University of California at Davis, Department of Medical Pathology, personal communication, July 1993.
13. Gardner, M., University of California at Davis, Department of Medical Pathology, personal communication, Aug. 23, 1994.
14. Gostin, L., "The AIDS Litigation Project: A National Review of Court and Human Rights Commission Decisions, Part II: Discrimination," *Journal of the American Medical Association* 263:2086-2093, 1990.
15. Karzon, D., "Potential for Adverse Reactions in the Development of an HIV-1 Vaccine," final draft report prepared for the Office of

Technology Assessment, U. S. Congress, Washington, DC, December 1994.

16. Katongole-Mbidde, E., "Expectations of Host Countries in HIV Vaccine Trials," *AIDS Research and Human Retroviruses* 9(suppl. 1): S17-S19, 1993.
17. Katongole-Mbidde, E., Director Uganda Cancer Institute, Kampala, Uganda, personal communication, Mar. 22, 1994.
18. Keystone Center, *Keystone AIDS Vaccine Liability Project: Final Report* (Keystone, CO: The Keystone Center, 1990).
19. Lawrence, D.N., Esparza, J., and Zoon, K.C., "Considerations on Criteria for Commencement of HIV Vaccine Efficacy Trials: a Working Group Summary," *AIDS Research and Human Retroviruses* 9(suppl. 1): S65-S69, 1993.
20. Levine, R.J., *Ethics and Regulation of Clinical Research* (New Haven, CT: Yale University Press, 1988).
21. Levine, R.J., "Applying Relevant International Ethical Principles," *AIDS Research and Human Retroviruses* 9(suppl. 1): S155-S156, 1993.
22. Louwagie, J., et al., "Genetic Subtypes of HIV-1," *AIDS Research and Human Retroviruses* 9(suppl. 1): S147-S150, 1993.
23. Lurie, P., et al., "Ethical, Behavioral, and Social Aspects of HIV Vaccine Trials in Developing Countries," *Journal of the American Medical Association* 271:295-301, 1994.
24. Mastroianni, A.C., Faden, R., and Federman, D. (eds.), *Women and Health Research* (Washington, DC: National Academy Press, 1994).
25. "The Nuremberg Code," *Trials of War Criminals Before the Nuremberg Military Tribunals Under Control Council Law No. 10* (Washington, DC: U.S. Government Printing Office, 2:181-182, 1949).
26. Public Health Service Act, S. 301(d), 42 U.S.C.
27. Serwadda, D., and Katongole-Mbidde, E., "AIDS in Africa: Problems for Research and Researchers," *Lancet* 335:842-843, 1990.
28. Sheon, A.R., "Overview: HIV Vaccine Feasibility Studies," *AIDS Research and Human Retroviruses* 10:S1-2, 1994.
29. Thomas, S.B., and Quinn, S.C., "The Tuskegee Syphilis Study, 1932 to 1972: Implications for HIV Education and AIDS Risk Education Programs in the Black Community," *American Journal of Public Health* 81:1498-1504, 1991.
30. U.S. Congress, Office of Technology Assessment, *Tools for Evaluating Health Technologies: Five Background Papers*, BP-H-142 (Washington, DC: U.S. Government Printing Office, February 1995).
31. Vermund, S.H., et al., "Building Partnerships Toward HIV Vaccine Trials," *AIDS Research and Human Retroviruses* 9(suppl. 1):S127-S132, 1993.
32. Wing, K.R., *The Law and the Public's Health* (Ann Arbor, MI: Health Administration Press, 1985), p. 224.
33. World Medical Assembly, "Declaration of Helsinki", adopted by the 18th World Medical Assembly, Helsinki, Finland, 1964; revised by 29th World Medical Assembly, Tokyo, Japan, 1975.

Liability and Compensation for Adverse Reactions to HIV Vaccines 4

by
Wendy Mariner
Boston University School of Medicine and School of Public Health
Boston, MA

Liability for personal injuries related to vaccines has been a matter of intermittent controversy for a quarter of a century (191, 201). Some pharmaceutical and biotechnology companies have said that the possibility of being liable for adverse reactions to vaccines or drugs may deter them from developing or distributing new products that could help reduce the spread of disease or its toll on the population (32, 160, 162, 209).

Although there is little evidence to prove or disprove the effect of potential liability on vaccine development, research on vaccines has lagged behind other pharmaceutical research, and several bodies have considered limiting the liability of vaccine makers in the hope of encouraging the continued development and sale of important vaccines (82, 140). Some have recommended a no-fault compensation system to largely replace liability litigation involving adverse reactions to vaccines (95). Congress enacted the National Childhood Vaccine Injury Act in 1986 (42 U.S.C. 300aa-10 et seq.) to establish a no-fault compensation program for injuries resulting from pediatric vaccines and to limit vaccine manufacturer liability for such injuries (115). Congressman Fortney "Pete" Stark circulated a proposal for a similar bill to create a no-fault compensation program for injuries arising from the use of any future vaccine to prevent AIDS (170).

In spite of decades of debate and several changes in state and federal laws, the controversy over liability for vaccine injuries has never been put to rest. In part, this may be because whether or how liability affects vaccine development has not been, and perhaps cannot be, measured empirically to reach reliable answers. But the controversy also reflects fundamental differences of opinion regarding responsibility for goods of social importance and responsibility for injury. Should government or private industry be responsible for ensuring the production of products that benefit society by preventing disease? Who should be responsible for injuries resulting from such products? Reasonable people may answer such questions quite differently. Even if they temporarily agree on a practical solution to a specific problem, the underlying political and ideological differences resurface with each new product that promises social benefit. Today they appear in a new debate over whether liability may deter companies from developing and marketing new vaccines to prevent HIV infection or progression to AIDS.

This chapter examines whether alternative injury compensation systems may facilitate the development and marketing of new vaccines to prevent HIV infection or AIDS. The first section of this chapter summarizes the possible goals of compensating people who experience adverse reactions to HIV vaccines. The second section reviews several factors that may deter private companies from developing an HIV vaccine and the possible influence of potential liability. The third section reviews basic concepts of tort liability applicable to personal injury and how they might apply to an HIV vaccine. The final section of this chapter considers alternatives for compensating adverse reactions to HIV vaccines and how they might affect the goals of HIV vaccine development and equitable compensation for injuries.

RESPONSIBILITY FOR INJURY AND COMPENSATION

Compensation systems can be classified into four broad categories on the basis of their organizational structure and the mechanism for determining who is entitled to what kind of compensation for what injuries and from whom: tort liability systems, voluntary contractual arrangements, public and private insurance systems, and administrative compensation programs. The choice of system depends upon the goals to be accomplished by compensation. A threshold decision, therefore, is the need for or desirability of compensating injuries. Obviously, if there is no need to compensate injuries, there is no need to establish a compensation system. This section describes the reasons most commonly put forth for compensating injuries.[1]

REASONS FOR COMPENSATING INJURIES

Injuries give rise to both physical and financial losses, as well as emotional turmoil. The injured person inevitably bears the physical consequences. Financial losses, however, may be shifted to someone else by requiring that party to compensate the victim with money.[2] These are the only choices available with respect to financial losses: leave them where they lie (with the injured person), or transfer all or part to someone else. With every type of injury, therefore, the question arises whether the financial losses should be shifted to someone else, and, if so, to whom. Compensation for injury has been justified for economic, philosophical or ethical, and pragmatic or social policy reasons.

Economic Reasons

Economists and legal scholars have argued both for and against compensating the victims of injury to achieve economic efficiency (26, 51, 80, 104, 161). The general idea is to minimize the total social costs of injury or maximize net social utility, taking into consideration both the benefits of a product or activity and the injuries it produces. Although opinions vary on what should be the optimal model, none necessarily requires that the number of injuries themselves be minimized. For example, it may be cheaper to pay compensation

[1] This section draws heavily upon Mariner, 1994 (116).

[2] Compensation may also take the form of in-kind services provided to the injured person, but because these have a monetary value and are ordinarily paid for with money, they will not be separately discussed.

for injuries than to modify a product to prevent the injuries.

Many conceptions of economic efficiency are difficult to apply in practice. Models based on perfect competition may not take into account how buyers and sellers behave in an imperfect world. Not everyone necessarily agrees on what counts as a benefit or a cost, especially where benefits and injuries fall on quite different segments of the population.

It is frequently assumed that companies can internalize the costs of injuries (recoup compensation payments) by raising the prices of their products, thereby spreading the costs over a large population. Even if compensation costs cannot be fully recouped from sales, the loss experienced by the company is relatively small when compared with the loss an uncompensated individual would suffer. Compensation then serves to spread the costs more equitably.

When injuries are frequent or severe enough to require a company to pay substantial costs that threaten its continued viability, it is ordinarily believed to be more economically efficient for a company to make the product safer, if possible, or cease producing the product. Some commentators have argued that this is economically inefficient if the product produces a significant social benefit (79). In theory, such an imbalance should not occur because the product's price should reflect its social benefit.

Economic analyses of loss allocation have influenced thinking about the nature of compensation, but have rarely been decisive on the question of whether compensation should be paid at all.[3] That question is more often answered with reference to moral arguments about who should bear responsibility for the consequences of injury.

Ethical Reasons

Injury compensation has long been justified as the moral duty of those who are responsible for causing injury. It is perhaps the most widely accepted basis for legal liability in tort (59). Principles of justice derived from the works of such diverse scholars as Kant, Bentham, and Locke support compensation for injury caused by an identifiable entity.

There is, however, room for debate on what counts as causing injury and the circumstances in which moral responsibility for injury, and therefore compensation, should be ascribed. Depending upon the circumstances, compensation may be:

1. morally required, so that not providing it is unjust;
2. morally desirable as an act of virtue, but not morally required; or
3. not morally required and possibly unjust.

Swazey and Glantz offer a useful paradigm to describe why society may apply different moral rules to different injuries (179). They argue that social conceptions of moral or ethical obligations to human research subjects may vary depending upon whether the subjects are seen as victims, heroes, or contractors.[4] Victims are characterized as those who have been misused or injured without their consent[5] (9). They may be especially vulnerable or targets of exploitation who have few

[3] For example, Philipson and Posner apply economic theory to the AIDS epidemic and conclude that the federal government "has no, or even a negative, stake in the development of treatments, such as the drug AZT, that merely prolong the lives of persons [with HIV because AZT] may increase the total medical costs by extending the period during which infected persons demand and receive treatment (138)." Fortunately, such reasoning has not halted AIDS treatment research.

[4] Their analysis is directed only to compensation for research injuries. It is pertinent to this discussion, however, because it describes generalizable theories and because the question whether human subjects in clinical trials of candidate HIV vaccines deserve compensation will necessarily have to be addressed first.

[5] Well-known research examples include subjects in the Tuskegee Syphilis Study (88), the Willowbrook Hepatitis B Study (90), and, more recently, radiation experiments conducted under the sponsorship of the Department of Energy (162, 188, 209).

means to avoid the injury in question. Victims have a strong moral claim to compensation, especially where society has facilitated the research or benefited by the use of a product (42, 200).

Heroes, in contrast, are seen as willing volunteers who assume risks in order to accomplish a goal, ordinarily for someone else's sake (179). Since heroes are not supposed to seek any reward, there is no obligation to compensate them. At the same time, society may wish to reward them voluntarily for their heroic efforts.

Contractors are often seen as businessmen striking a bargain (179). As long as the bargaining process is fair, contractors may be entitled to no more than they bargained for, and may be seen as seeking an unfair advantage if they later demand more. Thus, for example, those who voluntarily buy a product without initially contracting for compensation may have little, if any, moral claim to it later.

This paradigm offers some insight into why some people may view entitlement to compensation for vaccine-related injuries so differently. Those who focus on principles of distributive justice view vaccine recipients as benefiting society by preventing disease transmission. In this view, injured recipients who are perceived as victims are morally entitled to compensation and not providing it would be unjust. Recipients who are perceived as heroes, such as subjects of research in clinical trials, have a lesser claim, but compensation is a morally desirable act of caring for those who benefited society.

In contrast, those who focus on respect for persons and autonomous choices may perceive vaccine recipients as contractors with no moral claim to compensation. In this view, the recipient has agreed to assume the risks of vaccination (and has received its benefits), and providing compensation would be wrong because it does not respect the subject's autonomous choice. This is the effect of informed consent in tort law. A person who has agreed to vaccination with knowledge of any attendant risks (including the possibility of unknown risks) is not entitled to compensation if a disclosed risk materializes to his injury. As long as the initial contract discloses the risk so that the recipient can decide whether or not to accept it, the contract is fair. In moral discourse, society has, at best, a privilege to compensate such persons as an act of charity, and not doing so is not unjust.

The view based on autonomy can be criticized on two grounds. First, it may be wrong to believe that consent to assume the risks of vaccination necessarily includes consent to assume the financial costs of injury. Indeed, it may be unfair to ask anyone to assume such costs if the injury is severe. Second, as a practical matter, one may question whether the contract can be made on fair terms. The ideal of voluntary, understanding, informed consent is not always achieved in practice, especially in a research setting (10, 92).

We do not yet know whether people who take an HIV vaccine will appreciate the consequences of their decision. In particular, we do not know whether people would consent to waive compensation for injury because they are rarely given the option of compensation. Most research studies advise potential subjects that compensation is not available. People who take vaccines are rarely advised that their consent will be deemed to be an assumption of the risks of financial loss. Of course, people take many risks from driving automobiles to white water rafting for which no one else is financially responsible.

Tort law has taken a somewhat broader view of entitlement to compensation by basing it on responsibility for injury. In 1951, Glanville Williams identified four possible goals of tort law imposing liability for personal injury: 1) justice (imposing the cost of injury on the one who causes it); 2) compensation (replacing the victim's losses); 3) deterrence (creating disincentives for socially undesirable activity that could result in personal injury); and 4) appeasement (assuaging the victim's desire for vengeance through compensation) (210). Most discussions of tort liability goals have used the same or a similar formulation (59, 142). Although justice may provide tort law's primary moral justification, compensation and deterrence are its most commonly recognized functions.

Sunstein has noted that traditional principles of compensatory justice have found compensation appropriate when: 1) "[t]he event that produced the injury is both discrete and unitary"; 2) "[t]he injury is sharply defined in time and in space"; 3) an identifiable defendant has clearly caused the harm suffered by an identifiable plaintiff; and 4) the harm is not attributable to some third party or to "society"[6] (177). He argues that these criteria are not well suited to affording justifiable compensation where the relevant harm cannot be connected to a discrete event, where there is scientific uncertainty, where the risk is shared or collective, or where the defendant has an ambiguous relation to the harm, as in environmental hazards.[7]

Current tort law would not readily accommodate compensation for increased risks rather than actual injuries. This has obvious implications for injuries to those who are vaccinated because of possible uncertainties about the cause of some injuries and the degree to which any risk may have been avoidable. It suggests that there may be some circumstances in which compensation should be provided even if it would not be granted under tort principles.

Social Policy Reasons

Compensation for vaccine-related injury has been seen as a pragmatic solution to a social problem. That social problem is sometimes characterized as unfairness to those with vaccine-related injury who suffer significant financial losses as well as physical and emotional damage and who have no legal claim to compensation from others. Compensation may benefit society as a whole if injuries are deterred and injured persons are adequately provided for. More commonly, the problem is seen as a means to relieve vaccine producers from an unfair burden of liability for injuries that should not be compensated or are compensated excessively through product liability claims. If compensation costs less than litigation, society, as well as manufacturers, may benefit by reducing litigation expenses. If liability deters the production of socially beneficial products, society may benefit from the availability of those products if they are produced.[8]

Compensation and liability appear to be linked in discussions of vaccine-related injuries because of a general sense that injured vaccine recipients deserve compensation, but that vaccine producers should not be responsible for paying compensation for *all* the injuries. Compensation can be justified on the ground that society benefits from reduction in disease and those who are willing to join the disease prevention effort should be compensated if injury results, perhaps even if the injuries were unforeseeable. This would grant compensation in many cases in which tort principles would deny compensation.

The fact that injury compensation can be justified, and is even desirable, however, does not answer the question of who should be responsible for compensating the injury. If compensation is to be provided beyond that currently permitted under tort principles, should the vaccine producer, government, or someone else be responsible?

SOCIAL GOALS OF ALLOCATING RESPONSIBILITY FOR INJURY

If compensation is warranted for all vaccine-related injuries that are not caused by negligence,[9] the central questions are: who should provide the compensation, and how? Financial responsibility

[6] One might add that compensation is generally precluded if the plaintiff has effectively consented to the injury by assuming the risk.

[7] Many regulatory programs (environmental protection, occupational health and safety, and food and drug regulation) are intended to prevent or minimize social risks that may arise in the future, often to a class or group of people whose affected members cannot be identified in advance. Sunstein argues that these programs operate to provide a mechanism for deterring risks, but not for compensating actual injuries (177).

[8] Where law mandates vaccination, as with pediatric vaccines, people have little opportunity to refuse to be vaccinated. The social benefit conferred by mandatory childhood immunization was one reason for creating the federal National Vaccine Injury Compensation Program in 1986.

[9] Because negligence is a deviation from acceptable conduct, and is not an inherent vaccine risk, injuries resulting from the negligence of a vaccine producer or one who administers a vaccine are ordinarily believed to remain the responsibility of whoever caused the injury.

for adverse reactions to a future HIV vaccine may be structured to help achieve one or more of the following goals:

1. to assure the development of an effective vaccine to prevent HIV infection or AIDS;
2. to assure the marketing and distribution of an HIV vaccine;
3. to assure the marketing and distribution of an HIV vaccine at a reasonable cost to users;
4. to assure the use of HIV vaccine to prevent HIV infection or the development of AIDS;
5. to assure compensation to persons injured as a result of an HIV vaccine;
6. to minimize the total social costs of HIV vaccine development, marketing, and injuries; and
7. to minimize the total social costs of HIV infection, including prevention and transaction costs.

It should be noted that none of these goals can be achieved solely by assigning responsibility (or liability) for injuries. Rather, by assigning responsibility to different parties, society may encourage or discourage progress toward specific goals. The ways by which the allocation of responsibility affects progress towards each of these social goals is described below.

Development and Marketing

The first two goals—HIV vaccine development and marketing—might be achieved by assigning financial responsibility to government, the producer, or the injured person. The choice depends upon who is to develop and market vaccines and how responsibility for injury affects their decisions.

The federal government has both funded and conducted HIV vaccine research and might assume responsibility for product development, if not marketing. It is more likely, however, that the private sector, which has also conducted vaccine research, will pursue product development and marketing, as it has in the past. Responsibility for injury might encourage the type of vaccine desired or it might discourage vaccine development entirely.

In theory, the key goal of responsibility for injury is deterrence: to provide an incentive to produce products of acceptable quality and to deter the production of products with avoidable risks. But the degree to which responsibility for injury actually promotes product safety and effectiveness is debatable and difficult to verify (20, 61, 178). Other mechanisms, such as the U.S. Food and Drug Administration (FDA), may achieve the goal equally well.

Currently, it is impossible to predict the degree to which either FDA regulation or potential responsibility for injury may affect an HIV vaccine's safety and effectiveness. Some would argue that, in the absence of such knowledge, responsibility should be retained. Others would argue that it should not because it may discourage producers from developing or marketing any vaccine. This assumes that producers who are otherwise willing and able to develop a vaccine would refuse to do it if they retained financial responsibility for adverse reactions. As discussed in the next section of this chapter, it may be impossible to confirm or refute that assumption, although HIV vaccines development has not been halted by the potential for liability.

Reasonable Vaccine Costs and Vaccine Use

The third and fourth goals of allocating responsibility for injury—offering vaccines at a reasonable price and assuring vaccine use—address the need for access to HIV vaccines. The obvious purpose of developing an HIV vaccine is to prevent HIV infection and stop the AIDS epidemic. A safe and effective vaccine must not only be produced, it must be used by those at risk for HIV infection. Unless an HIV vaccine is to be given away free to anyone who wishes it, the cost to vaccine purchasers, whether private individuals or government entities, must be affordable. If the cost of injuries drives the price of vaccine too high, it will not be used.[10] In that event, it may be cheaper (in theory) to rely on behavioral education to help prevent some modes of HIV transmission. Thus, if responsibility for injury causes producers to set an unaffordable price on vaccines, many people may not be able to obtain it.

On the other hand, if individual vaccine recipients must bear the financial burden of adverse reactions, then they may be unwilling to use the vaccine. Either result undermines the goal of vaccine distribution and use. One alternative for government is to limit the price at which vaccine is sold, either by negotiating government prices with producers or by legislation limiting prices. However, vaccine makers may be unwilling to produce a vaccine that is subject to such price limitations.[11]

Compensation for Adverse Reactions

Responsibility for injury may be allocated so as to achieve the fifth social goal—to provide compensation to those injured in the most efficient, fairest or least costly manner. If the goal is to spend the fewest dollars on injuries, then the choice might be to leave injured people to pay for their injuries. This would avoid any administrative or transaction costs associated with transferring compensation to the injured, but not the burden on injured persons. This option has little appeal because the financial costs of injury are sometimes more than one person can bear. It also seems unfair to the individuals when society as a whole benefits from the vaccine's use. Moreover, if responsibility for injury has the effect of deterring injuries, then requiring compensation may reduce total costs by reducing the number of injuries. It may be more efficient to spread the cost of injuries across the population of vaccine users or the larger society by making government or vaccine producers financially responsible.

Minimizing Vaccine and Injury Costs

If responsibility for injury is to be allocated so as to provide compensation to injured people, then the responsible party may be selected so as to achieve the sixth social goal—to minimize the total social costs of vaccine development and marketing and the costs of injury. This takes into account the fact that injuries do impose costs on individuals, even though they may be less visible to society than the costs reflected in the price of products.

Often this goal is erroneously invoked by those who wish to achieve the narrower objective of minimizing the costs to one participant in an endeavor. For example, if only the costs to manufacturers were recognized, limiting liability and compensation would reduce manufacturers' costs. The remaining injury costs would not disappear, however; they would rest with injured people or government. If government wishes to minimize its own costs, then it would ordinarily impose financial responsibility on vaccine producers. However, if the price of vaccine rose higher than the cost to government of providing compensation, and government purchased a significant proportion of vaccine, government would incur much of the cost theoretically imposed on producers. The least costly option would depend upon whether government controlled the price of vaccine, either by regulation or negotiation.

Minimizing Total Social Costs of HIV Infection

The seventh goal of responsibility is to minimize the total social costs of HIV infection. In assessing the social costs and benefits of HIV vaccine development, production, and distribution, all of the social costs of HIV infection should be taken into account. Society is already paying a high price, in terms of human suffering as well as economic

[10] Of course, this ignores the human cost of not preventing HIV transmission if the vaccine is not used. It also assumes that vaccination is voluntary.

[11] It may be difficult to achieve both the goals of affordability and production if production is to remain entirely with the private sector.

losses, for the persistence of HIV infection. Moreover, current efforts to prevent HIV transmission also impose social costs. The benefits to be gained by preventing additional disease are likely to outweigh the costs of vaccine development, marketing, and injury compensation. If so, then the question is how to allocate responsibility for injury in order to maximize those benefits and minimize those costs.

Conclusion:

Any system for assigning responsibility for injury that satisfies one goal may undermine another. For example, a system that minimized the costs of compensation to vaccine makers might encourage vaccine development, but also reduce incentives to limit potential safety risks, and result in more injuries. A system that provided generous compensation to all injured parties might achieve the goal of equitable compensation, but might be too expensive for many companies that society wishes to attract to vaccine development to achieve other goals. Government assumption of responsibility for compensation might conflict with other goals to minimize government expenditures or to fund other important programs. The amount of compensation may also affect the price of marketed vaccines. At some point, high prices may deter potential vaccine recipients from taking the vaccine. Systems that discourage either vaccine development or vaccination may work against the goal of preventing HIV transmission and disease.

Most important, any system that limits compensation to injuries from one specific cause, like an HIV vaccine, raises questions of fairness to people with similar injuries caused by something else. A compensation system limited to persons with adverse reactions to an HIV vaccine invites the question why people living with HIV infection or AIDS (or any other illness or injury, for that matter) should not be compensated in the same manner.

POTENTIAL DETERRENTS TO HIV VACCINE DEVELOPMENT

As the first section of this chapter illustrates, who should bear responsibility for adverse reactions to HIV vaccines depends upon the goals of HIV vaccine development and compensation for injury and how responsibility for injury may affect vaccine producers' decisions about vaccine development. If society intends to rely on the private sector to develop and distribute an HIV vaccine, then private sector attitudes toward responsibility for injury must be considered. If private companies are unwilling or unable to distribute an HIV vaccine if they are charged with responsibility for injury, then arguments that they *should* have that responsibility will not suffice to produce a vaccine.[12] If, on the other hand, responsibility for injury has little impact on their decisions, then even elimination of responsibility for injury will not improve the prospects for private sector vaccine development.

This section examines the degree to which legal responsibility or liability for adverse reactions might affect private companies' decisions whether to develop and market an HIV vaccine.[13] Unfortunately, there is no empirical evidence that of-

[12] If government were to produce or distribute the vaccine, such concerns would be unnecessary.

[13] This examination is based on a literature review; an empirical study was beyond the scope of this report. The possible approaches to studying potential liability's effect on product development have inherent biases and limitations. These parallel the approaches to studying defensive medicine described in the Office of Technology Assessment's 1994 report *Defensive Medicine and Medical Malpractice* (195), and have similar limitations. One approach is to ask vaccine companies why they did or did not develop specific vaccines. Such surveys may elicit biased responses. If respondents believe that the survey is intended to measure sensitivity to liability, they may exaggerate liability's role in their decision making in the hope of gaining added protection against liability in general. If liability is not mentioned, respondents may underplay its role in favor of emphasizing purely scientific or other reasons. An alternative approach is to compare the products developed, marketed and abandoned by companies with their exposure to liability. Such a study requires access to information concerning products not marketed as well as data on companies' liability experience which companies are generally unwilling to disclose.

fers a clear answer to the question. There are no epidemiologic studies of the effect of liability like those ordinarily required to prove vaccine risks. Inferences might be drawn from past behavior but are highly speculative because the reasons underlying decisions about research and marketing are not independently verifiable. The available evidence consists largely of anecdotes.[14] Analyses of the effect of liability have been forced to rely on inferences from history and assumptions based on logic (and sometimes ideology).

Companies in private industry necessarily make choices about what business to pursue and what products to make. Because new biologic and pharmaceutical products require a substantial investment of both time and money, choices by companies in the pharmaceutical and biologic industry may have long-term consequences for their product line (194).

An initial fundamental decision is whether to invest in the production facilities and equipment, as well as human expertise, necessary to produce an HIV vaccine. Factors influencing such a decision include: whether the company already has (or has access to) adequate facilities that can be used or adapted for HIV vaccine purposes or financial resources to construct such facilities; whether existing or new facilities can be used or adapted to other purposes within the company's business if vaccine development is unsuccessful; whether the company has sufficient regulatory and clinical trials expertise, as well as financial resources, to pursue testing an investigational product in clinical trials with human subjects and applying for FDA approval; whether the market for the product is likely to support a price that will cover the costs of development and marketing and still produce an acceptable profit; the likely length of patent protection that will preclude other companies from marketing a similar product and competing on price; and whether other potential investments and products are more likely to produce the same or higher profit (82, 121, 194).

It seems logical that potential liability for product-related injuries can influence decisions about whether to pursue developing a specific product. Whether that influence becomes significant depends on its relative weight compared with other factors, especially the scientific and technical feasibility of HIV vaccine development and its expected financial return compared with alternative investments.

Scientific and Technical Feasibility

The major obstacle to developing an HIV vaccine is HIV itself.[15] Despite remarkable advances in scientific knowledge about HIV, too little is known about how to produce an immune response in human beings that would protect against infection or development of disease to be assured that an effective vaccine can be produced in the foreseeable future.[16] For example, it remains unclear how to protect against multiple or mutating strains of HIV, how to prevent mucosal infection or infection through sexual contact in addition to infection through the blood stream, whether cell mediated immunity is required in addition to

[14] Two Institute of Medicine committees attempted to evaluate existing evidence that certain adverse reactions were or were not caused by pediatric vaccines (85, 87, 174). They classified the evidence into 5 categories: 1) No evidence bearing on a causal relation; 2) The evidence is inadequate to accept or reject a causal relation; 3) The evidence favors rejection of a causal relation; 4) The evidence favors a causal relation; 5) The evidence establishes a causal relation (174). Applying their categories to the available evidence bearing on a causal relationship between liability for adverse reactions to vaccines and private industry's willingness to develop or distribute an HIV vaccine, one can at best conclude that the evidence is inadequate to accept or reject a causal relation.

[15] The journal *Science* surveyed "more than 100 of the [vaccine] field's leading researchers, public health officials, and manufacturers" for their opinion on why vaccines have not been developed for many serious infectious diseases, especially those considered priorities by the Institute of Medicine (37). The 67 respondents reported that the "Scientific unknowns are the highest hurdles...but they also stressed that the field lacks strong leadership and funding to speed progress (37)."

[16] For a description of current HIV vaccine research and development, see chapter 2.

humoral immunity (to free virus), and whether infection mediated by both cell-free and cell-associated virus can be prevented. Moreover, it is not known whether a vaccine that does not prevent initial infection by the virus could prevent the development of disease and reduce or prevent active HIV transmission to others. Promising research is beginning to answer such questions, but, historically, it has been especially difficult to develop vaccines to prevent viral infections—and HIV is an extraordinarily complex virus (99).

In April 1984, Secretary of Health, Education and Welfare Margaret Heckler optimistically announced that an HIV vaccine would be ready for testing in 1986 (151). A decade later, the scientific community may not be much closer to developing an effective vaccine, although it may better understand why. The difficulty of determining the precise mechanism by which the virus might be neutralized in human beings may discourage companies from mounting the research effort that is likely to be required to solve the problem.

Other technical considerations may affect vaccine development decisions. On the plus side, the technologies used to produce new recombinant vaccines may be adaptable to other promising products, like diagnostics (192). New recombinant vaccines can be produced in large quantities and, because they are usually stable for long periods, are generally less expensive to produce than other biologic products. At the same time, vaccines pose numerous technical challenges.[17] Animal testing requires special facilities and money to maintain the animals. Finding a suitable adjuvant to enhance the immunogenicity of a candidate vaccine has already proved difficult. Candidate vaccines produced from laboratory adapted strains in cell lines may not protect against other HIV strains that infect human beings in the real world, that is, field isolates.

One way to increase the effectiveness of vaccination may be to combine two or more candidate vaccines made by different companies. This requires the cooperation of different companies in a highly competitive industry. The difficulty of sharing technical information while protecting trade secrets and patents may make such joint ventures unattractive to some companies. Moreover, products that are developed in collaboration with governmental agencies, such as the National Institute of Allergy and Infectious Diseases (NIAID) or the National Cancer Institute (NCI), may give rise to disputes over patent ownership, such as that between Burroughs-Wellcome Co. and National Institutes of Health's (NIH's) licensee, Barr Laboratories, over Zidovudine (AZT) (55). Some companies prefer not to collaborate with the NIH because of the constraints imposed by its "reasonable price" requirements.

Another technical barrier is the need for dedicated product development facilities to produce vaccines. These must comply with FDA regulations specific to biologics, are estimated to cost as much as $10 million to construct, and may have to be updated periodically (121). They also must include expensive ongoing production and quality control processes conforming to Current Good Manufacturing Practice (CGMP) to ensure the potency and purity of each batch of vaccine. The cost of conducting large field trials has also been cited as a major obstacle to vaccine development (121). Large research-based vaccine manufacturers have an advantage in these respects, since few small biotechnology companies have large production facilities or clinical field trial capabilities. Those that can get the financing may prefer to pursue products with a higher probability of success.

It is encouraging that almost thirty candidate HIV vaccines are currently being tested in Phase I and II clinical trials[18] (207). According to public reports, most of these vaccines have been well tolerated and have produced few side effects so far, which supports predictions that they should be reasonably safe. Whether any of these candidate

[17] For a further discussion of difficulties with vaccine development, see chapter 2.

[18] For a description of current HIV vaccines in development, see chapter 2.

vaccines will prove to be effective enough to prevent HIV infection or disease progression in a significant proportion of human vaccine recipients remains to be seen. Indeed, the reported results are somewhat discouraging so far (34, 100).

Phase III trials, in which vaccine efficacy can be studied, remain in the proposal stage, with some companies and prospective study populations eager to begin large field trials with the candidate vaccines that have completed phases I and II trials (3, 133). In late 1993, NIAID expected to begin Phase III trials between 1994 and 1998, "as soon as promising candidates are available," and awarded two contracts to administer feasibility studies and multi-site phase III trials both in the United States and abroad (122). On June 17, 1994, however, an NIAID advisory committee voted to delay phase III clinical trials of the two vaccine candidates that have proceeded the furthest in clinical testing (40, 125).[19] Committee members were not convinced from prior test data that these candidate vaccines could prevent HIV infection in enough people to warrant their use in a large Phase III field trial. Ultimately, NIAID recommended proceeding with efficacy trials only if and when more compelling data could be produced. This is likely to delay such trials for one to three years (125).[20]

Regardless of the merits of the specific vaccines at issue, the decision not to go forward with phase III trials in 1994 may send a discouraging signal about the difficulty of surmounting the scientific obstacles to developing a suitable vaccine.

Some AIDS researchers argue that it would be worthwhile to proceed with the candidates that have already been tested, even if they are not expected to prevent disease transmission or progression in most recipients. They point out that some lives could be saved even if the vaccines are effective in only 30 percent of recipients or if they reduce (while not eliminating) clinical disease or the virulence of the virus and its likelihood of transmission to others.[21] This is of special concern in countries with rising rates of infection, such as Thailand, Uganda, and Zaire.[22]

Others would prefer to concentrate on developing new vaccine candidates with greater promise of effectiveness. They argue that using the tested candidates for immediate Phase III field trials could delay or deter the development of a more effective vaccine. The logistics of organizing a large field trial, especially overseas, are formidable (although perhaps less expensive than in the U.S.), and it may be difficult to use the same population for more than one vaccine. The combined difficulty and expense of mounting such trials may deter some companies from launching a later trial if another vaccine has already been tested and approved.

Researchers at a November 1994 meeting on Advances in AIDS Vaccine Development sponsored by NIAID heard additional discouraging news (126). Newborn monkeys who received a promising prototype simian immunodeficiency (SIV) vaccine derived from live attenuated virus exhibited symptoms of SIV disease and one

---

[19] Both candidates, one by Genentech, Inc., the other by Biocine Company, a joint venture of Chiron and CIBA-Geigy, are recombinant vaccines using gp120, an HIV-surface protein. For further discussion of these vaccines, see chapter 2.

[20] This does not mean that trials cannot go forward in other countries. The companies may try to persuade the World Health Organization or national governments that their vaccines deserve to be tested in phase III trials.

[21] Such a vaccine could not be counted on to prevent HIV infection, so a recipient would still have to practice safe behaviors to avoid becoming infected, or, if infected, to avoid infecting others.

[22] There may also be concern about imposing on private companies an obligation to provide any vaccine that is ultimately approved to the population of research subjects that were used to test it, a principle accepted by most, but not all, scholars of research ethics (110). Industry representatives have argued that this would mean giving the vaccine away free in foreign countries that cannot afford market prices or pay in hard currency. Their resistance persuaded the CIOMS not to include such a requirement in its 1993 International Ethical Guidelines for Biomedical Research Involving Human Subjects (42). For a discussion of the CIOMS Ethical Guidelines, see chapter 3.

monkey died. This may set back efforts to develop HIV vaccine using a similar model. In addition, eighteen human research subjects who received candidate HIV vaccines in clinical trials have become HIV infected despite having high titers of neutralizing anti-body (36). Although their infection may indicate only that the vaccine is ineffective or less than completely protective, the possibility that the vaccine might increase susceptibility to infection may be considered.[23] Some researchers worry that no vaccine that is currently in Phase II trials can achieve even very low levels of efficacy.

Current HIV vaccine research is both exciting and frustrating because so much has been learned yet progress toward an effective vaccine has been so slow. If a private company does not believe that research can identify an adequate vaccine candidate over the next decade, or if it does not have the resources to develop one, then it is not likely to pursue HIV vaccine development.

Market and Financial Factors

If scientific obstacles can be overcome and an HIV vaccine appears technically feasible, the major factor influencing vaccine development is its expected return on investment or profitability. Private industry must look to the potential market to predict the revenues it may yield in order to compare them to the predicted costs of development and marketing, and the potential profits from alternative investments.

The potential market for HIV vaccines is worldwide. However, from a company's perspective, the relevant market consists of paying purchasers. Potential HIV vaccine markets, then, include individual vaccine recipients who can pay for the vaccine either out-of-pocket or with insurance and government agencies which purchase vaccine for distribution to individuals. The paying market may include health care workers, people with hemophilia, and people at risk for HIV infection (such as employed men who have sex with men). This parallels the market for hepatitis B vaccine (HBV) and exists primarily in the United States, Europe, Australia, and possibly Japan. It may also exist in the "carriage trade" in other countries (like Thailand, India, and Egypt). This market may be quite profitable, even though it includes fewer people than the market for other vaccines, like those against polio and influenza.

It is possible, however, that not everyone in this market would be willing to buy an HIV vaccine, perhaps because they mistakenly do not consider themselves at risk for HIV infection, because they prefer to avoid risk behaviors instead of being vaccinated, or because they fear adverse reactions (or acquiring HIV infection) from a vaccine. Some people may fear being labeled as "at risk" if they seek vaccination or being stigmatized as having HIV infection if they become seropositve as a result of vaccination. National or local laws requiring vaccination would maximize the use (and purchase) of HIV vaccines. HIV vaccination appears unlikely to be made mandatory for the entire population, at least in industrialized countries. It might be possible to generate legislative support for mandatory vaccination of certain populations at high risk of HIV infection, such as newborns born to HIV-positive women or certain health care workers. But even targeted mandates are likely to face opposition and may depend upon the perceived safety and effectiveness of the vaccine to be used.

The market may also be affected by the price of the vaccine. Some potential purchasers may be unwilling to pay more than a certain price for the

[23] For a discussion of possible HIV vaccine enhancement of susceptibility to HIV infection, see chapter 2.

vaccine unless it is covered by health insurance.[24] Physicians in the U.S. have traditionally placed little emphasis on preventive care, other than the required childhood immunizations, perhaps because they, in turn, are paid comparatively little for such services (105).

The United States may be the most profitable market for vaccines in the world. Many foreign markets are not attractive because they are highly regulated and vaccine prices are often limited, either by governments (which purchase drugs and vaccines for national health programs) or by competition with foreign vaccine makers (who may receive government subsidies). Many developing countries have severely limited budgets for vaccine purchases and are unable to pay in the hard currency demanded for transnational sales (147).[25] U.S. companies are reluctant to sell at a lower price abroad than in the United States for fear of charges of price-gouging in this country.[26] Thus, the United States offers the most attractive market for HIV vaccines made by United States companies.

Federal, state, county, and city government purchasers may provide a secure market for HIV vaccine. The volume of government purchases may be higher than the total population willing to pay for vaccination because the government may provide vaccine for those unable to pay or not covered by insurance. The population at risk for HIV infection includes a disproportionate number of people who are uninsured for immunizations and who could not afford to pay for vaccination themselves. Government purchasers may not be willing to pay the price that private companies wish to charge for vaccine, however, especially if they purchase large volumes. There is precedent for governments demanding a lower-than-market price for vaccine. The federal government negotiates prices for pediatric vaccines that are significantly lower than "catalog" prices (121). It is also beginning to do the same for drugs,[27] which may make companies fearful that all governmental purchase prices may be regulated more strictly in the future (33).

At the same time, greater price regulation of drugs may make vaccines relatively less unattractive as compared with drugs, which historically and in general, have commanded significantly higher prices than vaccines. If government purchasers were unwilling to pay a high price for an HIV vaccine, companies might be unwilling to sell to them (172). However, it would be awkward for companies to sell a vaccine to private individuals and clinics or physicians while refusing to sell to government.

Vaccines suffer from the disadvantage of not being advertised to the public (as compared with over-the-counter drugs). This means that companies cannot build a market directly, but must rely

---

[24] Private health insurance policies in the U.S. rarely cover the cost of preventive vaccination. President Clinton's proposed Health Security Act would have included childhood and certain other immunizations in its comprehensive benefit package that must be covered by all health insurers. (U.S. Congress, Senate, S. 1757, Health Security Act, Sec. 1128, (Washington, DC: U.S. Government Printing Office, 1993).) Immunization against HIV has not been included in health reform proposals, presumably because no vaccine is available.

[25] The price of some U.S. vaccines is higher than the per capita budget for health care in some developing countries (147).

[26] In 1982 Congressional hearings, a vaccine maker was chastised for charging the U.S. government a higher price than that for foreign countries. After the hearing, U.S. companies no longer bid for UNICEF or PAHO contracts to sell vaccines at low prices in the developing world.

[27] The Medicaid program receives rebates on outpatient drug prices from manufacturers (Social Security Act, s.1927), and certain Public Health Service grantees and certain disproportionate share hospitals receive discounts on outpatient drug purchases (Public Health Service Act, s.340B). Many private health insurers, health maintenance organizations, and large hospitals have negotiated new, lower prices for bulk purchases to reduce health care costs. President Clinton's proposed Health Security Act would have encouraged negotiated price reductions and rebates on certain drugs purchased by Medicare. (U.S. Congress, Senate, S. 1757, Health Security Act, Sec 1128, (Washington, DC: U.S. Government Printing Office, 1993).)

on physicians and health agencies to buy the product and use it with their patients.[28] In addition, vaccines do not create a loyal market of users (105). Unlike drugs that are used repeatedly for chronic diseases, vaccines are used only once or a limited number of times per person. A highly successful vaccine would eliminate its own market by eradicating the disease. Indeed, this is the goal for an HIV vaccine. On the other hand, if only one HIV vaccine is approved, a company is likely to hold a monopoly for many years and will not need to spend money persuading physicians to use it. Government agencies may be counted on to encourage vaccine use, and fear of AIDS may be sufficient incentive for many people.

The most profitable product for a private pharmaceutical company is a patented product that is the only available or effective means to treat or prevent a serious disease.[29] An HIV vaccine would surely qualify in this category. This monopoly position, coupled with strong demand for the product, often allows pricing at whatever the market will bear, (61, 194) as experience with AZT (12) and Clozaril demonstrated. Market potential is ordinarily assessed by comparison with other products that a company might pursue instead of HIV vaccines. Because so few products ever emerge from the research and regulatory pipeline with FDA approval, it makes economic sense to invest in the product with the highest profit potential.

An HIV vaccine is likely to have considerable appeal to companies that believe that market demand will be strong, the price will not be regulated, and users will pay the price. HIV vaccine development may appear unattractive to companies that perceive any of these factors to be absent.

Potential Liability for Adverse Reactions

HIV Vaccine Experience

The evidence that fear of liability has dissuaded companies from pursuing HIV vaccine development comes from reports of companies that withdrew, some only temporarily, from research. A review of these cases, however, reveals that other factors typically were present—a disappointing product, lack of financing, poor market predictions, internal corporate restructuring, or potential patent problems—that could account for the action.

Genentech

Genentech stopped research on a preventive HIV vaccine in 1986, citing liability concerns as one reason. Observers close to the company noted that the vaccine was set aside after it failed to protect chimpanzees against HIV infection and the vaccine-producing cell line was suspected of having retroviral particles. Genentech has since resumed research with a different recombinant vaccine, now in clinical trials, which it hopes to take to market.

In 1986, before Genentech dropped its first vaccine, California had enacted legislation limiting the liability of California makers of an AIDS vaccine, with support from Genentech (Calif. Health & Safety Code 5. 199.49). In 1988, the California Supreme Court issued an opinion endorsing immunity from strict liability for prescription drug makers, which is thought to be equally applicable to vaccine makers, (225) and California repealed its statutory protection against liability (Calif. Stats. 1988, ch. 1555, 5.3). The company also be-

[28] Recently, some pharmaceutical companies have begun advertising prescription drugs directly to consumers. It is possible that vaccines could be advertised directly to consumers in the future.

[29] It is not known whether any vaccine candidate would not qualify for patent protection.

came part of Hoffman-La Roche, a large Swiss pharmaceutical company, which may provide it with financial backing to pursue expensive vaccine development. Large companies with substantial assets, however, are often thought to be more vulnerable to liability claims than small companies with few assets because of their deeper pockets (61).

Finally, the company apparently clarified or resolved earlier scientific questions about vaccine production, safety and efficacy. Which, if any, of these factors persuaded the company to proceed with a new HIV vaccine is unknown outside the company. By mid-1994, Genentech and Biocine were prepared to test their candidate vaccines in the first U.S. phase III field trials. After the NIAID decided not to proceed in June 1994, the companies were reportedly disappointed, and ready to seek alternative ways to pursue the trials without NIAID support (40).

Oncogen

Oncogen, a subsidiary of Bristol-Meyers Squibb, stopped producing preventive vaccine (using live vaccinia virus as a vector to express recombinant gp 160) in 1992 before testing its efficacy in human subjects. A researcher reportedly attributed the decision to "fear of lawsuits from injured vaccine trial subjects" together with "other commercial negatives like a questionable market and patent snafus" (32). Others note that lack of data indicating potential efficacy prompted discontinuation.

Immune Response Corp

Immune Response Corp., co-founded by Jonas Salk, was also reported to delay testing its whole, killed-virus vaccine in uninfected subjects because of liability concerns, but other reports said the company was willing to go forward if the vaccine showed evidence of effectiveness (32).

The vaccine has been tested, without liability issues, in HIV-positive people as a therapeutic means to prevent disease progression to AIDS. Although the whole, killed-virus approach has shown promise, (124) it has raised safety concerns it might cause HIV infection if any of the virus survived processing. Recent tests of live attenuated SIV vaccine in newborn monkeys lend weight to such fears (126).

MicroGeneSys

MicroGeneSys reportedly refused to conduct trials of its vaccine to prevent HIV transmission from HIV-positive pregnant women to their newborns, unless the state legislature granted it immunity from liability (172). Lobbyists for MicroGeneSys argued that children born to HIV positive mothers, many of whom had used illegal drugs, are at high risk for medical problems which might be blamed on the vaccine. The company's president reportedly claimed that a new law was needed to establish a parent's right to consent to involving a fetus in research (169).[30] The company refused to conduct trials in Tennessee which offered no special protection against liability.

Connecticut, the company's home state, enacted a statute in 1991 granting Connecticut manufacturers, research institutions, and researchers immunity from civil liability for personal injury to research subjects resulting from administration of any investigational AIDS vaccine (Conn. Gen. Stat. 19a-591-591, 1992c). The law, which offered no compensation to injured subjects, provides immunity from both strict liability and negligence in cases involving research subjects, but retains liability for gross negligence, and reckless, willful or wanton misconduct. At the same time, Connecticut provided substantial economic support to the company, which had no income-producing product and needed substantial capital to construct a plant to produce vaccine (17). MicroGeneSys insisted on conducting the

---

[30] It is questionable whether a company would be liable under existing common law for fetal injuries resulting from research to which the pregnant woman consented (31).

trial at Yale University only, rejecting other planned and proposed sites in Connecticut. After about a year, only two subjects were enrolled. The trial was then closed because it could not produce useful data.

Elsewhere, Genentech conducted trials of its vaccine to prevent maternal HIV transmission in the NIAID-supported sites around the country, although only California had statutory protection against manufacturer liability for injuries arising out of such trials. Preliminary results have not supported hopes for the vaccine effectiveness in pregnant women, and Genentech is dropping its therapeutic vaccine research to concentrate on preventive vaccines.

MicroGeneSys did not mention liability when it lobbied successfully for a $20-million congressional appropriation to the Department of Defense (DOD) to finance trials of its vaccine for therapeutic use in HIV-positive adults. The appropriation, for a specific project proposed by an individual company outside the usual peer review channels, created considerable controversy, was opposed by DOD, NIH, and FDA, and was ultimately rescinded (38). NIH, FDA, and DOD preferred a trial comparing several candidate vaccines chosen by peer review.

The first vaccine to be approved for testing in human beings (in 1987), MicroGeneSys's product might not fare well against the more recent generation of candidate vaccines. MicroGeneSys's corporate partner, American Home Products, Wyeth-Ayerst Laboratories, which had financed the company and acquired worldwide marketing rights to the vaccine, terminated its agreement with MicroGeneSys and its involvement with the vaccine's development in January 1994 without comment (39).

Abbott

Another report involved Abbott Laboratories' human immunodeficiency virus immune globulin (HIVIG), which was intended to stop the transmission of HIV from HIV-positive mothers to their newborns. Not a preventive vaccine, HIVIG contains antibody against HIV derived from the plasma of HIV-positive people with strong immune responses to the virus. Researchers hoped it would reduce the viral load in pregnant women with HIV and prevent infection of their children, either before or during delivery. A large multicenter trial of HIVIG had been planned under the sponsorship of Abbott and the National Heart Lung and Blood Institute, the NIAID and the National Institute of Child Health and Human Development. After two years of planning, Abbott suddenly withdrew in 1992, citing liability concerns (41). Researchers could not recall earlier mentions of liability, even though high-level company representatives had met with them to plan the trials.

Some participants and observers believed that Abbott was seeking to get rid of its blood products division in a reorganization to improve profitability and used the trial as the excuse to do so. According to news reports, Abbott's interest in the trial dropped after the head of its transfusion medicine branch left the company. Abbott first objected to certifying that its costs and prices to government were properly computed, a standard NIH requirement that NIH finally waived (41). Then Abbott objected to patent rights arrangements. Finally, Abbott asked for indemnification against liability (citing the Swine Flu Program[31] as precedent), which NIH could not provide without Congressional action. Other organizations that make immunoglobulin did not consider liability an ob-

[31] The Swine Flu Program, created by Congress in 1976 to encourage the development and marketing of a vaccine against a strain of swine flu which was expected that fall and winter, held manufacturers harmless from injuries arising from the swine flu vaccine, and permitted claims for vaccine-related injuries to be filed with the U.S. government. The program is discussed in more detail in the next section.

stacle.[32] One AIDS organizer opined that Abbott was trying to manipulate activists and researchers to lobby Congress for liability protection (41). Abbott employees active in transfusion medicine later formed their own company and successfully bid to produce HIVIG for the multi-center trials, which finally began in 1993.

Summary

These examples fail to clarify the role of potential liability in HIV vaccine development. It is plausible that liability was a concern. It is also plausible that liability was not a serious consideration. In all cases, other factors could explain not pursuing an HIV vaccine, most commonly lack of evidence of effectiveness, but also inadequate financing, poor market predictions, corporate restructuring, and potential patent problems.

Garber argues that when a company says it is withdrawing a socially beneficial product from the market because of fear of liability, such statements should have credibility (61). But vaccines may be an exception. If the primary reason for withdrawal is financial—such as a desire to focus on products with much higher returns—a company may be loath to state publicly that it is foregoing a socially beneficial product in order to make more profit. The public is likely to find ordinary concern for profits less acceptable when the product it loses is greatly needed, and more likely to tolerate the loss if it seems beyond a company's control.

Moreover, from the company's perspective, there is always the possibility that Congress might take action to limit liability, which would decrease expenses. The only risk in attributing withdrawal to liability is that Congress might require the company to guarantee production or to sell at a low price in return for limiting liability. But Congress has never imposed such a quid pro quo, so the risk is probably negligible.

Drugs Withdrawn from the Market

A look at drugs that have been the target of liability claims and whether they remained on the market may yield some clues as to whether potential liability is a serious threat to HIV vaccine development. Studies of product withdrawals recognize the impossibility of identifying the reasons for withdrawal in many cases (61, 178). It is often difficult to sort out whether producers acted out of concern for consumers, fear of regulatory action, actual regulatory action, disappointing financial returns, changing business opportunities, litigation experience, fear of liability, or some combination of these.

Relatively few drugs have been withdrawn after marketing.[33] Some undoubtedly were withdrawn or never marketed because risks materialized that made them too hazardous to use. Such withdrawals for safety reasons are sometimes attributed to liability. To be sure, a drug that turned out to be dangerous to use, especially if its benefits were limited, could be the subject of liability claims. As Bovbjerg notes, however, one must assume that "right-thinking" producers would withdraw a dangerous drug because they did not wish to subject consumers to its dangers, or their reputations to public wrath, not merely because of potential liability (21). To assume that liability is the sole cause of such withdrawal would mean that liability is the sole deterrent to marketing unsafe drugs.

Drugs that have been withdrawn from the market include Bendectin, DES (diethylstilbestrol), MER-29, Merital, Oraflex, Selacryn, Versed and Zomax. Bendectin and DES were the subject of mass tort claims in which thousands of claimants

[32] Burroughs Wellcome Co. jointly sponsored trials of AZT in pregnant women to determine whether it would reduce HIV transmission. Preliminary results are encouraging.

[33] Most medical products that have been withdrawn have been medical devices rather than pharmaceuticals: the Dalkon Shield; Copper-7 and other IUDs; Bjork-Shiley Heart Valve; and silicon-gel breast implants (61, 178).

have filed suit amid substantial publicity. The last five drugs were not involved in extensive liability claims and are rarely mentioned in discussions of liability effects on product marketing. Garber suggests that perhaps the fact that other alternatives were available mitigated their withdrawal (61).

The few studies of product liability claims for medical products indicate that the claims are highly product-specific, with Bendectin accounting for the majority (194).[34] Bendectin, the drug to prevent morning sickness during pregnancy, is the best example of a drug that can be said with any confidence to have been withdrawn for liability reasons. There is little, if any, evidence that the drug causes serious side effects. The producer, Merrell Dow Pharmaceutical, has won all but a few of the litigated cases.[35] The FDA did not require withdrawal of the product, although warnings were strengthened (61, 105). Yet the cost of defending or settling the more than 2,000 suits that have been filed may not have been worth the effort or expense.[36]

DES, a synthetic estrogen produced by several companies (including Abbott Laboratories, Eli Lilly & Co., Squibb Corp., and Upjohn Co.), is a more complicated example because it did cause cancer in the daughters of women who used the drug to prevent miscarriage. The FDA approved DES in 1941 and banned its use in 1971. Although many have decried its withdrawal (80) and no drugs to prevent miscarriage are being marketed now, no one suggests that withdrawal of DES itself is a great loss to society. One reason it has become a cautionary tale for liability seems to lie in the fact that the risk was latent, exposing several companies to lawsuits a generation after the drug was used.

It may be that the possibility for mass tort litigation involving risks to a fetus unknown at the time of marketing is a special case which deters marketing certain drugs. Bendectin and DES were both intended for use by pregnant women who wanted to have a child. Drugs used for pregnancy are more susceptible to claims alleging serious permanent harm to children than other drugs (194). Until quite recently, few drugs prescribed for pregnant women were tested in pregnant women before marketing (118), so that their effects on the fetus were often unknown.

Several drugs with recognized serious side effects (such as Accutane, Clozaril, and Cytotec) remain on the market in spite of successful claims of liability. The FDA reportedly estimated that Accutane, Hoffman-La Roche's drug to treat severe cystic acne, had caused perhaps 1,300 birth defects by 1986 (61, 164). Hoffman-La Roche has provided special information kits to prevent the drug's use in pregnant women, but has not withdrawn the product, as might be expected if liability claims determined product availability.

Similarly, Sandoz's Clozaril (used to treat schizophrenia) has potentially fatal side effects in perhaps two percent of patients (139). It requires careful monitoring of white blood cell counts to avoid agranulocytosis. It is possible that the potential for liability is diluted by the physician's involvement in supervising the drug's use.[37] Still, contrary to conventional wisdom, the severity of the side effects has not been sufficient to deter

[34] Although claims involving pharmaceuticals and medical devices have risen since the 1960's, there is no information on whether the baseline level of claims was too high, too low, or about right, because the merits of such claims were not (and probably could not be) investigated.

[35] Bendectin was the subject of *Daubert* v. *Merrell Dow Pharmaceutical, Inc.*, 113 S.Ct. 2786 (1993), in which the U.S. Supreme Court held that the *Frye* rule for admitting scientific evidence in Federal court was superseded by the Federal Rules of Evidence, which permits the admission of "all relevant evidence" unless specifically excepted by the Rules (8).

[36] One commentator suggests that mothers who had used Bendectin may have viewed the company with suspicion because it had acquired other problem products, including Thalidomide, MER-29, DES, and Agent Orange (154).

[37] The limited potential for damages in the case of people with severe schizophrenia who are unable to work, even while using the drug, may also reduce the financial exposure for liability, although it is unclear what proportion of patients would fall into that category. Damages for the death of an individual are typically less than damages for permanent injury.

marketing. Cytotec would appear to have even greater potential for withdrawal because its benefits have less dramatic social value. The drug is used to prevent ulcers in patients who take nonsteroidal anti-inflammatory drugs (like aspirin and ibuprofen) for arthritis, but can cause abnormal bleeding and miscarriage or abortion in pregnant patients (61, 139). G.D. Searle still markets Cytotec with strong warnings of the risks.

Another factor influencing product withdrawal may be the importance of the revenues it produces for a company. Prozac (an antidepressant) reportedly accounts for about 25 percent of Eli Lilly's drug sales, $1 billion in the United States. Lawsuits have claimed that the drug causes suicide, violence, and even murder, but the validity of such claims is uncertain at best. The background rate of such behavior among users means that some cases may be misattributed to the drug but that it will also be difficult to prove causation. Such circumstances appear to be precisely the sort that would prompt a manufacturer's withdrawal of a drug for fear of unfounded liability claims. Indeed, they parallel Bendectin's claims experience (61). Nonetheless, Lilly is not expected to withdraw Prozac and is vigorously defending all claims against it. The generally favorable publicity it has received suggests that a significant proportion of the population wants the drug on the market (102).

Halcion, the most widely prescribed sleeping pill in the United States, has also been the subject of claims that it causes suicide and violence.[38] The Upjohn Co. is keeping the drug on the market—it has reportedly produced about $2 billion in sales—although alternative medicines are available. The company recently brought a libel suit in England against the British Broadcasting Corporation and an expert witness who testified for plaintiffs and publicly criticized Upjohn (18).

In sum, it is difficult to generalize about the effect of liability concerns on marketing from these examples. In particular, they say nothing about products that were never marketed in the first place.[39] They do suggest, at a minimum, that whatever weight potential liability may have, it is balanced with other factors to predict the net social and financial returns that marketing a specific product may bring.

Different companies may give such factors different weights. Arguably, breakthrough drugs for diseases without any current cure, or drugs that offer a significant improvement over existing drugs, are more likely to be marketed (and remain on the market) than "me-too" drugs or those with only marginal additional benefits or fewer risks. Drugs that may harbor serious latent hazards, especially those that might become the subject of mass tort claims, might be considered more susceptible to withdrawal, before or after marketing; but all the drugs discussed fall into this category, yet not all were withdrawn.

Perhaps the higher financial returns from a large market can offset concerns about potential exposure to large numbers of claims. The severity of inherent risks may not be determinative, especially if the drug can produce substantial revenues. If the hazards can result from multiple causes, the probability of claims attributing injury to the drug is higher than when causation is clear, but the proportion of claims resulting in liability is lower.

Where the risks are known, some companies may feel they can protect themselves against inappropriate liability by ensuring that proper warn-

[38] One woman, criminally indicted for homicide for fatally shooting her mother after taking Halcion, Valium, and codeine, had the charges dropped on the grounds that she was intoxicated by the drug. She sued Upjohn for negligence and received an $8 million settlement (18). A decision by the Supreme Court of Utah (255) held that makers of FDA-approved drugs were immune from strict liability for defective design.

[39] Thalidomide may be an example of a drug that is not being marketed now because of its potential to cause severe birth defects when used by pregnant women to relieve nausea (105). Merrell reportedly settled claims that the drug caused birth defects among residents in Canada and the United States (154). Although the FDA had not approved thalidomide, it was distributed for investigational use. It is currently being investigated as a therapy for patients with leprosy or AIDS wasting.

ings are given, as they have with Accutane, Clozaril, and Cytotec.[40] Others may not. Where adverse reactions cannot reasonably be predicted, there is always the possibility that serious harm could materialize in the future and, with it, liability claims. Although lengthier and more sophisticated premarket testing has probably lowered the risk of unforeseen adverse reactions, no drug is free from that risk.

Vaccines Withdrawn from the Market

Conventional wisdom has held that, whatever the reasons for withdrawing particular drugs from the market, vaccines have been withdrawn primarily because of fear of liability for adverse reactions (13, 61, 79, 80, 105). As with drugs, there can be many reasons for withdrawing a vaccine; the lack of empirical data makes it difficult to draw generalizable conclusions.

The two examples of vaccines that were withdrawn or delayed to market are the swine flu and DPT (diphtheria-pertussis-tetanus) vaccines. In 1976, makers of swine flu vaccine said they would not produce or market the vaccine unless the Federal government assumed liability for adverse reactions. Their insurers would not provide liability insurance covering such reactions. The vaccine was developed hurriedly in response to public health officials' fears of a new influenza epidemic like the one that killed tens of thousands of people in 1918 (129). Amid substantial publicity, then President Gerald Ford encouraged everyone in the country to be vaccinated. There was insufficient time to test the swine flu vaccine in the same manner that other non-influenza vaccines were tested if the vaccine were to be available to vaccinate the entire American population by flu season. In response, Congress enacted the National Swine Flu Immunization Program, whereby the Federal government assumed legal liability for non-negligent adverse reactions to the vaccine (180).[41]

The lessons from swine flu are conflicting. On the one hand, vaccine makers could not get liability insurance for the vaccine,[42] and fear of liability apparently stopped vaccine production. Congress took such fears seriously enough to pass protective legislation (56). In addition, Guillain-Barré syndrome, an unexpected serious adverse reaction resulting in paralysis, did materialize, and with it, about 4,000 claims against the government. This gives credence to liability fears.

On the other hand, the government paid out less than $2 per dose of vaccine distributed in awards and settlements to claimants.[43] The government agreed to accept responsibility in any case in which the symptoms of Guillain-Barré syndrome appeared within ten weeks of vaccination (a generous assumption of causation that would probably not be accepted by any vaccine maker), so that it paid a larger proportion of claims than would have been paid had the cases been litigated under ordinary tort requirements.[44] In litigated cases involving Guillain-Barré syndrome appearing after ten weeks or other conditions, court decisions awarded compensation in only six reported cases (247, 260, 286, 305, 308, 315).

Swine flu probably represents a worst case scenario for vaccine liability. The legislation was enacted as a temporary measure and was not designed to resolve liability issues systematically

---

[40] The tobacco industry has succeeded in defeating claims of liability for the use of cigarettes largely by virtue of warnings.

[41] The federal government assumed responsibility for defending all claims and had a right of abrogation against the manufacturer in cases in which the manufacturer's negligence caused injury, allowing the government to obtain payment from the manufacturer for awards in negligence. However, the government also provided $230 million in liability insurance for vaccine manufacturers, thereby paying for its own indemnity.

[42] Most vaccine makers now self-insure in whole or in part.

[43] Total awards and settlements were approximately $76 million, excluding administrative costs.

[44] According to one court, the government agreed to liability in Guillain-Barré cases not only to provide compensation to those who could not prove negligence, but also because the syndrome was not mentioned as risk in the consent document (315).

(82). As the Institute of Medicine noted, the legislation "only changed the defendant" (82). Certainly Congress is not anxious to repeat the experience and would shy away from assuming liability for any new vaccine. At the same time, the total amount of awards may be manageable if the vaccine is appropriately priced. This suggests that the price at which a vaccine can be sold may determine how much room there is for liability payments.

Swine flu development also differed from the circumstances surrounding most other vaccines because of its necessarily hasty development and its immediate use in millions of people. Of course, the more deliberate pace of research possible with most vaccines does not ensure that all risks will be discovered before marketing. But the more a vaccine is studied, the more likely it is that adverse reactions will be discovered.

Wyeth Laboratories ceased DPT vaccine production in 1984, reportedly because of claims filed asserting adverse reactions to the pertussis component of DPT. It is entirely plausible that Wyeth could have decided that vaccine production would not be profitable enough to justify defending additional lawsuits. At the same time, Wyeth reportedly faced replacing its old vaccine production facilities if it were to continue selling the vaccine. If the company wanted to get out of the vaccine business, this would have been the time to do it, before it invested heavily in an expensive new plant. Wyeth did continue to produce the vaccine, but sold it to Lederle for distribution.

Also in 1984, Connaught Laboratories announced that it would stop producing DPT because it was having difficulty getting liability insurance at a reasonable price. The Centers for Disease Control and Prevention (CDC) recommended vaccinating only older children to conserve diminishing vaccine supplies. Connaught soon found acceptable insurance and continued to produce DPT. In 1986, prices for childhood vaccines rose dramatically.

CURRENT VACCINE RESEARCH AND DEVELOPMENT

Companies have few business incentives to produce vaccines at all. The number of U.S. vaccine makers has declined since the early 1970s. At that time, many vaccines were "me-too" vaccines, produced much like generic products and sold in high volume at very low prices (121). In the mid-1970s, the FDA began to require evidence of effectiveness of vaccines as a condition for continued marketing. Many vaccine makers may have dropped out of the business rather than conduct the expensive clinical trials necessary to demonstrate their vaccines' efficacy. The U.S. market for children's vaccines may not be large enough to support several competitors. The percentage of research and development (R&D) expenditures devoted to biologics (as opposed to pharmaceuticals) in the industry declined from 4 percent in 1973 to 2.1 percent in 1983 (121).[45] During that period, sales of biologics represented between 2.7 and 3.6 percent of total sales, including pharmaceuticals, of members of the Pharmaceutical Manufacturers Association (since renamed the Pharmaceutical Research and Manufacturers Association). Between 1973 and 1980, R&D expenditures for biologics ranged unevenly (between 12.9 and 23.1 percent of sales of biologics alone). In 1981, that percentage was 9.2 (121).

In recent years, however, vaccine research and development has increased in the United States. A recent report by the Institute of Medicine concludes that "the worldwide vaccine industry appears to be entering a new era of activity and innovation" (121). Applications submitted to the FDA to study new biologics rose from 66 in 1980 to 558 in 1992 (212). Most have been for thera-

[45] Total research and development for both pharmaceuticals and biologics increased gradually from 12.57 percent in 1973 to 15.32 percent of total sales in 1983 (121). Total R&D for 1990 was 17.4 percent of total sales.

peutics, but Investigational New Drug applications for vaccines have been increasing since 1990 (67 in 1990, 81 in 1992). Some established pharmaceutical companies in the United States have begun new investments in vaccine research.[46] Several U.S. companies are joining with foreign firms to develop or license vaccines.

The past four years have seen the introduction of a dozen new vaccines, including a new acellular pertussis component of the combination vaccine (DTaP) with diphtheria and tetanus toxoids by Lederle-Praxis and Connaught Laboratories, several new *Haemophilus influenzae* type b (Hib) vaccines, Japanese encephalitis virus vaccine, and a new typhoid vaccine. Other new or improved vaccines, including one to prevent chicken pox, are in clinical trials or expected to be approved by the FDA in the near future. It is possible that the industry went through a shaking-out period in the 1980s and is being restructured to meet the new scientific challenges posed by infectious diseases more efficiently.

The growth in biotechnology companies may have helped this trend. Biotechnology researchers are likely to be an important source of innovative products in the next few years (77). More than 75 biotechnology companies around the world were conducting vaccine research and development in 1992. Small companies may be able to invest in risky products because they have less to lose in the event of catastrophe.

At the same time, the biotechnology industry may experience a shake-out in the near future, with many of the estimated 1,300 companies going out of business. Few small companies have any FDA-approved products on the market, and thus have no product revenue. Most companies reportedly do not have enough financing to operate for more than two years (67, 77). The investment community may be wary of investing further in companies that face a low probability of producing a commercial product within the next several years, especially after news reports of the failure of eight companies' pharmaceutical products in clinical trials in 1994 (47). Small firms that are short of operating capital may sell or license their product rights or the entire company. Most are expected to be acquired by large pharmaceutical companies, including foreign companies.[47]

Other biotechnology companies may survive by concentrating on only one or two products, by licensing new products to large domestic or foreign companies, or by limiting themselves to one phase of product development and conducting joint ventures with other companies that specialize in clinical trials, manufacturing, or marketing (77). If the pharmaceutical industry scales back its investment in research and development, the biotechnology industry may fill the gap in research. Which companies will do so remains to be seen.

The modern vaccine industry looks more like the pharmaceutical industry and less like the earlier vaccine industry. The trend appears to be toward developing sophisticated products, often the result of recombinant DNA technology, that can be sold at prices approaching the higher prices of pharmaceuticals. Often the technology used influences the attractiveness of vaccine production. Technologies that can be used to produce other marketable products, such as diagnostic tests, are more likely to be pursued than technologies that have only one use. In view of the fact that only a small proportion of potential products are ultimately approved by the FDA and successfully

---

[46] For example, Merck & Co., Inc., maker of measles vaccine, created its Merck Vaccine Division in 1991, has invested in a new biotechnology facility in Pennsylvania, and has entered into joint or cooperative ventures with other companies, such as MedImmune. Lederle Laboratories, the target of DPT vaccine lawsuits, acquired Praxis Biologics, developer of a conjugate *Haemophilus influenzae* type b vaccine (Hib-CV). American Cyanamid made the resulting Lederle-Praxis Biologicals a regular business unit in 1992, giving it greater corporate weight (121).

[47] For example, Ciba-Geigy, Ltd. of Switzerland is reported to have agreed to buy 49.9% of Chiron Corporation, a profitable independent company and provide it with new financial and technical assistance (57). Ciba-Geigy and Chiron are also partners in Biocine which developed a candidate HIV vaccine.

marketed, companies may be reluctant to gamble a large investment on a single long-shot vaccine.

The National Childhood Vaccine Injury Act of 1986[48] may also have encouraged vaccine research because it limits producers' liability to a predictable amount (paid as a tax on vaccine sales) and frees them from defending claims. As originally enacted, however, the Act did not apply to investigational or newly approved vaccines. It was to cover only vaccines that children were required by law to take. A 1993 amendment permits the Secretary of Health and Human Services to extend coverage to new vaccines that are recommended for children; Hib and HBV vaccines are expected to be added soon. Vaccine makers may anticipate that other vaccines will be added. Most of the recently approved vaccines had been under development before the act took effect in 1988. If it does further encourage research, then an even larger increase in vaccine development should be expected in the future.

Research initiatives for HIV vaccine development are also encouraging. At least twelve companies are actively engaged in HIV vaccine research and development, and others are developing adjuvants and other supporting products.[49] This exceeds the number of companies developing a vaccine for any other disease. Almost 30 candidate vaccines are now in clinical trials (207). The debate over phase III field trials centers on scientific issues whether any of the candidate vaccines that have been tested show sufficient promise of effectiveness to warrant large=scale testing in human beings. Potential liability for adverse reactions does not appear to be a factor in these debates. There is a possibility that subjects injured in a foreign field trial might try to sue a U.S. vaccine maker in the United States (173). But the rarity of injuries in clinical trials in general (140) and the even greater rarity of claims arising out of such trials suggests that liability has not much influenced decision-making about whether to conduct field trials abroad.

Conclusion:

There is evidence that vaccine research and development is increasing and that a surprising number of companies are engaged in HIV vaccine research. Indeed, more companies are developing vaccines for HIV infection than for any other single disease. Potential liability may have concerned a few companies, but it has not prevented a strong research effort and appears unlikely to halt HIV vaccine development. The major stumbling blocks remain scientific. Even if new vaccine candidates show more promise than those currently in clinical trials, the likely market for an HIV vaccine is uncertain. Given the business disincentives to producing an HIV vaccine, the vigor of research is encouraging.

Decisions about HIV vaccine research and marketing are likely to vary from company to company and from product to product, as they have with other vaccines and drugs in the past. Fear of liability may influence a few companies' choice of vaccine type, so that they may avoid killed or live attenuated vaccines in favor of recombinant vaccines that are believed to pose little or no safety risk. If so, the array of possible vaccines could be limited to the more expensive recombinant types.

TORT LIABILITY FOR ADVERSE REACTIONS TO VACCINES

Overview of Product Liability

Like manufacturers of all products, vaccine makers are responsible under state law for personal injuries caused by their own negligence or by a de-

[48]The National Childhood Vaccine Injury Act of 1986 is discussed below under Public Compensation Systems.

[49]See chapter 2 for a discussion on the current state of HIV vaccine development.

fect in their products.[50] Tort law provides two categories of legal responsibility for personal injuries caused by products: negligence and strict liability (94).[51]

Negligence is conduct by the product maker that deviates from standards of acceptable conduct adhered to by the ordinary manufacturer of similar products and that results in harm to the product user. To succeed on a negligence claim, a plaintiff must prove that: 1) the manufacturer had a duty to the plaintiff, 2) the manufacturer breached that duty, 3) the plaintiff suffered an injury for which damages may be awarded by law, and 4) the injury was caused by the manufacturer's breach of duty (94).

Few cases for vaccine-related injury are brought in negligence alone. Before 1960, plaintiffs were generally unable to prove that a manufacturer had been negligent or that a vaccine had caused an injury (228, 295, 314). Strict liability developed in part because consumers were frequently unable to obtain the evidence that a manufacturer of consumer products had acted negligently.[52] By the mid 1960s, when more vaccines were being marketed widely in the United States, the state had begun to adopt the doctrine of strict liability for injuries caused by defective products, so that plaintiffs were able to apply that theory to vaccines as well as other consumer products (13, 168).

The concept of strict liability generally applied in the United States is summarized in Section 402A of the Restatement (Second) of Torts and holds "[o]ne who sells any product in a defective condition unreasonably dangerous to the user or consumer or to his property [liable] for physical harm thereby caused to the ultimate user or consumer...." (4).[53] Thus, strict liability is said to focus on the condition of the product itself, while negligence focuses on the behavior of the manufacturer (206). Because the manufacturer's actions or knowledge are often at issue in deciding whether a product is defective, however, the strict liability concept has increasingly mimicked aspects of ordinary negligence (72).

These rules would also apply in some cases involving adverse reactions to U.S. products that occur in developing countries and are ligated in the United States (see box 4-1).

PRODUCT DEFECTS

Traditionally, product defects have been divided into three categories: 1) manufacturing flaws, 2) defects in product design, and 3) errors or omissions in directions and warnings accompanying the product. Least controversial are manufacturing flaws or errors in the manufacturing process.[54] These produce something other than the product intended by the manufacturer, since the manufac-

[50] Although state laws vary to some degree, the basic principles are sufficiently similar to permit generalization for purposes of this report. There is no general federal tort law, although supporters of tort reform have sought enactment of a federal law governing product liability for many years. For a description of the National Vaccine Injury Compensation Program, see discussion below.

[51] Causes of action also exist for breach of express or implied warranty of fitness for a particular purpose, but because they are not based in tort law, tend to cover the same facts and duties as strict liability and are usually superseded by strict liability or negligence claims, they are not discussed herein.

[52] Strict liability combines elements of traditional actions in negligence (which do not require privity of contract) and warranty (which do not require proof of negligence). Warranty claims were available only to those who had purchased a product directly from a seller and were therefore in contractual privity (51, 52).

[53] Section 402A also specifies that the seller is liable if engaged in the business of selling the product and "it is expected to and does reach the user or consumer without substantial change in the condition in which it is sold." This rule "applies although (a) the seller has exercised all possible care in the preparation and sale of his product, and (b) the user or consumer has not bought the product from or entered into any contractual relation with the seller" (4).

[54] Liability for manufacturing errors dates back from the thirteenth century when those who supplied contaminated food were subject to criminal liability (4).

BOX 4-1: Liability for Adverse Reactions to HIV Vaccines in Developing Countries: The Doctrine of *Forum Non Conveniens*

Although the NIH has postponed Phase III clinical efficacy trials of HIV vaccines in the United States, some U.S. pharmaceutical manufacturers have begun large-scale clinical trials of HIV vaccines in developing countries. These U.S. pharmaceutical manufacturers are thus exposed to liability for adverse reactions to HIV vaccines that occur among trial participants in developing countries.

Plaintiffs may seek to bring a legal proceeding to the place of manufacture if they believe there is an opportunity for a larger recovery. Foreign trial participants who are injured by HIV vaccines manufactured in the United States may prefer to bring suit in U.S. courts, because U.S product liability law is considered more favorable to plaintiffs than product liability laws of most developing countries. For instance, U.S. law allows plaintiffs to hire attorneys on a contingency fee basis, so that the plaintiff's attorney is not paid unless there is a recovery. U.S. law allows for the award of punitive damages in product liability cases, whereas the laws of many developing countries do not. And unlike most countries, U.S. law permits jury trials in product liability cases; awards by juries have the reputation of being more generous.

The legal doctrine of *forum non conveniens*, however, substantially limits the ability of foreign plaintiffs to bring suit in U.S. courts. One of the original intents of this doctrine was to prevent "forum shopping" by plaintiffs, but the doctrine has increasingly been used as a means for "reverse" forum shopping by defendants who wish to dismiss cases brought by foreign plaintiffs in U S. courts. In analyzing whether to grant a *forum non conveniens* motion, courts considers a three-part test. The court first determines whether an appropriate alternative forum exists where the plaintiff can receive redress (usually the home country of the plaintiff, or the place where the injury occurred). In determining whether there is another suitable forum, the court is not to consider which forum would be more or less favorable to either of the parties.[1]

If the court finds that an acceptable alternative forum exists, then it determines whether the greater "convenience" of the alternative forum would warrant dismissal. In determining whether it is more appropriate to bring the suit in an alternative forum, the court is to balance the various public and private interests in the location of the suit.

In considering *forum non conveniens* motions, courts have emphasized the administrative burden of the case on U.S. courts. This concern was important in the courts decision to grant a *forum non conveniens* motion to dismiss in *In re Union Carbide Corporation*, (268), which followed an explosion at a chemical plant in Bhopal, India, with a large number of deaths and injuries. U.S. lawyers who were representing a number of injured individuals and their families in a tort action against Union Carbide sought to try the case in a United States Federal court. The court decided that India's legal system could provide an adequate forum. The court also decided that India's courts were the most appropriate forum, considering the location of the witnesses, the evidence, and the documentation for this case. The court weighed the public and private interests involved, and, in dismissing the case, placed the greatest emphasis on administrative concerns. The court reasoned that "the American interests are relatively minor. Indeed, a longer trial . . . would unduly burden an already burdened court, involve both injury and hardship and heavy expense." *Ibid*.

(continued)

[1] In *Piper Aircraft Co*. v. *Reyno,* (287) the Supreme Court held that the doctrine of *form non conveniens* applied despite the possibility that the plaintiff may face less favorable product liability laws in foreign courts. The court reasoned that U.S. courts, with their strict liability theory, potential choice of fifty jurisdictions, availability of jury trials, contingent attorney's fees, and rules allowing extensive discovery, are especially attractive to foreign plaintiffs, further congesting crowded U.S. dockets.

BOX 4-1: Liability for Adverse Reactions to HIV Vaccines in Developing Countries: The Doctrine of *Forum Non Conveniens* (Cont'd.)

The doctrine of *forum non conveniens* has been raised in a number of cases involving injuries from U.S. pharmaceutical products marketed abroad.[2] In some cases, especially involving injuries that may also have occurred to a large number of other persons as well, courts have granted *forum non conveniens* motions to dismiss the case. In *Dowling* v. *Hyland Therapeutics*, (237), the plaintiff, an Irish hemophiliac, brought suit in a Federal court in New York City against the U.S. manufacturer of HIV-infected blood clotting factor that he received. The blood product was manufactured in the United States, and the blood product was administered to the plaintiff in Ireland. The court dismissed the case, reasoning that "[t]he public interest in AIDS prevention is equally important in New York as in Ireland. However, in all other respects, the public interest clearly favors trial in Ireland. Irish law would apply since Dowling received treatment, allegedly contracted HIV, and at all times resided in Ireland." Ibid.[3]

However, in other cases involving individual injuries that were unlikely to have occurred to many others, courts have permitted foreigners injured by U.S. drugs and vaccines to bring their case into U.S. courts. See, e.g., *Carlenstope* v. *Merck*, (227); *Chan Tse Ming* v. *Cordis Corp.,* (230); *Corrigan* v. *Bjork Shiley Corp.,* (233); *Haddad* v. *Richardson-Merrell, Inc.* (256); *Hodson v. A.H. Robins Co., Inc.,* (261).

Given that the U.S. judicial system is overburdened, courts are expected to continue to use the doctrine of *forum non conveniens* to limit access of foreign plaintiffs to U.S. courts.

SOURCE: R. E. Stein, Blicker & Stein, Washington, DC, "Selected Issues of AIDS Vaccine Liability," unpublished contractor report prepared for the Office of Technology Assessment, U.S. Congress, Washington, DC, Sept. 30, 1994.

[2] All of the cases cited here involve drugs that have been approved and marketed. To date, there are no cases where a foreign plaintiff has been permitted to sue in the United States for injuries that occurred during a foreign trial of a U.S.-manufactured drug or vaccine.

[3] See also *De Melo* v. *Lederle Laboratories*, (236) (Eighth Circuit Court of Appeals upheld the dismissal by a federal district court of a lawsuit brought by a Brazilian woman permanently blinded in Brazil by a drug manufactured in the United States. While the U.S. labeling for the drug warned of permanent blindness, the Brazilian labeling warned only of temporary blindness).

turing process failed to conform to the manufacturer's own specifications, and are generally limited to particular units or batches of the product. Examples include adulterated or contaminated products and products in which a toxic element was not removed or rendered harmless by the manufacturing or quality control process. Claims based on manufacturing defects in vaccines are extremely rare, probably because such defects themselves are so rare.[55]

Defects in design are problems with the product specifications themselves, not an isolated manufacturing error. A design is defective if the product could have been developed so as to reduce its inherent danger to the user without significantly decreasing its effectiveness. Whether a design is defective depends upon a manufacturer's behavior in its research and testing activities and the state of scientific knowledge at the time of product development. Thus, although liability for design

[55] The so-called Cutter incident occurred when the manufacturing process for the Salk killed-virus polio vaccine failed to "kill" particles of live polio virus, the vaccine was used in a mass immunization program, and almost 100 people developed poliomyelitis (15). More than 60 lawsuits were filed. Plaintiffs in the lead case (250) ultimately won their action on the theory that the manufacturer had breached its implied warranty (302). Most of the remaining lawsuits were settled thereafter.

defects is theoretically part of strict liability, it is understood to apply in essentially the same way as liability for negligence. Few cases claiming that vaccines were defectively designed were brought until the 1980s (117).[56] More recently, several courts have rejected such claims and granted vaccine manufacturers effective immunity from strict liability for design defects, absent fraudulent conduct.

The vast majority of litigated claims involving vaccines are based on warning defects.[57] These are of two types: 1) a failure to provide warnings of risks inherent in the use of the product (failure to warn),[58] and 2) providing directions and warnings that fail to adequately describe product risks (inadequate warning). A defect in the warning is independent of any flaw in the product itself. A properly produced vaccine that is not accompanied by adequate warnings of possible side effects is a product that is defective *as marketed.*

Liability for Defectively Designed Vaccines

Most vaccine manufacturers and some commentators argue that drug and vaccine makers should be exempt from liability for defectively designed products (as long as they meet FDA requirements for approval) because of the benefits their products confer (159). Others argue that no exception should be made because not all drugs provide a significant social benefit and, because consumers are especially vulnerable to undetectable risks in pharmaceutical and biological products, their makers should be held to at least the same standards as manufacturers of ordinary consumer goods (211).

Courts have upheld both positions, although the trend appears to be against holding drug and vaccine makers liable for design defects (156). Almost all courts base their reasoning on Comment k to Section 402A of the *Restatement (Second) of Torts* (American Law Institute, 1977):[59]

> *Unavoidably Unsafe Products.* There are some products which, in the present state of human knowledge, are quite incapable of being made safe for their intended and ordinary use. These are especially common in the field of drugs. An outstanding example is the vaccine for the Pasteur treatment of rabies, which not uncommonly leads to very serious and damaging consequences when it is injected. Since the disease itself invariably leads to a dreadful death, both the marketing and use of the vaccine are fully justified, notwithstanding the unavoidably high degree of risk which they involve. Such a product, properly prepared, and accompanied by proper direction and warning, is not defective, nor is it unreasonably dangerous. The same is true of many other drugs, vaccines, and the like, many of which for this very reason cannot be legally sold except to physicians, or under the prescription of a physician. It is also true of many new or experimental drugs as to which, because of lack of time and opportunity for sufficient medical experience, there can be no assurance of safety, or perhaps even the purity of ingredients, but such experience as there is justifies the marketing and use of the drug notwithstanding a medically recognizable risk. The seller of such products, again with a qualifica-

---

[56] In 1985, a California Court of Appeals found only one case (224) in which strict liability had been applied to a prescription drug (oral contraceptives in that case) (273). No case involving vaccines was identified. The facts in *Brochu* may have permitted the plaintiff to recover in negligence without resorting to strict liability.

[57] Plaintiffs often bring claims in strict liability for both defects in design and warning defects, as well as claims in negligence, to ensure that their claim is not dismissed for failure to correct cause of action.

[58] This type of warning includes the failure to provide directions for the proper use of a product whose operation is not apparent to a consumer, but such directions are not relevant to the use of vaccines.

[59] The American Law Institute (ALI) prepares treatises that summarize several fields of law. Its *Restatement (Second) of Torts* is widely considered by the legal profession to be the most authoritative statement of tort law in the country. Most states have adopted its provisions, albeit not uniformly, and some states have interpreted its technical requirements slightly differently. In 1993, the ALI began preparing a new (third) restatement of the law which will include an updated volume on products liability (5).

> tion that they are properly prepared and marketed, and proper warning is given, when the situation calls for it, is not to be held to strict liability for unfortunate consequences attending their use, merely because he has undertaken to supply the public with an apparently useful and desirable product, attended with a known but apparently reasonable risk.

Comment k describes an exception to strict liability in the case of products that are "unavoidably unsafe." It was reportedly drafted in response to an unsuccessful proposal that all prescription drugs be exempt from Section 402A. The proposal was defeated, but Dean Prosser included language indicating that at least some drugs and vaccines should be exempt from strict liability for harms that could not be avoided if the product were to serve its beneficial purpose (132).

Most courts have refused to grant a blanket exemption for all drugs or vaccines (224, 229, 242, 251, 258, 273, 282, 284, 296, 300, 301, 303, 312, 318, 319). Instead they would exempt only those drugs and vaccines that are unavoidably unsafe, on a case by case basis.

However, other courts have held that makers of FDA-approved prescription drugs are entirely exempt from strict liability for defective drug design, regardless of the drug in question, because of the public interest in drug availability (255, 270, 277).[60] The California Supreme Court did so in 1988 in a case involving diethylstil bestrol (DES), even though the court doubted that DES could not have been redesigned to reduce its risks or replaced with a safer drug (225).

The American Law Institute is preparing a revised version of its *Restatement of Torts*, which will include a volume on products liability that is expected to become available in 1995. The September 1994 draft of the chapter on liability for defective products includes provisions specifically delineating and limiting the liability of pharmaceutical and biologics manufacturers for personal injuries caused by their products (5). In particular, the draft abandons the use of the term strict liability and instead sets slightly different standards for "liability" in tort for harm caused by a product defect, depending on whether the defect is a manufacturing error, a design defect, or a warning defect. This characterization does not significantly alter existing law with respect to manufacturing errors and warning defects; it does describe a more stringent standard of proof for design defects, however. If these provisions are accepted by the Institute, they may further support the trend against holding manufacturers strictly liable for alleged design defects in prescription drugs and vaccines. Whether the states adopt all the Institute's revisions remains to be seen.

Where defective design is a permissible basis for liability under current law, the plaintiff must prove that the product is defective because its risks render it unreasonably dangerous. The product's benefit or utility is balanced against the risks it poses. This requires proving that, on the basis of scientific knowledge known or available at the time the product was marketed, the manufacturer knew or should have known that the risks could have been avoided or reduced without jeopardizing the product's effectiveness and losing its benefit.[61] Several courts have described the factors that should be considered in this calculus in differ-

---

[60] This does not necessarily preclude liability for claims of negligent design.

[61] A few courts have applied a "consumer expectations" test, which required the plaintiff to prove only that the product was more dangerous than would be contemplated by an ordinary consumer possessing knowledge common in the community. This test appears to have been applied little outside the area of ordinary consumer products like automobiles and has little, if any, application to product liability claims involving drugs or vaccines (225). The consumer expectation test was used in the first formulation of a modern strict liability standard in *Greenman* v. *Yuba Power Products, Inc.*, (253), and its predecessor, *Escola* v. *Coca Cola Bottling Co. of Fresno,* (239) (Traynor, J., concurring). Both cases involved ordinary consumer products (a power tool in *Greenman*, a Coca Cola bottle in *Escola*), not drugs or vaccines. The consumer expectations test is also suggested in Comment g (to Section 402A), which defines a "defective condition" as "a condition not contemplated by the ultimate consumer, which will be unreasonably dangerous to him." Comment j also notes that Section 402A liability applies "where the product is...in a condition not contemplated by the ultimate consumer."

ent terms, sometimes creating uncertainty as to the precise evidence needed to prove or disprove a claim.[62] Often, the plaintiff must show that a safer alternative design was feasible and would have achieved at least the same benefits. Nonetheless, in all its formulations, the risk-utility test embodies fundamentally the same concept.

The proposed revision of the Restatement of Torts, if adopted, would further narrow the grounds for liability for design defects in prescription drugs, including vaccines, and devices. It would provide that a drug is not reasonably safe due to defective design only if its foreseeable risks of harm are "sufficiently great in relation to its foreseeable therapeutic benefits so that no reasonable health care provider . . . would prescribe the drug . . . for any class of patients" (5). This would limit liability for design defects to drugs that do not provide any benefit to any group of patients. If a reasonable, informed health care provider would prescribe the drug to his or her patients, then the drug would not be deemed to have a design defect and no liability would attach. The effect of this restatement appears to be to reduce the grounds for liability for design defect. It may simply reflect the practical results in reported cases, however, since products whose benefits outweigh their risks are used by reasonable providers and are not found to have design defects.

Because a design defect case turns on a manufacturer's knowledge and conduct, most courts have found that the cause of action is effectively one of negligence (225). Manufacturers are held to the knowledge of an expert in the field of drug or vaccine production. They have a duty to keep up with advances in scientific knowledge and to conform to ethical drug industry standards in research, development, and marketing (242, 255).

In the 1980s, there was some concern that manufacturers could be held liable for failing to eliminate a product risk that was unknown or unknowable at the time the product was developed and marketed (146, 158). The 1982 New Jersey case that sparked such concerns, *Beshada* v. *Johns-Manville Products Corp.*, however, was largely overruled in 1984 (242).[63] The Supreme Court of California concluded that drug manufacturers are not liable for hazards not foreseeable at the time of sale (225).

As a practical matter, no drug or vaccine manufacturer has been found liable for selling a product with risks that were unknowable when marketed. A few cases have upheld jury or court decisions that Quadrigen (a vaccine combining DPT and polio vaccine marketed between 1959 and 1962) was defective because the preservative used or combination of vaccines created a known risk of harm and resulted in more adverse reactions than using the separate vaccines (284, 311).

The requirement that the risk be one that the manufacturer knew or should have known on the basis of scientific knowledge at the time the product was produced creates a defense to liability based on the state of the art or the state of science.[64] This is essentially a negligence defense because it relies on industry standards, not on subsequently detected product risks.

Design defect claims are claims that a different (safer and at least as effective) product should

[62] These variations can add complexity to litigation, primarily for national companies that defend cases in several states.

[63] *Beshada* v. *Johns-Manville Products Corp.*, (223) involved asbestos, and *Feldman* v. *Lederle Laboratories*, (242), a failure to warn case, limited imputing knowledge of product hazards to asbestos cases. Other courts have not made any exception for asbestos, but require a showing that all manufacturers knew or should have known of the hazard to impose liability for failure to warn of a product's dangers. (*Anderson* v. *Owens Corning Fiberglass Corp.*, (220)) But, in cases involving baby oil and asbestos, one court interpreted Washington's tort reform statute to permit liability for design defects and failure to warn of unforeseen risks. (*Ayers* v. *Johnson & Johnson Baby Products Co.*, (221); *Falk* v. *Keene Corp.*, (241)).

[64] Some courts consider it an affirmative defense, requiring the manufacturer to carry the burden of proving the unavoidable nature of the risks and the fact that the benefits outweighed the risks at the time of distribution. (*Castrignano* v. *E.R. Squibb & Sons, Inc.*, (229); *Schackil* v. *Lederele Laboratories*, (297); *Taggart* v. *Richards Medical Company, Inc.*, (309); *Toner* v. *Lederle Laboratories*, (312).

have replaced the product that was sold. Some drug manufacturers have argued that all claims of liability are preempted by Federal law because product specifications may not be altered without FDA approval. Ordinarily, FDA regulation of particular products or classes of products does not bar states from imposing additional requirements or providing state law remedies in tort (259).

The vast majority of courts have followed this principle with respect to vaccines (214, 242, 244, 251, 276, 280, 297, 300, 312, 319).[65]

The fact that the FDA has approved one vaccine design does not mean that other vaccine designs might not be safer or more effective. However, FDA approval has often provided persuasive evidence that an approved vaccine was not defective. The Federal National Childhood Vaccine Injury Act does preempt manufacturer liability for failure to directly warn consumers but does not foreclose other state tort actions (*Abbott* v. *American Cyanamid Co.,* 844 F.2d 1108 (4th Cir.), cert. denied, 488 U.S. 908 (1988)).[66]

In summary, although concerns about design defect litigation surfaced in the 1980s, there are no reported decisions after 1969 upholding liability for a defectively designed vaccine.[67] The majority of states permit a cause of action claiming defective design of a particular vaccine. Such claims are not generally preempted by federal law, and compliance with FDA requirements is not a legally conclusive defense. Nonetheless, plaintiffs have not been able to sustain a claim that a vaccine was defectively designed.

Liability for Errors and Omissions in Warnings

In view of the impossibility of creating a risk-free vaccine, tort law imposes an obligation on the manufacturer to warn of inherent risk. The history of vaccine warning defects litigation parallels the history of litigation involving informed consent to medical care. The two differ, however, in *whom* must be warned: a vaccine manufacturer ordinarily has a duty only to warn the physician prescribing its vaccine, not the person taking the vaccine; a physician has a duty to inform the patient of any vaccine risks.

In the 1960s, the majority of medical consent cases involved a failure to warn a patient of the risk of undergoing a specific medical procedure (53). Physicians failed to mention even the inherent possibility of death or paralysis, often because they believed that the patients would refuse the therapy if advised of the risk (91).

Courts uniformly found that the patients' right of self-determination entitled them to accept or refuse any treatment, even if their choices were foolish, as long as they were competent to make medical decisions (226, 231, 281, 293). In order to exercise that right, patients needed information that only physicians could provide, so the law imposed a duty of disclosure upon physicians that required them to tell patients not only the benefits of alternative treatments but also their material risks. Similarly, the first vaccine cases involved the absence of warnings of the risk of contracting poliomyelitis from the oral polio vaccine (235, 290).

---

65 The proposed revision of the *Restatement* also continues this rule (5). But see Hurley v. Lederle Laboratories, (264), finding that the Food, Drug and Cosmetic Act and the Public Health Service Act preempted state claims as to the FDA's determination of the proper wording of a warning, provided that the manufacturer has not withheld any relevant information from the FDA.

66 The Medical Devices Act (21 U.S.C. 360g et seq.) expressly preempts state laws affecting most medical devices. Two federal courts have found the statute's language precludes strict liability actions under state tort law for medical devices that require premarket FDA approval (274); *Stamps* v. *Collagen Corp.,* (306) Other courts have reached different results depending upon the device's classification and requirements for premarket approval (58, 275, 278, 279, 304).

67 Design defect causes of action have been used primarily against commercial products, such as asbestos, consumer products, and medical devices, such as the Dalkon Shield, the Copper-7 IUD, the Bjork-Shiley heart valve, and silicon-gel breast implants (61).

A failure to warn can be prevented by providing a warning. But, as the next generation of informed consent cases showed, some warnings failed to mention material risks. Similarly, more recent vaccine cases have turned on the adequacy of the warning given. However, like informed consent cases, the majority of reported cases have been decided in favor of the defendant manufacturer or physician (238, 270, 289, 299).[68] This is primarily because vaccine makers have been exempted from the general duty of manufacturers to provide warnings directly to consumers.[69]

The exception, known as "the learned intermediary rule," holds that a manufacturer of prescription drugs or vaccines need only warn the prescribing physician, not the patient who receives the product (248, 255, 269, 310, 313). Courts have generally limited the manufacturer's duty to warn consumers directly to those circumstances in which a vaccine is given *without* the intervention of a "learned intermediary," generally a physician who makes a medical judgment that the vaccine is appropriate for an individual patient (63, 144).[70]

Thus, a vaccine manufacturer's duty to warn consumers directly applies only in mass immunization or routine public health programs where physicians are not making "individualized medical judgments" (235, 264, 286, 290). It has been applied to two vaccinations given in a private physician's office, where the physician testified that he acted like a public clinic employee, dispensing vaccine without evaluating individual recipients (249, 294). Two of these cases appear to have given rise to the fear in the 1970's and 1980's that manufacturers would have to warn all vaccine recipients directly (235, 290). Recent cases, however, have reiterated that a vaccine manufacturer's duty to warn is limited to the prescribing or dispensing physician alone because patients cannot obtain vaccines except from a physician or medical clinic (258, 285, 288, 292, 301, 307, 322).

To succeed on a claim of inadequate warning, the plaintiff must prove that an adequate warning to the physician would have prevented the injury. This entails proving that the warning would have persuaded the physician not to give the vaccine to the patient, as well as proving that the injury would not have occurred if the vaccine had not been given (246, 307, 310, 321).

Physicians and other providers do have an independent obligation to warn patients of vaccine risks as part of their duty to obtain informed consent to any vaccination, regardless of the manufacturer's action. Aside from patients with immunosuppression or allergies, however, it is often impossible to predict whether an individual patient is at risk of experiencing an adverse reaction to a vaccine, at least the first time it is given. Therefore, it is questionable whether an individualized medical evaluation would affect a physician's recommendation about vaccination in most cases, and several cases have been decided against plaintiffs on the ground that the warning did not or would not alter the physician's decision.

The National Childhood Vaccine Injury Act barred any cause of action for a manufacturer's failure to directly warn a recipient (or a recipient's parent or guardian) about the risks of any childhood vaccine covered by the compensation program. It also created a rebuttable presumption that warnings approved by FDA are adequate (42 U.S.C. 300aa-22(b), (c)). At the same time, the act required the Secretary of Health and Human Services to develop new written materials to provide

[68] Although the academic literature contains numerous articles debating the merits of the doctrine of informed consent to medical care, the number of cases actually claiming lack of informed consent remains very small and few such claims succeed.

[69] Section 402A of the *Restatement* imposes liability for inadequate warnings by sellers even if they do not sell directly to consumers. The duty was imposed on the manufacturer because it, not the retail seller, controlled the condition of the product, assuming it had not been altered after it left the manufacturer's hands. The proposed revision of the *Restatement* retains this general rule and the exception for prescription drugs. (5)

[70] A few cases have found that a nurse acted as a learned intermediary (*Rohrburgh* v. *Wyeth Laboratories, Inc.*, (292); *Walker* v. *Merck & Co.*,(317) (*Mazur* v. *Merck &Co., Inc.*, (276)). but others disagree on the grounds that nurses do not ordinarily make medical judgments.

parents with information about the benefits and risks of each childhood vaccine. Earlier, the CDC, which buys about half the domestic supply of pediatric vaccines, had prepared "Important Information Sheets" to serve as warnings, and the CDC played a primary role in drafting the materials required by the act.

Before the act took effect, most childhood vaccine manufacturers had required the CDC to assume responsibility for providing such warnings or alternatively to have a learned intermediary dispense the vaccine as a contractual condition of the sale of vaccines. One federal court of appeals recently held that a vaccine maker fulfilled its duty to warn by such a contract with the CDC, regardless of whether or not the warning actually reached the recipient (276). More recently, the Supreme Court of Nevada reached the opposite conclusion where the vaccine was distributed by a county health district with information sheets prepared by the CDC (219). The court found that the manufacturer cannot be relieved of ultimate responsibility for an inadequate warning where it knew that the contractor used warnings that omitted risk information the manufacturer had provided with the vaccine.

Liability based on inadequate warnings has been criticized on the ground that it is too difficult to describe vaccine risks in terms that patients can understand.[71] The legal doctrine does not require that patients understand the information included in the warning, although it is obviously better if they do. Instead, most courts require only that the risks be disclosed in ordinary language that is understandable by a reasonable lay person (226, 231). Because the learned intermediary rule applies in most vaccine cases, however, warnings are directed not to patients, but to physicians, who are presumed competent to understand technical information and its implications.

A few cases have found specific warnings inadequate because they failed to apprise physicians of the vaccine's known risks (240, 311). In most cases, warnings have been found adequate in that they disclosed all reasonably known risks (238, 270, 273, 288, 299). As with all cases alleging design defects, the state of scientific knowledge determines whether a risk should be disclosed (225, 242, 243, 255), and FDA approval of labeling information is often persuasive evidence of the adequacy of a warning (242, 296).

Most lawsuits claiming injury from vaccines allege several bases for liability, including defective design, inadequate warning, and negligence in manufacture, design, or risk disclosure. Because, except for manufacturing defects, strict liability requires proof similar to that required to prove liability for negligence, the specific cause of action may be less important than the possibility of any liability.[72] This means that where a vaccine maker is exempted from liability on one basis (such as design defects), it may be subject to claims of liability on other grounds. Specifically, the number of claims against vaccine makers may not be effectively reduced unless manufacturers are exempted not only from strict liability but also from liability for negligence.[73]

Practical Problems with Litigation

Even if the principles of product liability law are sensible in theory, there can be practical problems with product liability litigation. The lengthy and cumbersome process of discovery, trial, and sometimes appeal is a perennial subject of legiti-

[71] Similar concerns about the difficulty of describing risks have arisen with respect to informed consent to other medical procedures and informed consent to experimentation with human subjects. Sometimes such concerns mask a reluctance to disclose the risk at all or professionals' discomfort with revealing uncertainty about risks (91). Recently, radiation experiments conducted in the 1950s have been denounced primarily because the human subjects of the experiments (including residents at schools for the mentally retarded and terminally ill patients) were not necessarily told that they were to be part of an experiment or any risks that it might entail (11, 75).

[72] The cases finding a defective vaccine were based on an implied warranty of merchantability (284, 311).

[73] For further discussions about HIV vaccines and product liability see Rosenfeld, 1991 (149); Smith, 1992 (168); Arnold, 1991 (13).

mate complaint. This is true whether the basis for suit is strict liability or negligence. Determining whether a particular injury to an individual was caused by a particular vaccine and whether the risk could have been avoided is a complex, time-consuming, and expensive process for both sides of a dispute. Even if it is decided that the plaintiff should be compensated, determining the amount of damages has become a similarly complex matter. Although alternative dispute resolution procedures can be somewhat cheaper and faster than courtroom litigation, they do not eliminate the need to prepare a case. Thus, the very process of dispute resolution can discourage both the pursuit and defense of claims, as well as the thoughtful application of the law.

Studies of tort claims indicate that ten percent or less of claims are tried in court (46, 69, 73). The rest are withdrawn or settled before trial, with roughly half resulting in some payment to the plaintiff, although in lower amounts than average trial awards. This means that defendants have to deal with many more claims than wind up in court. There is no publicly available data showing whether similar figures apply to cases involving vaccines. If court awards influence settlements, as they are believed to do, then the low proportion of court decisions favoring plaintiffs may suggest that a lower-than-average proportion of claims are settled with payment to a plaintiff in vaccine cases.[74]

It may not be the number of claims, but the possibility of an expensive mistake that worries vaccine makers. One kind of mistake is when a jury makes an error of fact, reaching a verdict that is not supported by credible evidence. In principle, such a mistake can be remedied on appeal, although additional time and expense can turn even successful appeals into pyrrhic victories. Some factual mistakes are inevitable in any dispute resolution system, whether or not it employs litigation. Variations in each party's ability to produce credible evidence and present its case mean that some cases that ought to be won are lost and others that ought to be lost are won. Ideally, dispute resolution methods should be designed to minimize both types of errors but the ideal is not likely to be achievable without substantial additional expense.

A second type of problem is more difficult to avoid. These are mistakes arising out of the uncertainty of scientific knowledge that must be used to identify and categorize the possible risks and benefits of drugs and vaccines. If the essence of a defective design is the availability of knowledge indicating an unreasonable danger, at least in light of expected benefits, then information indicating that a drug might produce an adverse reaction is potential evidence of a design defect or a risk that should have been disclosed. It is, however, only *potential* evidence because it is a matter of knowledgeable interpretation whether and how the risk might materialize, and whether the possibility is sufficiently credible to warrant further investigation. A manufacturer might reasonably determine that the problem was a "fluke." But in a later lawsuit, the plaintiff might conclude that the manufacturer ignored an important potential risk. In some cases, it is impossible to know whether a drug or vaccine caused a particular injury in an individual or even whether it was capable of causing such an injury. In those cases, there may be no way to know whether a mistake was made, whatever the outcome might be.

If the law is not properly applied, then the process, not the law, stands indicted. But if the law cannot be properly applied at all in some circumstances, then it cannot serve its purpose. Unfortunately, there is no good information to determine what proportion of cases have been decided correctly or incorrectly, or what proportion cannot be decided correctly for lack of scientific

---

[74] Most reported court opinions that make final decisions in a case have dismissed a plaintiff's complaint or granted judgment for the defendant manufacturer (225, 255, 270, 271, 285, 288). However, few reported decisions contain final dispositions of a case. Most determine whether a plaintiff is entitled to go to trial. The outcome of any such trial or settlement in lieu of trial remains unreported.

knowledge (60, 153). Thus, we do not know whether litigation is producing good or bad decisions.

These types of uncertainties can give rise to fears of unwarranted liability on the part of vaccine makers. They can be compounded by fears of high damage awards, including punitive damages. Most punitive damages awards are in cases of intentional torts (like assault), unfair business practices, or fraud or bad faith in contracts.[75] Because liability for personal injury is rarely based on intentional or fraudulent conduct, but on negligence or strict liability, there should be little occasion for punitive damages.

The few studies that have been done have concluded that punitive damages are rarely awarded in personal injury actions and, where inappropriately awarded, are ordinarily reduced or reversed on appeal (45, 135, 185). The only known punitive damage award in a vaccine case was reversed on appeal and the vaccine maker found immune from liability (270). Punitive damages do not appear to be a significant factor in product liability (104).[76] In product liability cases, they are more likely to be awarded in cases involving defective automobiles or other consumer products than drugs or vaccines. Uncertainty surrounding inappropriate damage awards applies to almost all types of litigation.[77] Whether litigation itself is a necessary form of dispute resolution depends upon the feasibility of alternatives.

POTENTIAL LIABILITY FOR ADVERSE REACTIONS TO HIV VACCINES

Vaccines are ordinarily subject to liability for negligence, manufacturing defects, defects in design, and inadequate warnings of risks. However, liability is rarely found in specific cases. Why, then, is the perception of excessive liability for adverse reactions to vaccines so prevalent?

Vaccine Susceptibility to Liability Claims

Fear of liability may arise from several factors that distinguish vaccines from pharmaceuticals and other biologics and that may encourage people to pursue tort claims. Prophylactic vaccines are taken by healthy people to prevent disease. This means that adverse reactions are more noticeable and may be perceived as less tolerable than adverse reactions to a drug that a person takes to relieve the symptoms of illness. Vaccines may also be taken by sufficiently large numbers of people to permit the occurrence of a rare side effect that might not materialize in a smaller group.[78] When a healthy person who takes a vaccine suffers an illness or injury, there may be a natural desire to find a cause beyond random accident or one's own behavior. These factors are likely to encourage attributing the injury to the vaccine, correctly or incorrectly, especially when there has been no other change in the person's circumstances.

---

[75] The U.S. Supreme Court upheld a state punitive damage law as against a challenge that it was an unconstitutional violation of due process in *Pacific Mutual Life Insurance Company* v. *Haslip* (283). In their brief amicus curiae, the Pharmaceutical Manufacturers Association and the American Medical Association cited two instances in which punitive damages had been awarded with respect to drugs (an oral contraceptive and Coumadin) (136).

[76] Plaintiffs may include *claims* for punitive damages in their complaints, but they are rarely awarded. Similarly, the amount a plaintiff may claim for compensatory damages often bears little relationship to the amount, if any, actually awarded or collected. There is some evidence that, in cases in which compensatory damages are awarded, the amount of damages correlates with the severity of the injury (46).

[77] Physicians and scientists may empathize with vaccine makers' fear of liability in light of the widespread fear of medical malpractice litigation among medical practitioners. In both instances, the actual risk of being sued (and of losing a lawsuit) appears to be significantly lower than is believed by those who might be the target of a lawsuit (25, 109, 182).

[78] Of course, some drugs (like Valium and aspirin) are taken by millions of people.

When adverse reactions are suffered by children, the financial consequences can be severe. In cases of serious permanent injury, inability to work and the need for expensive rehabilitative or custodial care over a lifetime generate substantial costs that may not be covered by private or public insurance. A lawsuit for substantial damages may be the only source of payment for needed services. This may account for relatively more concern about potential liability for adverse reactions to vaccines administered to children than for those given to adults. Of course, the potential for large damages also exists with most drugs used by children and pregnant women.[79]

Latent hazards that may not have been detectable before marketing may materialize ten or twenty years after a vaccine (or drug) is used. There is a greater chance of discovering such hazards when vaccines are used in children and young adults with longer subsequent life spans than those expected for older adults.

Thus, even if tort principles make it difficult for a plaintiff to win a lawsuit, there may be more claims brought with respect to vaccines than with respect to ordinary drugs.

Potential Adverse Reactions to HIV Vaccines

The risks of HIV vaccines most commonly mentioned are: 1) low levels of effectiveness (so that not every vaccine recipient is protected); 2) enhanced susceptibility to HIV infection (increased risk of acquiring infection upon exposure); 3) more rapid than normal (enhanced) progression of disease if HIV infection is acquired; 4) the development of cancer many years after vaccination; and 5) direct vaccine-induced HIV infection from inadequately attenuated or inactivated virus in vaccines made from killed or attenuated HIV. In addition, HIV vaccination may result in social harms.

Low Levels of Effectiveness

There has been speculation among researchers that some candidate HIV vaccines now in clinical trials may ultimately prove effective in less than half of the vaccinated population.[80] If the vaccinated population is at risk for HIV infection, as anticipated, then some proportion may become infected after taking a vaccine of limited efficacy, even if the vaccine is not defective. Claims based on low levels (or lack) of effectiveness have not been brought against existing vaccines. The likelihood of success of a claim of lack of effectiveness of an HIV vaccine is speculative, but probably small as long as those who take the vaccine are warned of its limited efficacy and advised to take precautions against exposure to HIV infection.

A claim based on defective design would have to demonstrate either that a more effective vaccine was feasible or that the level of efficacy was so low that the vaccine should not have been marketed at all.[81] Given the difficulties of finding a vaccine that works at all, and the need for a vaccine to prevent any additional HIV infection, neither requirement would be easy to meet. The more likely basis for a claim would be inadequate warning of the vaccine's limited effectiveness and the need for the recipient to take appropriate precautions. Ordinarily, a plaintiff would have to prove that any warning to the physician was inadequate and that an adequate warning would have caused the phy-

[79] This has fueled fears of large claims for contraceptive products and drugs used by pregnant women (31). The number of successful claims, however, appears to be smaller than the perception (44).

[80] For a discussion of effectiveness of current vaccines in development, see chapter 2.

[81] The latter theory raised the possibility of a claim against the FDA for approving a vaccine in violation of its own standards of safety and effectiveness, although it would be difficult to prove that the level of effectiveness was too low in light of the need for a preventive vaccine. The United States Supreme Court has found that, under the Federal Tort Claims Act, the FDA may be subject to suit if it fails to follow its own governing statute and regulations, unless it is performing a discretionary function (222, 266). In the absence of any statutory or regulatory requirement for any minimum level of effectiveness, the balancing of risks and benefits in the approval of a new HIV vaccine is likely to be treated as a discretionary function which is exempt from challenge.

sician either not to recommend the vaccine or to warn the plaintiff more strongly against risk behaviors (119). If physicians are properly warned of a vaccine's limited effectiveness, the plaintiff would have no cause of action against the manufacturer. Rather, any claim would be against the physician for lack of informed consent.

In addition, a plaintiff would have to prove that he or she failed to take appropriate precautions against infection *solely* because of the inadequate warning. If the infection were acquired through sexual contact, the plaintiff would have to prove that he or she would have abstained from sex or used barrier protection in most, if not all, relationships. If the transmission occurred through intravenous (IV) drug use, it may be especially hard to prove that the plaintiff would have abstained or used precautions, like sterile needles.[82] Alternatively, a plaintiff would have to prove that he or she would not have taken the vaccine had an adequate warning been given, and that *not* taking the vaccine would have prevented infection. Both alternatives would entail proving the somewhat implausible: continuous use of precautions against infection or complete avoidance of exposure to HIV infection.

Enhanced Susceptibility to Infection or Disease Progression

Some researchers have theorized that candidate vaccines might have the potential to increase one's susceptibility to infection with HIV or other organisms (24). Others have speculated that a vaccine might increase the rate of disease progression in people who become infected with HIV in spite of vaccination.[83] Both hypotheses raise the possibility of a claim for defective design if they are not investigated, or a claim for inadequate warning if they are not disclosed. Such a claim would face the same difficulties as a vaccine with low levels of effectiveness, discussed above. In addition, a plaintiff would have to prove that the manufacturer knew or should have known that the vaccine was capable of causing the reaction. The strongest case against a manufacturer would be one in which the vaccine was demonstrated to cause the susceptibility in controlled clinical trials. This suggests that such hypotheses should be studied, at least to attempt to determine whether they are realistic concerns or merely theoretical.[84] Potential liability may provide an incentive to vaccine makers to invest in additional vaccine research, which may both clarify the vaccine's safety profile and increase the eventual cost of development. In this respect, however, HIV vaccines do not differ from other vaccines or drugs.

Development of Cancer

There has been speculation that, because HIV is a retrovirus, an HIV vaccine might cause cancer many years after vaccination.[85] The likelihood of a claim for vaccine-induced cancer is also similar to the claims for other potential adverse reactions. It differs primarily in the length of time it may take for the reaction to be discovered. This means that, in the absence of feasible studies that could predict the risk, if any, of cancer, neither manufacturers nor vaccine recipients would know whether the vaccine posed any such risk for perhaps two decades. Although a manufacturer is not liable for injuries caused by unforeseeable dangers in its products, there may be some question as to whether a manufacturer adequately investigated a suggested risk. Given the need for an HIV vaccine, however, it seems unlikely that a manufacturer would be held responsible for distributing a vaccine with a risk that could not be verified at the time it was released.

[82] As a practical matter, juries may have little sympathy for habitual drug users.

[83] For a discussion of vaccine-induced enhancement of disease susceptibility, see chapter 2.

[84] Since some subjects who received investigational preventive vaccines have become infected, there is renewed attention to examining whether the vaccine simply failed to prevent HIV infection or might have enhanced the risk of infection upon exposure.

[85] The potential of an HIV vaccine to cause cancer is discussed in chapter 2.

Vaccine-Induced HIV Infection

Non-recombinant vaccines that use killed, inactivated, or attenuated virus have been reported to hold some promise (124). Concern about such vaccines arises from the possibility, albeit remote, that the manufacturing process might inadvertently fail to remove or render harmless part of the virus that could actively infect a person, or that an attenuated virus could revert to an infectious state.[86] Reports of newborn monkeys that became ill after inoculation with a live attenuated virus vaccine to prevent SIV may increase such concerns. A person who became infected with HIV from such a vaccine would have a claim against the manufacturer for injury caused by a manufacturing error.

It is unlikely that a claim for design defect would be possible, except in the unlikely event that the manufacturer knew or should have known that its manufacturing process could not render the virus incapable of infection. Although claims of vaccine manufacturing errors have been rare in the past, the consequences of a batch of vaccine accidentally escaping inactivation are sufficiently serious to make this type of vaccine unappealing to many vaccine makers. Thus, potential liability for manufacturing errors may discourage companies from developing this type of vaccine, and provide relatively greater incentive to pursue recombinant vaccines. At the same time, companies may not wish to pursue a type of vaccine that might produce HIV infection, regardless of exposure to liability, especially if they believe that they cannot eliminate the risk of manufacturing error.

Social Harms

HIV vaccines may pose risks of social harm that are not ordinarily linked with other vaccines or drugs. People who receive HIV vaccines will test positive on screening tests, making them especially vulnerable to denials of health or life insurance,[87] permission to travel abroad,[88] loss of employment or housing,[89] segregation in institutions, or rejection by family and friends (2) (98, 114).[90] People institutionalized in prisons or mental health facilities may be segregated or victimized. Other forms of discrimination and stigmatization are also possible. The possibilities remain largely unexamined.

An HIV vaccine may produce an antibody reaction that may be difficult to distinguish from a positive test for HIV infection, so that vaccine recipients may be mistakenly believed to be HIV positive. But vaccine recipients (and subjects in vaccine clinical trials) may be targeted for discrimination on the assumption that they are members of a risk group, regardless of whether they are shown to have HIV infection. Moreover, most such harms result from lawful conduct for which the vaccine recipient would have no legal recourse. Although job loss might violate the Americans with Disabilities Act (42 U.S.C. 12101 et seq.), most other forms of discrimination would not, and no law prevents family members, lovers, and friends from abandoning someone stigmatized as at risk for HIV infection.

Although such risks should be made clear to anyone who takes a vaccine, there is no precedent

---

[86] The potential for whole killed virus or attenuated virus vaccines to cause infection is discussed in chapter 2.

[87] Many health, life, and disability carriers now require an HIV test for individual coverage or extended coverage (173).

[88] The Department of State lists 45 countries that have restrictions on entry of HIV-infected individuals to their countries and require HIV tests of all or some people entering their countries (202).

[89] The U.S. armed forces, the Department of State, Job Corps and some other employers either require or urge employees to have HIV tests as a conditions of employment.

[90] These social harms are discussed in further detail in chapter 3.

for holding a vaccine maker liable for their occurrence, and it is unlikely that a claim would be successful on such grounds. Manufacturers are not responsible for the bigotry of others. Product liability is intended to impose responsibility for physical injury caused by defective products, not personal insults resulting from discriminatory actions. There does not appear to be any basis for counting social harm as either a manufacturing defect or a design defect.

It might be possible to claim that an adequate warning *should* include the risk of social harms.[91] A successful cause of action would require the plaintiff to prove that he or she would not have been identified as at risk for HIV infection but for the vaccination. But, ordinarily it would be the act of vaccination, not the vaccine itself, that confers any stigma. Moreover, it is unlikely that a vaccine maker would be responsible for specifying social risks, since such risks are not necessarily within the realm of expertise of vaccine manufacturing. Physicians who administer HIV vaccines may be the more likely target for any claims that a vaccine recipient was not adequately warned about possible discrimination.

Different Uses of Vaccines

The same principles of liability apply to manufacturers of all vaccines, regardless of whether they are preventive (intended to prevent) or therapeutic (intended to treat or cure infection or disease), and regardless of whether the vaccines are experimental (investigational) or approved and licensed. The likelihood of adverse reactions and liability claims occurring may differ, however, depending upon the way in which a vaccine is used.

Preventive HIV Vaccines

Preventive HIV vaccines have most of the factors that make vaccines more susceptible to liability claims than drugs. They are intended for use by healthy individuals who may be sensitive to the appearance of adverse reactions. At the same time, HIV vaccines are likely to be given to people at risk for HIV infection for the foreseeable future. Several risk groups are also at risk for other diseases, such as Hepatitis B and other blood-borne and sexually transmitted diseases. It may be difficult to distinguish some symptoms or illnesses from other causes from adverse reactions to vaccination, at least until sufficient years of experience with the vaccine have produced reliable data identifying vaccine-related risks.

Uncertainty about the cause of illnesses following vaccination may encourage vaccinees to attribute injuries to the vaccine and seek legal redress against manufacturers. On the other hand, the difficulty of demonstrating that the vaccine caused the injury is likely to discourage or defeat product liability claims. In other words, the very uncertainty that may increase the likelihood of lawsuits also decreases the probability of plaintiffs' success on the claims.

The characteristics of the populations that use an HIV vaccine may influence the potential for liability. Most people at risk of HIV infection are young adults with a relatively long life expectancy. Potential damages for permanent injury arising from vaccination could be substantial, although less than those for young children. A growing proportion of people at risk, however, are IV drug users, many of whom are not working and may not be able to claim lost income as damages. However, if the majority of people who actually take an HIV vaccine are middle-class workers, then permanent injury that deprives them of the ability to work will give rise to potential damages for lost income, as well as medical expenses. If HIV vaccines are given to newborns and young children, the potential damages increase proportionately with life expectancy. Pregnant women who are HIV-positive and take a vaccine to prevent transmission to their children can expect very limited damages because of their preexisting condition and shorter life expectancy.

---

[91] Ethical principles would certainly require such warning in careful counseling sessions, but ethical principles go beyond legal duties. For a discussion of ethical duties to warn about adverse reactions to HIV vaccines, see chapter 3.

The number of vaccinations may also affect potential liability. If an HIV vaccine's effectiveness is limited over time and requires several doses and booster vaccinations, there are more opportunities per vaccinee for adverse reactions and for injuries following vaccination to be attributed to the vaccine. The costs involved may be balanced to some degree by the increased sales generated by a multiple dose vaccine.

In summary, the potential for liability arising from the use of an approved HIV vaccine appears to be similar to what might be expected from any new vaccine intended for use by adults. Although the possible damages from a successful lawsuit may be large in the case of a permanently disabled young adult or child, the probability of a successful lawsuit appears to be quite low. Although an HIV vaccine might carry unknown latent risks that portend a DES-like future, that possibility probably exists for every new drug and vaccine marketed. HIV vaccines are not unique in this respect. Currently, the most likely basis for liability claims is an inadequate warning of low levels of effectiveness or limited protection against HIV infection. Yet it would be very difficult for anyone who became HIV positive to prove that his or her infection was caused by either the vaccine or an inadequate warning of the vaccine's limited protection. Physicians are likely to be more vulnerable to such claims than vaccine makers.

Investigational HIV Vaccines

The potential for liability for adverse reactions to investigational preventive HIV vaccines is less than that for marketed vaccines. The legal grounds for liability are the same for both investigational and approved vaccines. But the nature of investigational vaccines and clinical trials reduces both the likelihood of claims and the probability of successful claims in practice.

It is generally understood that the purpose of clinical trials is to determine how safe and effective an experimental vaccine may be and whether unpredictable adverse reactions may occur. There are more protections for subjects in clinical trials than for patients in ordinary medical care settings. Federal regulations governing both federally funded research with human subjects and research intended for submission to the FDA require that subjects' informed consent be in writing in a document approved by an institutional review board (21 U.S.C. Parts 50 and 56). Regardless of the merits of the document itself, prospective subjects are likely to be made aware that they will be part of a research experiment and that the vaccine has not been approved by the FDA. The subject's consent has the legal effect of making the subject assume responsibility for any disclosed risks that materialize. Since most informed consent documents note that not all risks can be predicted and unknown adverse reactions might occur, there is little basis for a claim that the subject was not properly warned.

Historically, there have been no cases of product liability claims involving research, probably because there has been a very low incidence of observed or reported injury among research subjects (27, 118, 200).[92] Rare adverse reactions may not materialize in a small cohort of research subjects and side effects may be reversed or minimized promptly where the subjects are being monitored by research investigators. Design defect claims are also minimized, if not precluded entirely, by the fact that the trial is being conducted to find out whether the vaccine works and whether it has dangerous side effects. Not until such trials are concluded and a risk is discovered or confirmed is there any significant basis for claiming that the vaccine was defectively designed.

It is possible that a vaccine might be too dangerous to test in human subjects at all. But this could only be inferred from prior laboratory research which should be reviewed by the FDA and an institutional review board. Those bodies serve

[92] There have been several cases in which people were not told they were being used as human subjects in a research study or that the research could produce serious harm (9, 188, 265, 183).

as a safeguard against proceeding with unjustifiable research and, although imperfect, they ordinarily should prevent unreasonably dangerous research from going forward.

The most likely risk of a preventive vaccine trial is that a research subject may believe that the vaccine is effective to prevent HIV infection, fail to take precautions, and become infected. (In a blinded, randomized trial, the subjects are not told whether they have received the investigational vaccine or a placebo, although they can find out by getting tested, even if they are asked not to do so.) As with marketed vaccines, the subject might claim that he or she was not adequately cautioned against risk behaviors, but would probably find that especially difficult to prove in a research setting. The written informed consent document would provide evidence that the information was given. Such documents have proved sufficient to defeat claims of lack of informed consent by patients in medical settings (320). The best solution to such a problem is to prevent it, by making clear the uncertainty about the candidate vaccine before a subject agrees to participate in the trial.

Another potential, but probably remote, risk is that use of an early candidate vaccine would preclude a subject from participating in a later investigational study of a newer vaccine, perhaps one that proved to be more effective. Again, the most likely basis for a claim would be lack of informed consent, with results similar to those described above. It may be more difficult to explain the nature of this type of risk unless there is some laboratory basis for predicting the effectiveness of vaccines that have not yet been fully developed.

Finally, subjects who experience some of the social risks of participating in a vaccine trial may claim lack of informed consent to such risks. Merely volunteering for a vaccine trial can expose the subject to discrimination. Research subjects may be more vulnerable to social harms than the recipient of a marketed vaccine, because participation in a vaccine trial may be discovered more easily than receipt of a vaccine from a private physician or public clinic. As with physiologic reactions, the precise social risks that may befall a vaccine recipient may not be predictable in advance. Indeed, vaccine trials may gather as much information about such risks as they do about vaccine safety and effectiveness. Thus, the risk of liability again depends upon the clarity with which the risk of social harm is presented, and the responsibility for warning prospective research subjects would lie with the investigators rather than the vaccine manufacturers.

Therapeutic HIV Vaccines

Therapeutic HIV vaccines that are used to treat people already infected with HIV are comparable to drugs. The special concerns surrounding the use of preventive vaccines do not apply. Patients and research subjects who take therapeutic vaccines may be willing to accept accompanying risks in order to receive any benefit the therapeutic vaccine might afford, as they have with drugs like Zidovudine, ddI, ddC, and d4T. Adverse reactions to the vaccine may be especially difficult to distinguish from other symptoms related to HIV infection and opportunistic infections and illnesses. Moreover, the potential for damages is quite limited because of the perceived limited life expectancy of people with AIDS. Perhaps this is why there have been no reports of fear of liability for adverse reactions to therapeutic vaccines. Even companies that reported fear of liability for their preventive vaccines actively pursued clinical trials of their therapeutic candidate vaccines without mentioning liability as a concern.

Conclusion

Preventive vaccines may be more susceptible to claims of liability than most drugs and biologics, primarily because they are ordinarily used in large numbers of healthy people. Their extensive use can permit even rare adverse reactions to materialize and people who expected vaccines to prevent disease may be less tolerant of such reactions than sick patients. As with drugs, the majority of claims have been directed against only a few vaccines. Despite the increased probability of claims, the proportion of reported cases that impose liability on the vaccine maker is very small. There is no publicly available evidence on the number or result of claims that were withdrawn or settled before a court decision. Thus, although the probability of *claims* of liability may be relatively high, the probability of actual *liability* is relatively low.

The main causes of action against a vaccine maker are claims of a defectively designed vaccine and an inadequate warning of vaccine risks. Plaintiffs have not succeeded on a claim of defective design, probably because of the improbability of demonstrating that a safer, equally effective vaccine could have replaced a vaccine approved by the FDA.[93] Few courts have found a vaccine maker liable for an inadequate warning of risks. More extensive and sophisticated warning statements may have improved vaccine makers' protection against such claims. In addition, a vaccine maker's duty to warn is ordinarily limited to the prescribing physician, who bears responsibility for disclosing vaccine risks to patients. Thus, physicians may now be more vulnerable to claims (of lack of informed consent) than vaccine makers.

The probability of future claims of adverse reactions to an HIV vaccine is impossible to predict because it depends upon what, if any, adverse reactions occur and whether they could be plausibly attributed to the vaccine. The probability of courts imposing liability in the case of an HIV vaccine appears to be about the same or lower than in the case of existing vaccines. This is primarily because of the difficulty of demonstrating that an adverse reaction was caused by the vaccine. Also important is the possibility that the most predictable risk of vaccination is discrimination against the person vaccinated for which manufacturers are not likely to be responsible.

Fear of liability for adverse reactions to vaccines may have been based on a perception in the 1970s and early 1980s that courts were expanding the grounds for liability. That expansion appears to have halted and, although there is no guarantee that it could not recur, there is no reason to assume that it will.[94] More important, it is difficult to argue that the principles of product liability are unfair in theory. Rather, the major concern lies with the time, expense and uncertainty of the litigation process and the fear that the law will not be applied correctly, so that a vaccine maker is mistakenly held liable where it should not be.

Since liability itself is so rarely imposed, fear of liability may be more accurately described as fear of having to litigate at all. This is understandable, but not limited to cases involving HIV vaccines. Therefore, there appears to be little, if any, basis for claiming that HIV vaccines present a special or increased risk of liability. This does not mean that an alternative means of allocating responsibility for injury and compensation is not warranted for other reasons. It does mean that any alternative that is intended to remedy tort litigation's inefficiencies would have application beyond HIV vaccines.

ALTERNATIVE COMPENSATION POLICY OPTIONS

People who are injured as a result of vaccination with an HIV vaccine could receive compensation in a variety of ways. Currently, their only option, apart from private health and disability insurance, is likely to be a product liability claim against the vaccine maker, or a claim of professional negligence (medical malpractice) against the physician or other health care provider who vaccinated the individual, if the circumstances support a legal cause of action[95]

This section summarizes several major policy options for compensating HIV vaccine-related injury—reforms in tort liability, voluntary contrac-

[93] The only reported decisions (in 1969) finding a vaccine (Quadrigen) defective were based on warranty, not tort law (284, 311). Whether any vaccine maker has settled any claims with payment to the plaintiff on this basis is unknown.

[94] If the revised version of the *Restatement of Torts* volume on product liability is accepted, the grounds for liability for design defects will be narrower than current legal principles in states that permit the cause of the action at all (5).

[95] Some recourse may be available with respect to California vaccines under a California statute, described below.

tual arrangements, government-financed insurance systems, and public no-fault compensation programs—and their advantages and disadvantages.[96] It also considers several alternative approaches to encouraging HIV vaccine development that focus on overcoming financial and scientific difficulties. Which option is best depends upon the goals to be achieved by compensation and how alternative approaches affect the achievement of other important goals like prevention of disease, deterrence of injury, and the just distribution of resources.

TORT LIABILITY REFORM

Tort liability functions as a compensation system by imposing legal responsibility for compensating certain specified injuries. It is also justified as a means of retributive justice or risk deterrence (51, 59, 210). Whether or not it serves adequately as a deterrent to risk, it is widely criticized as either ineffective or inefficient in providing equitable compensation. The tort system does not provide compensation to all victims of injury. In theory, compensation is allowed only in cases in which a plaintiff can prove another party's legal responsibility for an injury. In practice, many people who might have a valid cause of action in tort do not file a claim or receive compensation, and others who may not have a legitimate claim may pursue a cause of action and receive compensation (69, 74, 109).

The most common criticisms are that tort litigation is unreasonably time-consuming and expensive and often unpredictable or inconsistent, with some plaintiffs seeming to receive undeserved windfalls and others receiving nothing in spite of a legitimate claim (82, 131). Even those who do not support specific tort reform proposals often voice these criticisms (156).

Others argue that product liability principles make manufacturers responsible for injuries that are unavoidable (80, 158, 203). Sometimes the objection is that the law itself grants plaintiffs a cause of action where, it is argued, it should not be permitted, such as for an injury caused by a design defect. More often, perhaps, the objection is that, in practice, judges and juries apply the law incorrectly, so that a defendant is mistakenly found liable. Of course, judges and juries make mistakes that operate in favor of, as well as against, defendants. But it is the prospect of mistaken liability, not mistaken absence of liability, that most often gives rise to calls for tort reform.

Almost all tort reform proposals seek to limit the liability of potential defendants. Limitations on liability, however, are cost control measures, not compensation mechanisms. Such limitations are ordinarily intended to decrease the number of people who seek and obtain compensation through litigation or the amount of compensation they receive. Such proposals may be justifiable if the goal is to save defendants money and if providing compensation to those who would not qualify under the reformed system is not relevant or desirable. If other goals are important, however, the specific limitations must be analyzed to see whether there is good reason to restrict compensation to a smaller population.

Reforms Granting Immunity from Strict Liability

Some vaccine manufacturers and legal commentators have argued that manufacturers should not be held strictly liable for a defectively designed vaccine. Several jurisdictions have, by court decision, already granted manufacturers immunity from strict liability for all vaccines (and drugs) (225, 255, 270, 277). The trend in other jurisdictions, while not granting complete immunity from liability, is for courts to reject claims for drug and vaccine design defects on a case-by-case basis, generally because the product is not found to be defective or the claimed defect was not avoidable (156).

One may draw conflicting conclusions from this trend. One is that the courts that have rejected

[96] Similar policy options have been reviewed by several groups (82, 95, 191, 201).

strict liability claims are applying the law correctly and as intended to sort out good products from bad ones, and good products are not being found defective. Another is that the courts have applied the law incorrectly, and companies are not being held liable for defective products. Finally, it could be argued that if most reported cases are being found correctly in favor of the defendant, then liability is not needed; drug and vaccine makers should be granted complete immunity from all strict liability, at least for defective design. This assumes that tort law has no deterrent effect. While everyone hopes that no drug or vaccine could ever be defective, it is probably an unrealistic assumption.

The argument for exempting all vaccines from strict liability is basically an argument that drugs and vaccines are special or differ from other products in significant ways that warrant protecting their producers from responsibility for injuries.[97] The California Supreme Court, for example, distinguished between drugs and ordinary consumer products on the grounds that the latter are used to "make work easier or to provide pleasure, while the . . . former . . . may be necessary to alleviate pain and suffering or to sustain life" (225). Of course, not all drugs have such valuable purposes,[98] and many ordinary consumer products provide important benefits.[99] If drugs and vaccines deserve immunity from strict liability, then they must be distinguished from other products on more precise grounds. In the absence of any such distinction, this argument requires exempting not just drugs and vaccines, but all equally beneficial products from strict liability. The alternative is to exempt only those particular drugs and vaccines, as well as other products, that confer special benefits on humankind. This is the kind of risk-benefit analysis adopted by courts that require case-by-case evaluation of strict liability claims.

A second argument for exempting drugs and vaccines from strict liability (again, excluding manufacturing errors) is that federal regulations provide sufficient incentives to ensure safe and effective products. One reason for the adoption of strict liability was to deter manufacturers from marketing products that are unsafe. Here, the fact that most, if not all, drugs and vaccines are intended to prevent or alleviate suffering is not advanced as a reason to dispense with liability. The importance of drugs and vaccines does not explain why their manufacturers should not be deterred from marketing unsafe products. Rather, drugs and vaccines differ from ordinary consumer products because they cannot be marketed without FDA approval based on substantial evidence of safety and effectiveness.

Federal regulation is said to serve the deterrence function of tort liability, so that liability is superfluous and unnecessarily costly. This is a practical argument with considerable basis in fact. Although FDA approval has not generally been sufficient to preempt a claim, it has often provided convincing evidence to reject a claim that a product could have been made safer. Thus, even if it is appropriate to permit strict liability claims against specific drugs or vaccines, few can be successful where the manufacturer has complied with FDA testing requirements and the product remains approved. If FDA requirements for approval are diluted or its standards for evaluating the safety and effectiveness of vaccines are reduced in order to speed up the availability of an HIV vaccine, the argument loses some of its force. Expedited review by the FDA thus may undermine reliance on regulatory standards. In any event, in reviewing new

[97] This would leave manufacturers responsible for product injuries that, in theory at least, they could not prevent, while exempting them from liability for errors in design that, again in theory, could have been corrected. In practice, the argument is advanced selectively to seek immunity from liability for design defects and inadequate warnings, not from liability for manufacturing errors.

[98] Aspirin is intended to relieve pain, but its importance to the public may diminish when it is used to relieve a slight headache.

[99] Automatic electrical current shut-off devices or furnaces to heat homes, for example, provide important safety benefits and relief from suffering.

drugs and vaccines for approval, the FDA does not explicitly examine whether they might be made safer.

Reforms Limiting Liability

Where liability should not be removed entirely, numerous reform proposals are intended to reduce the number (frequency) of claims made, the number of claims in which a plaintiff can succeed (awards), or the amount of compensation payable to a successful plaintiff. Other reforms are intended to expedite the litigation process or make it more accurate or less expensive. A growing number of studies have begun to evaluate tort reforms adopted by the states, primarily those directed to reducing medical malpractice insurance premiums by reducing malpractice litigation (20, 185, 186).[100] In many cases, the generalizability of research results has been hampered by limitations on the data available and variations in study design (193). The studies show that reforms have had somewhat mixed results to date. Few reforms have had a significant effect on the price of insurance, the frequency of claims, or the amount of awards.

A limitation or cap on the amount of damages that can be awarded to a successful plaintiff has been the most effective type of reform to date. As might be expected, caps have been found to reduce the average amount of awards in successful cases in several studies (193). But they have not been found to affect the frequency of claims consistently (46, 213), perhaps because they apply to only a small proportion of claims made. Caps have been enacted to limit either non-economic damages (pain and suffering) or total damages (including incurred medical expenses and lost income).

Different studies have reached different conclusions with respect to the effect of different types of caps. One study of reforms and malpractice insurance premiums found that premiums were reduced most successfully by a cap on total damages (213). This is consistent with conventional wisdom that insurers are best able to set premiums when they have a fixed ceiling on future expenditures. Caps on total damages, however, have been criticized as disadvantaging the most severely injured plaintiffs with the largest losses. One study found that an increased proportion of awards granted the maximum amount after a damage cap was enacted (66).

Limitations on the amount of plaintiffs' attorneys' fees, usually by placing a ceiling on the percentage of an award that can be paid as a contingency fee, are intended to limit claims made by discouraging attorneys from accepting cases, and to increase the proportion of the award that the plaintiff can keep.[101] Danzon found such contingency fee limits had no effect on the number of malpractice claims made or the amount paid per claim (46), while another study found that they increased the amount paid per claim (213). Fee limits may have little effect where they are about the same as the prevailing customary percentage of awards.

Shortening the statute of limitations (the time within which a claim must be filed) to bar claims submitted long after an injury occurs also produced mixed results, with several studies finding no significant effect (193). Shorter statutes of limitations may encourage claims to be filed earlier (193).

Pretrial screening panels are intended to screen out nonmeritorious claims, expedite settlement, and reduce the costs of litigation. They have been difficult to evaluate because panel types vary from state to state and voluntary panels are not used frequently. Studies have found both increased pay-

[100] The Robert Wood Johnson Foundation and the Agency for Health Care Policy and Research, for example, support ongoing studies, of medical malpractice and the US General Accounting Office has conducted several studies (184). The Office of Technology Assessment summarized much of the published research in a 1993 report (193).

[101] There has been little interest in limiting the amount of defendants' attorneys' fees, presumably because they do not affect plaintiffs' decisions to make claims. Legal defense costs do contribute to total litigation expenses.

ments for successful claims using mandatory panels (213), and decreased payments per claim using voluntary panels (193). Another study found that panels had no effect on the probability that a plaintiff would be awarded payment (166). Some may increase costs by adding another layer of procedure. One study found that panels were associated with reduced malpractice insurance premiums for obstetrics/gynecology but not for general surgery or general practice (213).

Collateral source offsets are intended to reduce the amount of awards and, indirectly, the number of claims, by prohibiting plaintiffs from collecting payment for insured losses, such as medical expenses.[102] Again, study results are mixed, with two studies finding no significant effect on the frequency of claims in the case of mandatory offsets, one finding a significant reduction in claim frequency when discretionary offsets were included, and both finding a significant reduction in amount of payment in successful cases (46, 213).

Requiring the losing party to pay the successful party's attorneys' fees and costs also has had little demonstrable effect on claim frequency, payment per claim, or premium prices. This may be explained by the fact that this type of reform has generally been limited to rare cases in which a court finds the claim to be frivolous or fraudulent, and few cases have been found to fall into that category (193).

In summary, tort reforms intended to reduce claims and payments have had spotty success to date. Most types of reform adopted in the past are unlikely to make a dramatic difference in the frequency of future claims. Since most such reforms are intended to reduce litigation and the amount paid to plaintiffs, without improving the probability of "correct" results, they do little to make compensation more equitable. Studies of product liability claims have not yet been able to determine whether the distribution of claims and payments comports with actual legal responsibility for injury (60). Thus, there has been no way to determine whether the number of claims and number and amount of awards are "correct." In the absence of any baseline knowledge of how many claims and awards would be warranted in an error-free system, it is impossible to know whether there are currently too many, too few, or about the right number of claims and awards (153).

Reforms Favoring Compensation

Four different types of tort reform may address the goal of equitable compensation. The first is to change the substantive law governing compensatory damages to make them more consistent across plaintiffs with similar injuries. This might be accomplished by a schedule of injuries, ranked by severity, loss of function, or other criteria, each with an assigned dollar value or range of values. The amounts of compensation could be determined by calculating appropriate medical expenses for each injury and adding expected lost income or expenses for continuing care. It may be difficult to reach agreement on what values should be used in each category. For example, should lost income be calculated by reference to the individual's own income (which awards more to those with higher incomes, as is done now), or should the same rate, such as average non-farm wages, be applied to everyone? How, if at all, should the amounts be adjusted for inflation or geographic area? Such technical problems should not be minimized.[103] In addition, there is the question of the whether the amount of awards can be set at a level that is sufficiently high to meet the reasonable

[102] A health or disability insurer may require the insured/plaintiff to reimburse it for health care and other expenses paid by the insurer if the insured receives compensation covering such expenses.

[103] Officials in the Division of Vaccine Injury Compensation note that children with neurological injuries have such different needs that it may be impossible to establish a schedule that would be fair to all. However, it may be possible to schedule non-economic damages more easily (20).

needs of injured people, but still affordable by those who have to pay.[104]

If such problems are surmountable, a schedule would offer some measure of consistency in compensation for the same type of injury. The schedule could be enacted by state legislatures, although a regulatory agency might be delegated responsibility for updating the award amounts periodically. Alternatively, courts could adopt the schedule to guide jury deliberations.

One advantage of scheduling compensation is that it makes defendants' exposure more predictable, and probably more insurable. Some counsel for vaccine makers have noted that it is not routine litigation, but the possibility of one multimillion dollar judgment that makes their employers nervous. If potential or maximum awards could be estimated on the basis of a schedule, they could more easily be accounted for in pricing. Of course, this does not eliminate the need for predicting the number of possible claims in the future; but that is true for all products.

A second type of reform is alternative dispute resolution, which is intended to expedite settlements in litigated cases and reduce expenditures. Although such procedures hold some promise for speeding up the resolution of disputes, they do not alter the law governing the cases they resolve. Their advantage is that they can be used with almost any type of dispute, regardless of how compensation is calculated. They may also produce more consistent decisions, especially if they are inexpensive enough to be used by more potential claimants and defendants.

A third type of reform would expand potential plaintiffs' opportunities to recover compensation; for example, by granting them a cause of action in instances that tort law currently forbids or by easing standards of proof for existing causes of action. This option would be unattractive to defendants. It is directly contrary to the current trend among courts to limit defendants' liability (50). Some countries in the European Union, however, are moving in the opposite direction from the United States, toward strict liability for product injuries, in their harmonization of laws effort (175). Some countries may not allow a "state of the art" defense, called developmental risk, but would make companies liable for risks that were not discovered or foreseen. The justification appears to be that drugs and vaccines are too important to people's health to permit anything less than the most stringent safeguards against product risks. Japan is considering replacing negligence with strict liability for defective products, although opposition has reduced the likelihood of reform (43).

Some Northern European countries have patient compensation funds to assist those with adverse reactions to drugs and vaccines (23, 165). Others have compensation funds specific to adverse reactions to vaccines recommended for children (112). These countries have a longer tradition of government provision of social assistance to their residents than the United States. Their relatively more extensive programs of health and disability insurance leave injured people with fewer unreimbursed expenses, so there may be less need for other sources of compensation than in the United States.

A fourth type of reform would encourage more people to bring claims under existing law. Several studies have found that only a small proportion of people who are injured as the result of another's negligence actually file tort claims, and an even smaller proportion (perhaps half of those who file claims) eventually recover any compensation (46, 69, 74). The Harvard Medical Practice Study, for example, estimated that about 28 percent of all adverse events experienced by hospitalized patients in New York in 1984 were attributable to medical negligence (one percent of all patients discharged)

[104] The workers compensation system has been criticized for offering too little compensation, and this has been thought to encourage product liability claims as an alternative source of compensation, as in the litigation involving asbestos.

(109). Yet for every eight negligently injured patients, only one patient filed any claim of medical malpractice.[105] Tort reform designed to provide equitable compensation would encourage more, not fewer claims, as well as more accurate claims determination.

Summary

If the goal of reform is to minimize costs to government and vaccine makers, then tort reforms limiting the liability of vaccine makers would be the best choice. It does have disadvantages, however. Most important, it is difficult to justify withdrawing a legal remedy from one class of injured people (those with adverse reactions to HIV vaccines) while it is preserved for other classes. In the past, when liability has been limited, those injured have sometimes been provided an alternative compensation system, such as workers compensation or the National Vaccine Injury Compensation Program. Other reforms, such as most of those intended to limit medical malpractice liability, have not included any alternative compensation system.

As a practical matter, however, even granting vaccine makers immunity from strict liability for design defects may not change the litigation climate significantly. Such claims are effectively litigated like negligence claims and would not be eliminated without granting vaccine makers immunity from liability for their own negligence.[106] Protection against liability, whether in strict liability or negligence, for design defects would not foreclose claims for inadequate warnings of product risks.[107] Elimination of product liability may result in shifting claims that would have been brought against vaccine makers to physicians and clinics that administer vaccines.[108] Such actions would probably be limited to claims of lack of informed consent, which may be difficult to prove. Nonetheless, physicians are not likely to welcome becoming a more visible target of complaints.

Tort reforms limiting liability are not likely to improve compensation for injured persons or make it more equitable. If the goal is to provide compensation within the tort arena to a larger proportion of people with injuries, then mechanisms to increase the number who file claims are needed.

Few reforms have the potential to correct the most pressing problems of tort litigation—its time and expense, and the possibility of inconsistent results. Of course, those problems are not unique to litigation involving vaccines. If tort reform is considered for vaccine-related injuries, it may have to be considered for all other types of injuries. This raises the question whether a Federal tort law should preempt state tort law. Although the advantages and disadvantages of such a change are beyond the scope of this paper, they should be studied if tort reform is thought to be an otherwise desirable option for HIV vaccines.

VOLUNTARY CONTRACTUAL ARRANGEMENTS

Private companies are free to reduce the time and expense of resolving claims by voluntarily agreeing to provide compensation without the necessity of litigation or legislation. The voluntary contract

---

105 Patients who filed claims were not necessarily among those that the study identified as negligently injured (109). It is not known whether such cases involved negligence that was outside the scope of the study (such as outpatient incidents or incidents in years not studied) or whether such cases did not involve negligence at all, or both.

106 See "Tort Liability for Adverse Reactions to Vaccines," above. Connecticut enacted a statute limiting HIV vaccine makers and researchers' liability for product defects and ordinarily negligence to encourage testing candidate HIV vaccines in human subjects.

107 The revised *Restatement of Torts* on product liability, if adopted, may effectively eliminate most causes of action for design defects in the case of prescription drugs and vaccines (See "Tort Liability for Adverse Reactions to Vaccines," above). One justification for reducing the scope of liability for design defects is to permit physicians to decide whether to use a specific vaccine. Warnings then become an important source of information about the vaccine's risks and benefits that affect the decision whether to recommend the vaccine (5).

108 For manufacturers that are owned by foreign companies, some part of any financial savings to the manufacturer is likely to accrue to the foreign owner.

model, such as that developed by Professor Jeffrey O'Connell and used by some schools with respect to football injuries, encourages such private agreements (130). A variant has been introduced in Congress, but never passed, in the Moore-Gephardt bill (99th Cong., 1st Sess., 1985). Applied to HIV vaccine use, it would have a vaccine maker or administrator contractually agree, at the time of vaccination, to promptly pay the vaccine recipient compensation for medical care and other specified financial losses in the event of an adverse reaction to the vaccine. Ordinarily, the vaccine maker or physician would agree to make an offer of compensation within a specified period of time, perhaps two to six months, following notification of injury. If the recipient agreed to accept the offer, he or she would ordinarily waive any right to pursue a tort claim. If a qualifying offer were refused, the recipient would forfeit certain tort remedies or be entitled to limited damages.

The advantage to the injured person is that a reasonable amount of compensation could be provided promptly following injury. The vaccine maker could limit its payments to actual out-of-pocket expenses (compensation for pain and suffering and for insured expenses is generally excluded) and incur few transaction costs, thereby improving the predictability and limiting the amount of liability expenses.

By itself, the contract approach does not affect tort law, and could be used voluntarily with or without tort reform. It could also be required by state or Federal legislation. A contract could be offered voluntarily by any vaccine maker, or any physician or clinic that administers vaccinations. It may be most attractive to companies that believe that they are likely to receive a substantial number of claims that would be successful under existing tort law. Companies that expect few such claims probably have little incentive to assume a voluntary burden of compensation, unless the contract can effectively limit claims to cases in which the company would have legal liability for the injury.

The contract model may work reasonably well in circumstances in which the payor and payee agree to the arrangement before any injury occurs and where causation is relatively easy to establish. It may be attractive to physicians who administer vaccines to their patients and to investigators who give investigational vaccines to subjects in clinical trials. Physicians and researchers are better able to monitor adverse reactions among people who take vaccines, although it may be difficult to identify the cause of many adverse reactions, especially when the vaccine is investigational.

Vaccine makers have no personal relationship to those who take their vaccines. It is doubtful that a standard form contract offered by a vaccine maker prior to vaccination would work as well. Vaccine recipients may reject the contract as self-serving on the part of the vaccine maker, or they might agree to it on the mistaken assumption that it was required in order to receive the vaccine. The utility of the contract depends upon whether vaccine makers could produce a realistic offer in a limited amount of time. Deciding whether to offer compensation requires investigating the merits of a claim that a vaccine caused injury, a complex undertaking. This process is similar to that used in deciding whether to settle a tort claim. The most salient obstacle to using the contract approach with a new HIV vaccine would be the difficulty in determining whether the vaccine caused the injury and, therefore, whether an offer should be made.

Some hospitals have adopted similar compensation programs for injuries resulting from medical research, although there are few reports of their use. Whether this is attributable to lack of knowledge of the availability of compensation or lack of injuries or both is not known. Where the program is voluntary, compensation is not assured to all injured persons. Those institutions and companies that do adopt a program may have different policies that produce inconsistent results.

GOVERNMENT-FUNDED INSURANCE ARRANGEMENTS

Government-financed insurance programs could fund compensation for injuries, with or without any change in tort law, in several ways.

Government-Funded Excess Insurance

If the only problem with relying on tort compensation were its cost, and that cost dissuaded vaccine makers from pursuing vaccine development, then one alternative would be to shift at least some costs to government by having government assume the obligation for liability costs in excess of a fixed amount. A state or the Federal government could purchase excess insurance or reinsurance policies or use government funds to pay excess amounts out of general or special revenues. Such a program could be adopted whether or not tort liability were altered. If government wished to change the number and amount or distribution of its payments, however, it could modify tort law either to increase or decrease the number or amount of awards to claimants. In the absence of any change in the way damages awards are calculated, it would not affect the possibility of inconsistent awards for similar injuries. Although individual states could adopt a reinsurance or excess insurance program, consistency could not be achieved unless all states adopted a substantially similar system.

The primary disadvantage of creating such a program for HIV vaccine injuries is that it may be impossible to predict the amount of excess insurance needed until there have been many years of experience with the vaccine. It is unlikely that the federal (or any state) government would commit to expenditures with no ceiling. It will also be especially difficult to determine the amount at which liability costs to vaccine makers should be deemed excessive. That question involves complex social policy decisions about the degree to which government and private industry should be responsible for HIV vaccine-related injuries, as well as the fairness of liability determinations.

Other more practical questions would have to be resolved. For example, should such costs be limited to awards to plaintiffs, or should they also include the costs of defending claims? If defense costs are included, how would they be verified? Would companies be willing to allow government to audit their records? Should government accept cost certification as sufficient proof of expenditures? Such questions are not insoluble. A more sensitive question is whether an excess insurance program would set a precedent for government reinsurance of liability expenses for other tort claims, from medical malpractice to automobile injuries.

Government-Funded Disability Benefits

Vaccine-related injuries could be compensated through a state or Federal disability insurance program that covers only adverse reactions to HIV vaccines or one that covers many or all injuries. For example, the Social Security program could be amended to specifically include coverage of injuries resulting from HIV vaccines. A more general expansion of disability insurance to cover injuries regardless of cause would be more in keeping with the purpose of Social Security, however, which bases eligibility on disability and age and already covers AIDS-related disabilities.

The only compensation mechanism that avoids serious questions of horizontal justice is a program that compensates all injuries regardless of their cause. This is because every program that provides compensation only for injuries from one cause requires a justification why those injuries deserve special compensation when injuries from other causes do not. The need for financial assistance is not a sufficient reason to provide compensation to some injured persons but not others with similar needs. The desire to encourage the production of important products by protecting them from liability is also not a sufficient justification when the makers of equally important products are not similarly protected. The cost and inefficiency of the tort system is not a sufficient reason to replace it with a special compensation program for only some people but not others. Other reasons specific to injuries from one cause are required to justify a special compensation system for those injuries. Although justifications may exist, they are often complex and difficult to identify.

Other countries, like Germany, have had general disability insurance programs in place for decades. The New Zealand Accidental Injury program provides compensation for injuries from almost all causes (62). The Commission established to study accidental injuries concluded that limiting the program to injuries from particular causes was both illogical and unfair and recommended universal coverage as the only defensible approach (1).

In the United States, a federal general disability insurance program may be more feasible if future health care reform achieves universal coverage of health insurance. Health insurance takes care of one significant cost of injuries. The remaining expenses are those needed to replace lost income to pay for living expenses and, in cases of permanent disability, rehabilitation or long-term care. These latter expenses can be paid for with disability benefits funded by insurance or general revenues.

Establishing such a program would require answering many of the questions raised for a cause-based compensation program, such as the seriousness of injuries covered, how much and what type of compensation would be available, and whether those responsible for certain injuries should contribute to financing the system.[109] The cost of such a program may require new government revenues, although it could be financed in part by taxes on products and services that caused injury. The existence of a compensation program may encourage a larger proportion of injured people to seek compensation. Because the costs of disability for the entire national population are relatively consistent over time, unlike the costs of injuries from specific products, they are likely to be more predictable than the cost of compensating injuries caused by new HIV vaccines. Moreover, a general disability insurance system would avoid the administrative expenses of resolving disputes over causation. There would be no need for separate administrative programs for injuries from different causes, each with its own fixed costs.

A general disability benefits program could exist with or without tort liability. A program that provided only compensation, however, could not purport to serve any deterrence function. If deterring unsafe products and services continued to be an important social goal, additional mechanisms would be needed, such as regulation of products and services, or requiring providers of products and services to help finance the program in accordance with the proportion of injuries attributed to their products.

PUBLIC COMPENSATION SYSTEMS

Federal and state governments have created several publicly administered injury compensation programs. Examples include state workers compensation programs, Virginia's Birth-Related Neurological Injury Compensation Act (Va. Code Ann. 38.2-5001 et seq.), Florida's Birth-Related Neurological Injury Compensation Act (Fla. Stat. 766.301 et seq.), the Federal National Vaccine Injury Compensation Program (42 U.S.C. 300aa-10 et seq.), the Federal Black Lung Benefits Act (30 U.S.C. 901 et seq.), and, most recently, the Radiation Exposure Compensation Act (42 U.S.C. 2210 et seq.).

Most such compensation programs are limited to specific injuries from specific causes (cause-based), but provide compensation on a no-fault basis. As long as the injury is demonstrated to result from the specified cause, compensation can be granted without the need to prove negligence or other traditional legal responsibility for the injury.

No-fault compensation systems have advantages over tort litigation. The most salient is that a larger proportion of injured people are entitled to compensation. There are ordinarily no defendants, so that parties that might otherwise be liable for injury need not participate in the claims deter-

[109] See Elements of a Compensation Program, below.

mination process or pay compensation.[110] The costs of administering the compensation system can be less that the total costs of litigation so that a larger proportion of funds go to injured people. Costs are ordinarily spread over a large population or society as a whole, rather than falling on individual companies or organizations. Compensation can be funded from different sources to achieve different goals. General tax revenues can be used where the program benefits society. Special taxes on entities that create the risk (such as employers in workers compensation, or vaccine makers in the National Vaccine Injury Compensation Program) can be used to link the benefits and risks of specific products or actions.

No-fault compensation systems have two main disadvantages. A cause-based system must satisfy the requirements of horizontal justice by justifying different or special treatment for one class of people or injuries. The more compensation programs that exist for specific causes, the more difficult it becomes to defend excluding other injuries from a no-fault system. This can be seen in the tendency to call for a special compensation program to remedy social problems.[111]

No-fault systems (whether or not cause-based) may also generate more, rather than less, cost, either in compensation awards or administrative expenses. Because no-fault systems compensate more people than would receive compensation (or even file a claim) in tort law, a system's cost depends upon who is eligible for compensation and the level of compensation awarded.[112] Per-capita compensation at the level of average tort awards would generate higher costs. Very low levels of compensation may be inadequate or unfair and generate dissatisfaction, as seen in some worker compensation programs. In the absence of reliable estimates of the number of compensable injuries, it is difficult to predict system costs.

Most important, no cause-based system can avoid disputes over the cause of injuries. Determining causation is often difficult and time-consuming, especially where the scientific and medical evidence is uncertain or conflicting (115).[113] Yet no-fault systems are often recommended in order to provide needed compensation in circumstances where causation is unclear or controversial. Thus, the same complexities that make litigation frustrating and expensive are often necessarily part of no-fault compensation proceedings.

Health care reform proposals debated in the 103rd Congress included provisions affecting compensation and liability for adverse reactions to HIV vaccines (see box 4-2).

The National Vaccine Injury Compensation Program

The National Vaccine Injury Compensation Program (42 U.S.C. 300aa-10 et seq.) was enacted in 1986 as part of the National Childhood Vaccine Injury Act in response to concerns that vaccine makers would not continue to produce childhood vaccines or to develop new ones if the pressure of liability for adverse reactions were not abated and the need for financial assistance to families whose children suffered permanent injury or death following vaccination (115). In August, 1992, Con-

---

[110] Most systems provide that the compensation program is subrogated to the rights of the claimant so that it may seek reimbursement for compensation paid from anyone who is legally liable for the injury. This is most often provided with respect to injuries caused by negligence.

[111] In 1986, Congressman Edward Markey called for compensating human subjects in radiation experiments sponsored by the Department of Energy's predecessors (190). Recent publicity has renewed interest in the proposal.

[112] The Harvard Medical Practice Study estimated that a compensation system for medical malpractice in New York State could be financed for approximately the same amount as current malpractice insurance premiums if it limited compensation to serious permanent injury or death, and excluded injuries lasting less than six months and medical expenses covered by Medicaid (70).

[113] For example, in workers compensation cases, it is generally far more difficult to determine the cause of a worker's chronic disease than the cause of a traumatic injury.

BOX 4-2: Health Care Reform and HIV Vaccines

Health care reform proposals that were debated in the 103rd Congress and ultimately defeated would have had implications on compensation for adverse reactions to HIV vaccines. Each of the proposals, to the extent that they expanded access to health insurance coverage, would have better ensured access to medical care for HIV vaccine trial participants. However, none of the proposals addressed needs for long-term care.

President Clinton's Health Security Act provided for coverage for investigative medical treatments.[1] Decisions about which investigative medical treatments to cover, however, were left to the discretion of the individual health plans. In addition, coverage only applied to investigative treatments that are qualifying, meaning that investigational treatment has been given as part of an approved clinical trial, and that another treatment would have been provided as routine care if the participant were not receiving the investigational treatment. Approved clinical trials were those sponsored by government agencies such as the National Institutes of Health, the Food and Drug Administration, the Department of Veterans Affairs, the Department of Defense, or a qualified nongovernmental research entity or a peer reviewed and approved program.

Other proposals that were presented to Congress did not specifically address these issues. The "single payor" approach (Wellstone) would provide universal coverage for medical care, including medical care for adverse reactions to HIV vaccines.[2] The plan did not detail whether the costs of experimental therapies would be covered under the plan.

HIV vaccine liability would also have been affected by health reform proposals that included provisions reforming medical malpractice liability. Clinton's Health Security Act included provisions reforming medical malpractice and strict liability for injuries from pharmaceuticals, including vaccines (Health Security Act, secs. 5501 *et seq.*). However, the Act left in place current product liability rules for injuries from pharmaceuticals due to negligence.

SOURCE: R. E. Stein, Blicker & Stein, Washington, DC, "Selected Issues of AIDS Vaccine Liability," unpublished contractor report prepared for the Office of Technology Assessment, U.S. Congress, Washington, DC, Sept. 30, 1994.

[1]U.S. Congress, Senate, S. 1757, *Health Security Act*, Sec. 1128 (Washington, DC: U.S. Government Printing Office, 1993).
[2]U.S. Congress, Senate, S. 491, *American Health Security Act of 1993* (Washington, DC: U.S. Government Printing Office, 1993).

gressman Fortney "Pete" Stark introduced the National Vaccine Development and Compensation Act, patterned after the National Childhood Injury Compensation Act, which would create a compensation program for injuries occurring in the development and marketing of an HIV vaccine (170). Because the National Childhood Vaccine Injury Act has been suggested as a model for compensating injuries following future vaccination with HIV vaccines, (Stark) it is described in some detail here.

The program, which took effect October 1, 1988, provides compensation on a "no-fault" basis for injuries resulting from vaccines to prevent poliomyelitis, diphtheria, pertussis (whooping cough), tetanus, measles, mumps, and rubella. These were the vaccinations then ordinarily required in all states to permit children to enter school or day care.[114] The program is a "no-fault" system because it does not condition eligibility for compensation on any party's legal liability for the

[114] The Act was amended in 1993 to permit coverage of vaccines recommended by the CDC for routine administration to children. (42 U.S.C. 300aa-14(e))

injury. Claimants (called petitioners) are entitled to compensation if they demonstrate either that the injury is listed in a statutory Vaccine Injury Table or that the injury was actually caused by a covered vaccine, and also meet other eligibility requirements.[115] There is no requirement that the vaccine be shown to have been defective or negligently administered or warnings inadequate. Neither vaccine makers nor health care providers are parties to the proceedings.

The program has been lauded for reducing tort claims against vaccine makers. This is undoubtedly because the act postpones and effectively precludes most lawsuits in two ways. First, it forbids tort claims against vaccine makers unless a petitioner has filed a claim with the Program. Only if a petitioner rejects the Program's decision may he or she commence a lawsuit.[116] The likelihood of succeeding in court on a claim that has been rejected by the program is probably too small to encourage petitioners to proceed. Only if a petitioner has a very strong claim and believes that a court would award much more than the program would a lawsuit be worth the effort.

Second, the act also bars liability on the part of vaccine manufacturers for failure to issue a direct warning of risks to the petitioner (42 U.S.C. 300aa-22(c)). However, most courts have reached the same result by finding that the manufacturer has no duty to warn the vaccine recipient. This leaves petitioners with a possible claim that the manufacturer's warning to the prescribing physician was inadequate, but the act provides that the warning shall be presumed adequate if the vaccine maker complied with all FDA requirements (42 U.S.C. 300aa-22(b)(2)). This represents a nominal change in the law; however, few cases have found FDA-approved labeling to be inadequate. Although petitioners may prefer the compensation system to litigation, in effect, they have little alternative. It should not be surprising that there are few liability claims against manufacturers for adverse reactions to the covered vaccines.

Parents or guardians of injured children[117] file petitions for compensation with the United States Court of Federal Claims (formerly the United States Claims Court) in Washington, DC. A special master in the Court's Office of Special Masters[118] reviews the petition and makes two determinations: whether the petitioner is eligible for compensation and, if so, how much compensation is to be awarded. The Secretary of Health and Human Services is named Respondent in the proceedings. The Department's Division of Vaccine Injury Compensation[119] reviews petitions and offers its opinion on whether the injury was in fact caused by a vaccine. Compensation may be denied if the Special Master determines that, on the

---

[115] Petitioners have the burden of proving entitlement to compensation. The vaccine must have been received in the United States or as a U.S. government employee or dependent overseas; the injury must last more than 6 months and result in more than $1000 in unreimbursable expenses, or death; the petition must be filed within a specified time period; and the petitioner must not have collected an award or settlement for the injury.

[116] Petitioners with retrospective claims who have recovered compensation in an earlier lawsuit are not eligible for the program. Those who had commenced a lawsuit before the Program took effect were not permitted to file a petition unless their lawsuit was suspended pending the Program's determination. A recent decision by the federal court of appeals for the First Circuit, however, held that the husband and daughter of a woman who received compensation from the Program (for contact polio) were entitled to commence a tort action for their own loss of the woman's consortium, because the husband and daughter were not eligible for compensation from the Program (54, 298). The Court of Federal Claims has also held that a prior tort recovery by a parent for her own losses did not bar a petition on behalf of the child for compensation from the program (215).

[117] Eligibility is not limited to children, and specifically includes polio contracted from someone who was vaccinated with OPV.

[118] There are currently seven Special Masters who work exclusively for the program.

[119] The division is part of the Bureau of Health Professions, Health Resources and Services Administration, U.S. Department of Health and Human Services.

basis of a preponderance of the evidence, the injury was not the result of the vaccine in question.[120]

There are actually two programs, one for vaccinations that occurred before October 1, 1988 (retrospective cases), and another for vaccinations on or after October 1, 1988 (prospective cases). All petitions for retrospective cases had to be filed by January 31, 1991. Compensation for permanent injury in retrospective cases is limited to unreimbursed medical and rehabilitation expenses incurred after judgment; past expenses are not covered.[121] Awards in retrospective cases are paid from general revenues appropriated by Congress. Until 1993, appropriations were $80 million per year; for FY 1993, they were $110 million and are authorized to continue at that level for future years.

Prospective cases may be filed within three years after the injury materializes,[122] and have no limit on the amount of compensation payable, except that compensation for death is fixed at $250,000 as in retrospective cases, and non-economic compensation may not exceed $250,000.[123] Awards are paid from a trust fund financed by excise taxes on sales of the covered vaccines.[124] The fund had approximately $700 million in unallocated, unawarded funds as of March 30, 1994.

Like most compensation systems in the United States, the program is cause-based. Only injuries or deaths caused or aggravated by a covered vaccine are compensable. Congress sought to avoid litigation-like disputes over causation by providing a list of medical conditions that are statutorily presumed to be caused by a covered vaccine in a Vaccine Injury Table, shown in table 4-1 (42 U.S.C. 300aa-15). The table lists conditions, such as anaphylaxis and residual seizure disorder, and the time period following vaccination within which the injury must have occurred to be presumptively compensable. However, in the majority of cases, causation has been disputed.

Many disputes, especially those involving the pertussis component of DPT,[125] were disagreements over whether a child actually experienced a condition listed in the table 4-1. These included disputes over whether the medical evidence demonstrated an injury covered in the table or whether factors unrelated to vaccination caused the injury. In addition, there were disagreements about whether a death resulted from a qualifying injury. The table did not eliminate difficult, time-consuming disputes over eligibility for compensation.

---

[120] Determinations may be made with or without a hearing including petitioners, their attorneys and witnesses, and medical reviewers from the Division of Vaccine Injury Compensation, which is represented by attorneys from the Department of Justice. The majority of cases to date have involved hearings, either in person or by telephone conference call.

[121] In the case of death, compensation is fixed at $250,000. A maximum of $30,000 may be awarded for the combined cost of lost income, pain and suffering, and attorneys' fees and costs.

[122] In the case of death, the period is two years after the date of death, but not later than four years after the initial injury.

[123] Compensation for injury may include past and future medical expenses and rehabilitative and custodial care (to the extent not paid for by insurance, other than Medicaid), lost income, pain and suffering (up to $250,000), and reasonable attorneys' fees and costs.

[124] The excise taxes per dose of vaccine currently in effect are: DPT- $4.56; MMR (measles-mumps-rubella)- $4.44; polio- $0.29; and DT (diphtheria-tetanus)- $0.06.

[125] Which, if any, adverse reactions to the pertussis component result in permanent neurological damage or death has been at the center of controversy for decades (85). Parents of children who suffered serious injuries or death following DPT vaccination were instrumental in initially advocating a compensation Program. (They also pressed for the adverse reaction monitoring Program and efforts to improve the safety of vaccines, which were provided for in companion legislation creating the National Vaccine Program. That Program, however, may soon be phased out). Not surprisingly, pertussis is the cited vaccine in the majority of petitions filed with the Program. But the Program has not settled the scientific controversy over the cause of many adverse reactions; nor was it designed to do so. The Secretary of Health and Human Services proposed revising the Vaccine Injury Table to add, modify, and remove several conditions presumed to result from rubella and pertussis vaccines. After publication of a follow-up study of the National Childhood Encephalopathy Study (111, 120) and the Institute of Medicine's analysis of the new data (87), however, the Secretary postponed action on the regulations in order to allow time for additional public comment. (59 Fed. Reg. 13916, Mar. 24, 1994).

TABLE 4-1: Vaccine Injury Table, National Vaccine Injury Compensation Program

Illness, disability, injury, or condition covered and time period for first symptom or manifestation of onset or of significant aggravation after vaccine administration, by vaccine.

Diphtheria-tetanus-pertussis (DPT); pertussis; DTP/polio combination; or any other vaccine containing whole cell pertussis bacteria, extracted or partial cell bacteria, or specific pertussis antigen(s)

- Anaphylaxis or anaphylactic shock, within 24 hours
- Encephalopathy (or encephalitis), within 24 hours
- Shock-collapse or hypotonic-hyporesponsive collapse, within 3 days
- Residual seizure disorder in accordance with subsection (b)(2), within 3 days
- Any acute complication or sequela (including death) of an illness, disability, injury, or condition referred to above which illness, disability, injury, or condition arose within the time period prescribed

Measles, mumps, rubella, or any vaccine containing the foregoing as a component; DT; Td; or texanus toxoid

- Anaphylaxis or anaphylactic shock, within 24 hours
- Encephalopathy (or encephalitis), within 15 days for mumps, rubella, measles, or any vaccine containing any of the foregoing as a component, within 3 days for DT, Td, or tetanus toxoid
- Residual seizure disorder in accordance with subsection (b)(2), within 15 days for mumps, rubella, measles, or any vaccine containing any of the foregoing as a component, within 3 days for DT, Td, or tetanus toxoid
- Any acute complication or sequela (including death) of an illness, disability, injury, or condition referred to above which illness, disability, injury, or condition arose within the time period prescribed

Polio vaccines (other than inactivated polio vaccine)

- Paralytic polio: in a nonimmunodeficient recipient, within 30 days; in an immunodeficient recipient, within 6 months; in a vaccine-associated community case, no time limit
- Any acute complication or sequela (including death) of an illness, ability, injury, or condition referred to above which illness, disability, injury, or condition arose within the time period prescribed

Inactivated polio vaccine

- Anaphylaxis or anaphylactic shock
- Any acute complication or sequela (including death) of an illness, disability, injury, or condition referred to above which illness, disability, injury, or condition arose within the time period prescribed

SOURCE: 42 U.S.C. 300aa-14(1)(a).

In its early years, the program suffered from inadequate funding and had difficulty developing an efficient mode of operating (115). The statute has been amended almost every year to correct technical problems. Now, however, the Program appears to be functioning relatively smoothly (198) and has been reauthorized as a permanent program.

As of September 7, 1994, the Program had received 4,069 petitions for retrospective injuries and 574 petitions for prospective injuries (table 4-2). Since retrospective petitions cover any injury or death resulting from a vaccination before 1988, they may indicate the number of adverse reactions that were believed by parents to be vaccine-related for each covered vaccine since it was first introduced, beginning with IPV (injected polio vaccine) in the mid-1950s. The number of petitions exceeds the number of lawsuits involving DPT brought against vaccine makers during the same period reported to the CDC. Some petitioners who did not file lawsuits may have believed that they did not have a cause of action in tort law. Others may not have been aware of the possibility that their children's injuries might be connected to vaccination until publicity about the program reached them.

TABLE 4-2: Number of Petitions Filed (as of Sept. 7, 1994), National Vaccine Injury Compensation Program

Fiscal year	Vaccination before October 1988	Vaccination after October 1988	Total
1988	24	0	24
1989	146	1	147
1990	3,060	31	3,091
1991	839[a]	119	958
1992	0[b]	191	191
1993	0	137	137
1994	0	95	95
Totals	**4,069**	**574**	**4,643**

[a]An additional 26 petitions filed were not accepted as timely filings.
[b]The deadline for filing retrospective petitions was Jan. 31, 1991. No retrospective petitions may be filed after that date.

SOURCE: Division of Vaccine Injury Compensation U.S. Department of Health and Human Services, 1994.

About 45 percent of the retrospective petitions filed between October 1, 1988 (when the Program became effective) and January 31, 1991 (the deadline for filing retrospective claims) had been finally decided by the United States Court of Federal Claims by September 7, 1994 (table 4-3). Of these, only 32 percent were determined to be entitled to compensation.[126] Payments totaling $417.2 million have been made to petitioners in about two-thirds (67 percent) of the adjudicated cases.[127] In fiscal year 1992, many awards could not be paid on a timely basis because the revenues appropriated to fund them were not sufficient. The average award in a retrospective case involving permanent injury is about $1 million, although awards in 1994 average $750,749.[128]

Prospective petitions are more representative of the number and type of claims that could be made annually on an ongoing basis. An average of 96 prospective petitions per year were filed during the six-year period 1989 through 1994 (table 4-2). More than a third (38 percent) of the 574 prospective petitions have been decided (table 4-4). Of decided cases, 44 percent have been determined to be compensable. Awards (including attorneys' fees in noncompensable cases) have been paid out to petitioners in 145 (67 percent) of the 217 adjudicated cases for a total of $53.8 million (table 4-5).[129] Awards for permanent injury are highly variable, but tend to exceed awards in retrospective cases because the children are younger and are eligible for past as well as future losses, and higher lost wages and pain and suffering awards.[130] The trust fund for prospective awards has always had a surplus. If prospective petitions continue to be filed and compensation awarded at the same rate

[126] This contrasts with the Program's experience during its first two years of operation (1989 and 1990), in which 73 percent of retrospective claims were awarded compensation. Since the majority of the retrospective claims were filed in late 1990 and January 1991, the earlier claims may have involved different or stronger facts.

[127] Award amounts also include "reasonable attorneys' fees" for petitioners' attorneys, which may be awarded in cases brought in good faith even if the petitioner is determined to not be eligible for compensation.

[128] Awards in the case of death are limited to $250,000. About 12 percent of all petitions filed have involved death. Awards in cases of permanent injury have ranged from $120 to $4,000,000 (Division of Vaccine Injury Compensation).

[129] An Institute of Medicine informal survey in 1984 found that the four responding vaccine makers had paid a total of about $2 million for all liability claims closed or settled in the previous ten years and an additional $1.8 million in defense costs (82). Even adjusting for inflation, the Program appears to provide substantially more compensation than did tort litigation.

[130] As of March 1, 1994, 51 percent of awards (34 out of 67) were for the death of a vaccine recipient, totaling $8.6 million. Awards for injuries totaled $32.8 million for 33 cases, or just under $1 million per compensable claim.

TABLE 4-3: Results of Adjudicated Claims (as of September 7, 1994), National Vaccine Injury Compensation Program For Vaccines Before October 1988

Fiscal year	Award granted # (%)	Claim denied # (%)	Claim dismissed # (%)	Total
1989	9 (41)	0	13 (59)	22
1990	98 (79)	10 (8)	16 (13)	124
1991	132 (29)	65 (14)	256 (56)	453
1992	135 (29)	51 (11)	280 (60)	466
1993	102 (21)	63 (13)	316 (66)	481
1994	102 (36)	36 (13)	147 (52)	285
Totals	**578 (32)**	**225 (12)**	**1,028 (56)**	**1,831**

SOURCE: Division of Vaccine Injury Compensation, U.S. Department of Health and Human Services, 1994.

as they have been during the last six years, the trust fund will continue to accumulate surplus funds. This would suggest that the surtax on vaccines is set at too high a level and could be reduced.[131]

The program's major advantages are the relative speed with which it can make decisions (compared with litigation) and the fact that it compensates a much larger proportion of children than would receive any recovery otherwise. The Program's ability to make speedy decisions was hampered by an unexpected influx of retrospective petitions in late 1990 and January 1991, as well as by funding disruptions; many retrospective cases have taken years to resolve. Prospective cases have generally been decided within the statutory period of 14 months.

Administrative costs appear reasonable for the services rendered. The Court of Federal Claims and its Office of Special Masters, the Division of Vaccine Injury Compensation, and the Vaccine Injury Claims Division of the Department of Justice have received a total of between $4.5 and $9 million annually in appropriations to pay for staff and resources.[132]

Although the program was not originally intended to be a model for replacing tort liability with no-fault compensation, it has been suggested as one for HIV vaccine-related injury. Congressman Stark circulated a proposal for legislation to create a no-fault compensation program for such injuries patterned after the legislation creating the program (170). The major technical difficulty with developing a compensation program for HIV vaccines lies in determining what types of injuries should be deemed compensable before sufficient experience with a vaccine permits causation to be reasonably determined.[133]

It may not be necessary to create another independent compensation system. HIV vaccines might be added to the vaccines covered by the existing program. The statute now provides for covering new vaccines when they are recommended for routine administration to children. In the near future, the Secretary of Health and Human Ser-

[131] It may also suggest that the estimates for liability, which were higher than the surtax amounts, were too high. The Public Health Service is contemplating recommending changing the amount of the excise tax to generate only about $60 million per year, which should be adequate to fund prospective awards.

[132] Over the five-year period 1989-1993, $7.5 million per year would total $37.5 million to decide 1,768 cases yielding total awards of $424.6 million. This represents about 8% of total awards plus administrative costs. In the future, a smaller number of petitions are likely to be filed and decided.

[133] Another important technical difficulty with the proposal involved the manufacturer's bond, the mechanism used to provide indemnity during the clinical trials stage. Some manufacturers objected that a bond would be difficult for a small company to raise. In addition, some manufacturers did not want their bond to be used to pay for adverse reactions attributable to other companies' vaccine candidates (173).

TABLE 4-4: Results of Adjudicated Claims (as of September 7, 1994), National Vaccine Injury Compensation Program For Vaccinations After October 1988

Fiscal year	Award granted # (%)	Claim denied # (%)	Claim dismissed # (%)	Total
1989	0 (0)	0	0 (0)	0
1990	2 (67)	0 (0)	1 (33)	3
1991	10 (37)	4 (15)	13 (48)	27
1992	28 (42)	6 (9)	33 (49)	67
1993	22 (35)	10 (16)	30 (48)	62
1994	33 (57)	7 (12)	18 (31)	58
Totals	**95 (44)**	**27 (12)**	**95 (44)**	**217**

SOURCE: Division of Vaccine Injury Compensation, U.S. Department of Health and Human Services,1994.

vices is likely to recommend adding Hepatitis B vaccine and hemophilus influenza type b vaccine to the list of covered vaccines. These additions would be consistent with the purpose of covering vaccines that are recommended, if not required, for children. It is unlikely that an HIV vaccine would be required for children or adults, although it might be recommended for people at high risk of HIV infection, including newborns whose mothers are HIV positive. Adding HIV vaccines to the program would represent a larger break with the origina purpose of the program than adding vaccines recommended for children. It raises the question why other vaccines taken primarily by adults should not be covered.

Beyond the program itself, attention to the larger question of horizontal justice may require asking why injuries from other causes should not be covered. If the most anticipated adverse reaction to an HIV vaccine is HIV infection, covering adverse reactions to HIV vaccines would treat people differently depending upon how they became infected. People who became infected as a result of vaccination would be eligible for special compensation, but those who became infected in other ways would not. This is true for any cause-based compensation program, of course, but it may be particularly sensitive in view of the limited resources often available to people living with HIV infection and AIDS.

State Compensation Programs

Two states, California and Connecticut, have adopted special measures pertaining to HIV vaccines that are described briefly below. In addition, Virginia and Florida have operated compensation programs for birth-related injuries that may suggest some lessons for the creation of cause-based compensation programs.

California

In 1986, California created the AIDS Vaccine Victims Compensation Fund as a source of future no-fault compensation (Cal. Health & Safety Code, Ch. 1.14, s. 199.50). The program is limited to people who suffer personal injury caused by an HIV vaccine that is developed by a California company and approved by the FDA or the state. It does not cover research-related injuries or injuries resulting from vaccines from non-California companies. Compensation (for medical expenses, lost earnings, and up to $550,000 in non-economic damages) is to be awarded by the California Board of Control out of funds collected from a surcharge on future HIV vaccine sales. Claimants remain free to pursue any tort claim they may have for the injury, but the state is entitled to recoup any damages that duplicate a program award. Since no vaccine has yet been approved for marketing, the program has not become operational. The authorizing legislation is relatively general, leaving details to be worked out by a task force.

TABLE 4-5: Awards Paid to Petitioners (as of September 7, 1994), National Vaccine Injury Compensation Program

For Vaccinations Before October 1988

Fiscal year	Number	Amount ($millions)
1990	91	$71.9
1991	149	75.4
1992	215	84.5
1993	390	110.4
1994	396	75.0
Subtotals	1,241	$417.2

For Vaccinations After October 1988

Fiscal year	Number	Amount ($millions)
1990	0	0
1991	14	$4.2
1992	33	13.1
1993	40	15.0
1994	58	21.5
Subtotals	145	53.8
Totals	1,386	$471.0

SOURCE: Division of Vaccine Injury Compensation, U.S. Department of Health and Human Services, 1994.

The AIDS Vaccine Victims Compensation Fund was part of legislation that was intended to remove three obstacles to AIDS vaccine development identified by California vaccine companies to the legislature: the high cost of testing investigational vaccines, an uncertain market, and strict liability for adverse reactions to vaccines. The legislation provides for grants to California vaccine makers for research and testing investigational vaccines and guaranteed state purchases of up to 500,000 units of an approved vaccine (at up to $20 per dose if fewer than 500,000 doses are sold within three years after FDA approval) (Calif. Health & Safety Code, s.199.45-51, 199.55-60). The state has provided almost $2 million dollars in research grants to two California companies. Under the statute, grants are to be repaid from sales of an approved HIV vaccine; California is also to receive royalties from such sales after the grant is repaid, with the royalty to be negotiated at the time of the grant award. In the absence of any licensed HIV vaccine, the state has not had to appropriate any funds to fulfill its purchase commitment. Because the statute gives the state discretion to choose among competing vaccines on the basis of their safety, effectiveness, and cost, it is not clear whether the guaranteed purchase is sufficiently precise to offer manufacturers a reliable market.

The 1986 legislation also limited the liability of manufacturers, in effect, to liability for negligence. In 1988, the California Supreme Court issued its decision in *Brown* v. *Superior Court* (225) which effectively precluded strict liability based on design defects caused by FDA-approved prescription drugs. The decision, which is considered to apply to FDA-approved vaccines as well as drugs, provided more protection against liability than the legislation, and the provisions limiting liability were repealed the same year (Calif. Statutes 1988, ch. 1555 s.3).[134]

California had already adopted a limited compensation program for severe adverse reactions to mandatory childhood vaccines in 1977 (Calif. Health & Safety Code, s. 429.35-.36, 1977; (112)). That program, however, provided compensation only for medical and institutional care up to a maximum of $25,000. California's Medi-Cal and other programs for disabled children were expected to provide other assistance. Children with severe injuries requiring extensive medical care could seek compensation from the fund in addition to pursuing any tort remedy they might have against a vaccine manufacturer. The legislation provided immunity from liability for physicians and others who administered the required vaccines. Perhaps because of its narrow scope, the program has received only a handful of claims. It was created in the aftermath of the swine flu program in the hope of encouraging continued vaccine development and marketing, but it was not considered an adequate model for the later AIDS Vaccine Victims Compensation Fund or the National Vaccine Injury Compensation Program, and has had little, if any, influence on vaccine development or compensation policy.

Connecticut

Connecticut adopted a statute protecting manufacturers, research institutions and researchers from liability for personal injury resulting from the administration of any HIV vaccine to a research subject (Conn. Gen. Stat. ss. 19a-591-591b) (172). The law exempts those involved in clinical trials of an HIV vaccine from all liability, including liability for negligence, unless the person provided false information to the FDA in connection with an Investigational New Drug application, or caused injury by gross negligence or reckless, willful or wanton misconduct. It was enacted after MicroGeneSys said it would not test its vaccine to prevent maternal-fetal HIV transmission in HIV-positive pregnant women. The trial was closed when it failed to enroll enough subjects to permit conclusions about the effect of vaccination to be drawn. MicroGeneSys is no longer pursuing those trials.

Virginia

The Virginia Birth-Related Neurological Injury Compensation Act (Va. Code Ann. 38.2-5001 et seq.) was enacted in 1987 in an attempt to reduce the cost of medical malpractice insurance on the theory that tort claims against obstetricians for birth-related injuries were driving up the price of insurance, limiting available coverage, and threatening the availability of obstetric services. It protects participating physicians from tort liability for medical malpractice for specific, narrowly defined birth-related injuries to newborns, and offers compensation in very restricted circumstances.

The Virginia program is limited to severe neurological injuries to a newborn that are caused by a physician who participated in the program and which render the infant "permanently in need of assistance in *all* activities of daily living." (Va. Code Ann. s. 38.2-5001 (emphasis added)).[135] Given the narrow definition, it should not be surprising that the program had received only ten

---

[134] In 1992, California enacted a law limiting the liability of HIV vaccine manufacturers, research institutions, and researchers participating in clinical trials of vaccines intended to prevent HIV transmission from a pregnant woman to her baby. (Calif. Health & Safety Code, s. 199.89) Liability is expressly limited as in the *Brown* decision. The law does not preclude liability for negligence, gross negligence, or reckless, willful or wanton misconduct, or for providing false information to the FDA.

[135] Birth-related neurological injury was redefined in 1990 as "injury to the brain or spinal cord of an infant caused by the deprivation of oxygen or mechanical injury occurring in the course of labor, delivery or resuscitation in the immediate post-delivery period in a hospital which renders the infant permanently motorically disabled and (i) developmentally disabled or (ii) for infants sufficiently developed to be cognitively evaluated, cognitively disabled. In order to constitute a 'birth-related neurological injury' ..., such disability shall cause the infant to be permanently in need of assistance in all activities of daily living. This definition shall apply to live births only and shall not include disability or death caused by genetic or congenital abnormality, degenerative neurological disease, or maternal substance abuse." Va. Code Ann. s. 38.2-5001.

claims by mid-1994,[136] although the Virginia State Medical Society had predicted at least 40 claims per year (118). Of these claims, seven were awarded compensation, two were denied and one was pending in August 1994.[137]

Claims against participating physicians and hospitals must be brought to the program exclusively. Physicians are protected against liability for the injuries covered by the program (Va. Code Ann. 38.2-508). The Virginia Worker Compensation Commission makes decisions on claims. Physicians (primarily obstetricians) and hospitals elect to participate in the program and pay an annual assessment. Assessments on non-participating physicians have been suspended because of surplus revenues in the compensation fund.

Florida

The Florida Birth-Related Neurological Injury Compensation Act (Fla. Stat. 766.301 et seq.) was modeled after the Virginia program. It has received more claims, presumably because it defines a compensable injury slightly more broadly.[138] The Neurological Injury Compensation Association (NICA) had received 108 claims through fiscal year 1993.[139] Of these claims, 31 received an award, 42 were denied as noncompensable by a judge (of which 4 were on appeal), and 22 were denied by the NICA and pending judicial determination. Total awards, which are paid throughout the child's lifetime as expenses as incurred, are estimated to be about $73 million, with about $5 million having been paid out.

It is not known whether either the Virginia or the Florida program has had any effect on malpractice claims or insurance rates for obstetricians in those states. In its recent report on defensive medicine, the Office of Technology Assessment speculated that the "subset of injuries is so small and the link between these injuries and physician practices so unclear, removing personal liability for the specified birth-related injuries probably has very little impact on defensive medicine and . . . impact on malpractice premiums is unclear" (195). No study has documented increased access to obstetrical care, one of the goals of the Virginia and Florida statutes.

ELEMENTS OF A NO-FAULT COMPENSATION PROGRAM

If a no-fault compensation program for HIV vaccine-related injuries is desirable, it can be constructed in different ways to suit different purposes. If the choices made are already part of an ongoing program, HIV vaccine-related injuries might be added to that program. The following pages summarize key elements of a no-fault compensation program and how they might be adapted to adverse reactions to HIV vaccines.

■ Eligibility

The first question to be decided is who should be eligible for compensation. Should the program be limited to United States citizens or residents, or should anyone who receives an HIV vaccine be eligible? In the National Vaccine Injury Compensation Program, people who are employed by the Federal government, such as diplomats and military personnel and their dependents, are covered if they receive a U.S.-made vaccine abroad, like all individuals who receive a vaccine in the United States. Should the program cover foreign citizens residing in their own countries who receive vaccine made by a U.S. manufacturer? Obviously, the

[136] Eleanor Pyles, Virginia Office of Birth-Related Compensation Claims, Richmond, VA personal communication, Aug. 8, 1994.

[137] Ibid.

[138] " 'Birth-related neurological injury' means injury to the brain or spinal cord of a live infant weighing at least 2,500 grams at birth caused by oxygen deprivation or mechanical injury occurring in the course of labor, delivery, or resuscitation in the immediate post-delivery period in a hospital, which renders the infant permanently and substantially mentally and physically impaired. This definition shall apply to live births only and shall not include disability or death caused by genetic or congenital abnormality." (Fla. Stat. 766.302(2)). Florida's definition does not require that an infant require assistance in *all* activities of daily living.

[139] NICA claims office, Tallahassee, FL personal communication, Aug. 8, 1994.

broader the eligible population, the more expensive the program. But if the program is to encourage HIV vaccine development for overseas use, as in Africa and Asia, it may wish to include foreign vaccinees, although potential liability claims from foreign vaccinees does not appear to threaten vaccine development. A different question may arise as to what counts as a U.S. vaccine if the company that makes it is owned or controlled by a foreign company.

It is customary to fix a time within which claims must be filed (a statute of limitations). Ordinarily, this would be several years after an injury manifests itself. If adverse reactions to HIV vaccines are not expected to occur for many years after vaccination and if they are difficult to identify, the first claims might not be expected for many years after the program begins.

Programs have often distinguished between investigational and marketed products, reserving compensation to those injured as a result of a marketed product. If a compensation program is to encourage research, as well as provide compensation, it may wish to cover injuries to research subjects. However, research-related injuries raise special questions in most of the categories discussed below.

The National Vaccine Injury Compensation Program was originally justified because it covered childhood vaccines required by law. An HIV vaccine is not likely to be required for any specific population, at least not in the near future. If a compensation program covers vaccines that are recommended or voluntary, then it may set a precedent for expanding the program to cover all recommended or voluntary vaccines.

Compensable Injuries

The question of what injuries to cover may be the most difficult and the least capable of resolution before an HIV vaccine acquires several years of experience. Three threshold questions could be answered sooner, however. The first is whether all injuries should be covered, regardless of seriousness, or whether there should be a minimum level of severity, defined in either physical or financial terms. If the compensation program is to make compensation more equitable, then, arguably, even transient injuries should be covered. After all, the less serious the injury, the less likely it is to be compensated in the tort system. If resources for compensation are limited, however, it may be necessary to restrict compensable injuries to those for which people are unlikely to be able to pay themselves. This could be done by specifying the particular injuries, by requiring injuries to be permanent or last more than six months, for example, by covering only uninsured or unreimbursed expenses, or by requiring that the injury cost more than a minimum amount in medical expenses or lost earnings or both. The particular choice might be balanced with the amount of compensation payable. More injuries could be compensated if the amount of compensation per injury were limited. It should be recognized, however, that if insured expenses are not covered, those costs remain with the health or accident insurer.

The second threshold question is whether to include HIV infection as a compensable injury. The possibility that vaccine recipients might become infected as a result of vaccination (because of enhanced susceptibility to infection, limited efficacy of the vaccine, or a manufacturing defect) poses an initial difficulty. If it is impossible to determine whether a person's HIV infection resulted from a vaccine or from other causes, it might be impractical to include HIV infection as a compensable injury. In many cases, it is likely to be quite difficult to attribute HIV infection to lack of vaccine efficacy rather than risk behavior. On the other hand, if HIV infection is the most common injury among vaccine recipients, then a compensation program that excludes HIV infection will compensate very few people.

A third question is whether social harms, such as discrimination in housing, employment, insurance, and personal relationships, should count as compensable injuries. Although compensation systems have traditionally been limited to cases involving physical injury for which someone could be legally liable, social harms, including lawful discrimination, may injure many HIV vaccine recipients. Social harm also serves to distinguish HIV vaccines from other vaccines. It may be difficult to determine whether discrimination resulted from taking an HIV vaccine or from other factors. At the same time, the cost of compensating lost earnings, housing, insurance, and even personal relationships, may be no higher than compensating similar losses resulting from permanent physical injuries.

Finally, injuries do not always appear in a single episode. Thus, it will be necessary to determine whether adverse reactions that aggravate or worsen existing health conditions should be compensable. Some adverse reactions result in death, although death may not be immediate. It may be impossible to determine whether death resulted from another compensable injury until more is known about adverse reactions to HIV vaccines.

Causation

If a compensation program is limited to injuries that are caused by an HIV vaccine, then causation must be determined. In the absence of a list of compensable injuries (and no complete list will be available immediately) and for injuries that do not appear on such a list, a procedure for deciding causation in individual cases is needed. Like tort law, most compensation programs place the burden of proving causation on the injured person. As a practical matter, however, the injured person is the least likely to be able to find the evidence needed to prove causation. The same factors that make a list of compensable injuries impossible may preclude proving causation. Some presumptions could be used to overcome this difficulty, such as presuming causation for any injury that cannot be explained by credible scientific or medical evidence as caused by something other than the vaccine. Alternatively, a reduced amount of compensation might be provided in some circumstances in which causation cannot be established.

The standard of proof, applicable to all requirements for compensation, affects decision making about causation in particular. Most programs use the preponderance of the evidence standard, which may be the standard most favorable to claimants. More stringent standards, like clear and convincing evidence, may be too difficult to meet, at least for many years. The standard of beyond a reasonable doubt, ordinarily reserved for criminal prosecutions and, in some states, for civil commitment, seems inappropriate and probably would be met very rarely whether one was trying to prove or disprove causation.

The type of evidence that should be admissible to prove or disprove causation may create problems. How much weight should be given to the opinion of individual treating physicians? Should epidemiological studies be admitted and, if so, how might they inform individual cases? Should the testimony of the injured person be sufficient to prove causation or must it be corroborated? What type of evidence should be required, permitted, and excluded to prove causation of social harms?

Compensation Benefits

The type and amount of compensation available affect both the program's attractiveness to potential claimants and its overall cost. If claimants retain the option to file lawsuits as an alternative to using the compensation program, then awards may have to be reasonably comparable to those available after litigation in order to attract claimants away from court. Of course, other program features, such as expeditious decisions, may offer sufficient attractions, but they may not be fully operational in the early years of a program.

Compensation may be provided for several types of losses. Medical expenses are the most common. These may include hospital and physician expenses, rehabilitative expenses, special education, vocational training, behavioral therapy, case management, residential and custodial care, medical and special equipment, adaptive construction to refit a home, and travel expenses related to obtaining care. It is difficult to justify limiting most of these expenses, especially those paid out of pocket. Many compensation programs do not compensate expenses that are paid for by health or accident insurance.[140] Whether such reimbursed expenses should be compensated depends upon who should bear the ultimate loss, the compensation program or the health or accident insurer. If it is appropriate for the health insurer to bear the loss, then the program might enroll the injured person in a health insurance program (if not already enrolled) rather than attempt to estimate and compensate future medical expenses.

If any health care reform succeeded in providing universal health insurance coverage, then a compensation program that did not cover insured expenses would be able to minimize payments in this category. It should be noted, however, that no health reform proposal contemplates covering long term care for permanent disabilities, so that the compensation program might be expected to do so.

Compensation for lost earnings is intended to enable an injured person to pay daily living expenses. Lost earnings can be calculated on the basis of an individual's actual losses, which pays high income people more than low wage earners, or on the basis of a standard formula independent of actual income. The use of actual losses is consistent with tort litigation practice but generally fails to compensate those who have no earnings, especially women with children who are not in the paid workforce. Standard formulas have been used in the case of young disabled children who will never be able to work, and could be applied to others.

In the case of death, many compensation systems pay a fixed dollar benefit in lieu of other forms of compensation. The size of the benefit varies with the nature of the program, although it is ordinarily less than the amount payable in the case of permanent injury which is intended to provide for living expenses. If the benefit were intended to replace the earnings that would have supported the decedent's family, however, it might be calculated in the same manner as lost earnings. If an injured person who has received compensation for the injury later dies, a death benefit could be paid or not, depending upon the purpose of the payment.

Compensation for social harms could be limited to actual losses, such as lost earnings, medical expenses that would have been covered by lost health insurance (or the amount of a more expensive policy, if obtainable), the increased cost of housing, and similar expenses. Additional amounts to compensate for any damage to one's reputation might also be considered, although these could be included in non-economic damages.

Noneconomic damages are intended to provide some compensation for the pain and suffering occasioned by injury. In tort practice, such compensation is often used to pay attorneys' fees in contingency fee arrangements, so that a plaintiff can at least be reimbursed for out-of-pocket expenses (although some fees can exceed the amount of noneconomic damages). If attorneys' fees are separately compensated, there may be less financial need for non-economic damages. But there may be reasons to compensate for pain and suffering, especially in cases of permanent injury and if the program intends to compete with litigation. Programs like the National Vaccine Injury Compensation Program limit noneconomic damages to a maximum amount, presumably to control at least one program cost.

It is also possible to provide fixed-dollar benefit payments in lieu of itemized compensation for losses and expenses, as does the Radiation Exposure Compensation Act (42 U.S.C. 2210 et seq.) and the United Kingdom's Vaccine Damage Payments Act (Current Law Statutes Anno. 1979, Ch.17). Fixing awards at a uniform amount obviously simplifies decision making and reduces administrative costs, but it does not purport to compensate for actual individual losses.

---

[140]Currently, some health insurance plans cover treatment for adverse reactions from investigative treatments. Other insurance plans, however, do not cover ordinary and necessary care that is required as a result of participating in an experimental activity such as a vaccine trial, reasoning that the care would not have been required but for the experimental procedure (173).

If claimants are permitted to be represented by attorneys, then the program will have to pay something toward their attorneys' fees, at least in the case of those who cannot afford to hire an attorney. Attorneys may be seen as necessary by claimants who are unfamiliar with the system and unprepared to prove causation. It may be cheaper to grant attorneys' fees to all claimants than to implement an income or means test to determine who can and cannot afford to pay themselves. The amount payable for attorneys' fees affects the willingness of attorneys to represent claimants. The amount can be determined on a case-by-case basis by the decisionmaker. Although this requires additional administrative time, there is precedent for determining what is reasonable. Alternatively, a fee schedule could be used if one could be developed that was sufficiently flexible to account for variations in the type of cases expected under the program.

Mode of Payment

Traditionally, payments have been made in lump sums which require predicting future losses and reducing them to a present value. More recently, periodic payments have been used to spread out payments, reduce immediate costs, and minimize the chance that the recipient will use or invest the whole amount unwisely and be left indigent. An alternative is for the compensation program to purchase an annuity or pension that provides periodic income to cover anticipated expenses. This approach is generally less expensive than periodic payments because the premiums are often less than the total payouts. If annuities are used and the injured person later dies, a decision will have to be made concerning who—the program or the injured person's survivors—should be entitled to any death benefit. As noted above, an alternative to making payments for medical expenses would be to purchase health or long term care insurance for the injured person, which would function in much the same way as annuities, although future premiums would not necessarily be fixed at the time of purchase.

Decisionmaking Authority

A compensation program can be organized and operated in many different ways. The most important administrative decisions are who has the authority to make decisions about claimant eligibility and awards, and how it is exercised. In the administrative agency model, such as Social Security, the authority to make decisions is vested with an administrative agency. Proceedings are often informal and recourse is limited. An independent agency or review board can perform the same functions, as do some worker compensation commissions. This may be preferred when there is a reason to avoid linking compensation decisions to a particular government agency.

Alternatively, decisionmaking authority can be exercised by one or more federal or state courts. Federal courts created under Article III of the U.S. Constitution require a "case or controversy" as a condition of jurisdiction, so that the decision making process may have to have both a claimant and a respondent or defendant, increasing the likelihood of creating a litigation-like atmosphere. An Article I court, like the U.S. Court of Federal Claims that hears National Vaccine Injury Compensation cases, does not necessarily require an identified defendant; the federal government is identified as the respondent and is presumed to be the target of a claim for payment. Special masters, like those who decide cases in the National Vaccine Injury Compensation Program, could be used to expedite decision making in proceedings that are less formal that court hearings. With respect to HIV vaccine related injuries, the simplest means of creating a compensation program may be to add HIV vaccines to the list of vaccines covered by the National Vaccine Injury Compensation Program.

The degree of discretion granted to decision makers can affect the efficiency of the program. The more specific the legislation governing the program, the less freedom decision makers have. Specificity is often used to prevent arbitrariness. But it may also require frequent amendments to the legislation to adjust to unanticipated problems or changing conditions. If the administering agency has the confidence of those who participate in the program, it might be granted the authority to make regulations governing many administrative procedures in order to reduce the rigidity that detailed legislation can produce.

Many compensation programs specify time limits for deciding claims in order to promote expeditious decisionmaking. Speed and informality may be a program's main advantages over litigation. Realistic time limits depend upon the complexity of the decisions to be made. More time is required to establish causation where there is scientific uncertainty than where there is clear evidence. More time is required to prove what is needed to compensate an individual when compensation is calculated on the basis of actual losses than when it is computed according to a schedule. If time limits are imposed, then the program should specify the consequences of exceeding a time limit, such as automatic payment or denial of compensation. Both alternatives can create incentives to delay dispute resolution and can operate unfairly in circumstances of unavoidable delay.

Not everyone will agree with the decisions of a compensation program. Should determinations of eligibility and compensation be appealable? Administrative programs ordinarily have an internal review mechanism, with appeals possible in at least some cases to the courts. The availability and extent of appeals may take into account the amount of compensation permitted by the program and whether claimants have the option of taking their case to court instead of the compensation program.

Relationship to Tort Law

A compensation program can be an exclusive source of compensation or an optional alternative to tort litigation. If the program's major goal is to eliminate tort litigation, then exclusivity may be preferred. If the program intends to make compensation more equitable and also retain any deterrent effect, then making the program optional may be preferable. The program could still be made a required "first resort" that must be used before proceeding in tort.

Many compensation programs have a right of subrogation that grants to the program any rights that a successful claimant might have against a third party who would be legally liable for the claimant's injuries. The program is then entitled to sue the third party for reimbursement of the compensation paid to the claimant. This both replenishes the program's funds for awards (although the cost of litigation may increase other expenditures) and shifts the cost of compensation (but not administration) to the responsible party. This is useful where it is beneficial to retain the link between responsibility for injury and financial loss. As a practical matter, however, proving that a third party is liable is difficult in vaccine cases, and is likely to be especially difficult in HIV vaccine cases, so the opportunities for subrogation may be limited.

Conditions on Program Operation

When the effects of a new program are uncertain, the authorizing legislation sometimes limits its period of operation with a sunset clause. If at the end of the time period the program is operating successfully, it may be reauthorized; if not, it may expire without doing further damage. Continued authorization may be contingent on the occurrence of certain conditions, such as the initial or continued marketing of an HIV vaccine or pricing. For example, the program might be continued only if an acceptable vaccine remains on the market and its price does not exceed a specified amount, or only if vaccines are sold to government at below-market prices for distribution to indigent persons.

If the costs of the program are not reasonably predictable when it begins operation, the continuation of the program may be made conditional on the availability of funds for either administration or compensation or both. A program that risks termination, however, may be unable to attract sufficient support to achieve its goals.

Financing

A compensation program may be financed by society as a whole, by those who produce, sell or administer the vaccines that result in injury, or by those who purchase or benefit from the vaccines. Compensation may be funded from the same or different sources as administrative expenses. Financing by society generally means government funding from general tax revenues. The feasibility of such funding may depend upon budget limitations. If the program wishes to incorporate an element of risk deterrence, then it may prefer to have those who produce vaccines fund the program. This can be done by levying a tax on each dose of vaccine sold or distributed or by assessing vaccine makers according to the awards paid that involve their vaccines. In this way, vaccine makers retain some financial responsibility for the injuries caused by their vaccines, but are relieved of the burden of litigation. Of course, some or all of the assessments or taxes will be passed on to vaccine purchasers as part of the vaccine price. Where government buys significant quantities of the vaccine, government will bear a significant share of the ultimate cost of the compensation program.

Supplements to Compensation Programs

Compensation programs deal only with compensating injuries. They do not prevent injuries. Thus, if a no-fault compensation system supplants all or part of tort liability, other mechanisms must be in place to prevent or deter avoidable risks.

ALTERNATIVE INCENTIVES FOR HIV VACCINE DEVELOPMENT

Compensation programs deal with the consequences of vaccine use after a vaccine is developed. By themselves, they cannot guarantee that any vaccine is developed. Thus, if HIV vaccines are insufficiently attractive to private industry for reasons of the difficulty and expense of research or an unrewarding market, other initiatives will be necessary to encourage vaccine development (100).

An Institute of Medicine committee, formed to study ways to foster U.S. industry participation in vaccine development for the Children's Vaccine Initiative, concluded that the most significant disincentives to producing new and better vaccines primarily for use in the developing world were the cost of research and clinical trials and the expected limitations on the price at which vaccines could be sold (121).[141]

The Committee recommended that the fderal government create a National Vaccine Authority to support new vaccine product development (121). This type of initiative could be used to foster research and development of HIV vaccines. A National Vaccine Authority or similar entity could provide grants to private industry to develop HIV vaccines. It could also reduce the risks and costs to industry by establishing product development programs, production facilities to make investigational vaccines for clinical trials, and assistance in complying with FDA regulations. In addition, the authority might arrange procurement contracts to create a guaranteed market for approved vaccines. Estimates of the annual operating costs of a National Vaccine Authority ($55 to $75 million) for all vaccines, including HIV vaccines, are about the same as estimates of annual future compensation awards for the National Vaccine Injury Compensation Program (about $60 million).

California created a research assistance program to provide grants to California vaccine makers to test candidate HIV vaccines in clinical trials.[142] In order to ensure a market, the state also agreed to purchase a minimum number of doses of an approved HIV vaccine from a California HIV vaccine maker and to subsidize the price of vaccines to guarantee a price of $20 per dose. Establishing a purchase price before a vaccine has even

[141] The author served as a member of that committee.

[142] See State Compensation Programs above.

TABLE 4-6: Incentives to HIV Vaccine Research and Development
Mechanisms for increased collaboration and information sharing among vaccine researchers to increase productivity and expedite research.
Simplification of collaborative arrangements between government and industry researchers.
Expanded access to preclinical nonhuman animal models for testing investigational vaccines.
▪ Tax deductions or credits for investments in vaccine development.
▪ Expedited review by the FDA of applications for vaccine licenses.
▪ International harmonization of national vaccine licensing standards.
▪ Expanded patent protection for approved vaccines.
▪ Guaranteed purchases of vaccine supplies by government.
▪ National coordination of vaccine research and distribution policies.

SOURCE: Office of Technology Assessment, 1995.

been tested in field trials is difficult. A future licensed HIV vaccine might be sold at a more than $20 per dose, and vaccine companies may be unable or unwilling to agree to any specific price before a vaccine is approved. Nonetheless, such efforts are examples of policy innovations that might be considered, with appropriate modifications, at the national level.

Other actions, such as those listed in Table 4-6, may facilitate scientific research or encourage HIV vaccine development. Although beyond the scope of this report, they target specific points in the vaccine research and development process and are likely to have a more direct effect on HIV vaccine development than future compensation programs.

Conclusion

The initiatives supporting vaccine research and development recognize that neither limitations on liability nor compensation for injury can produce new HIV vaccines. It is not clear that a new compensation program is needed to abate fears of liability on the part of most companies engaged in HIV vaccine research. A compensation program cannot guarantee that important research will be done, that new products will be brought to market, or that any new products will be affordable to those who need them.

This is not to suggest that a compensation system should not be considered. But a compensation program can and should be adopted on its own merits. Society might feel an ethical obligation to compensate those who take an HIV vaccine in an effort to abate the epidemic. Even if society does not feel an ethical obligation itself, it might conclude that compensation is nonetheless desirable as a means of rewarding those who suffer adverse reactions in an effort to prevent the continuing spread of HIV infection and the tragic toll of AIDS. The reasons for providing compensation, however, should be carefully considered in light of their application to other types of injuries.

It will be especially important to consider why people who have adverse reactions to a vaccine to prevent HIV infection or progression to AIDS should receive special compensation when people who have adverse reactions to drugs like Zidovudine, ddI and ddC, do not. Special compensation for HIV-negative people may give the appearance of social indifference to the needs of people living with HIV infection. A public debate about the justification for compensating specific injuries may offer a valuable opportunity to reconsider the ways in which responsibility for injuries and illnesses of all kinds should be allocated.

CHAPTER 4 REFERENCES

1. Accident Compensation Corporation, *Unintentional Injury: New Zealand's Accident Compensation Scheme* (Wellington, New Zealand: Accident Compensation Corporation, 1988).

2. AIDS Action Foundation, *HIV Preventive Vaccines: Social, Ethical, and Political Considerations for Domestic Efficacy Trials,* Report of a Working Group Convened by the AIDS Action Foundation (Washington, DC, July 1994).
3. Altman, L.K., "After Setback, First Large AIDS Vaccine Trials Are Planned," *New York Times,* p.C3, Nov. 29, 1994.
4. American Law Institute, *Restatement (Second) of Torts* (Philadelphia, PA: 1977).
5. American Law Institute, *Restatement of the Law of Torts: Product Liability,* Council Draft 2 (Philadelphia, PA: Sept. 2, 1994).
6. American Law Institute's Reporters' Study on Enterprise Responsibility for Personal Injury, *San Diego Law Review* 30:371-404, 1993.
7. Anders, G., "Vital Statistics: Disputed Cost of Creating a Drug," *Wall Street Journal,* p.B1, Nov. 9, 1993.
8. Annas, G.J., "Scientific Evidence in the Courtroom: The Death of the *Frye* Rule," *New England Journal of Medicine* 330: 1018-21, 1994.
9. Annas, G.J., and Grodin, M.A., *The Nazi Doctors and the Nuremberg Code: Human Rights in Human Experimentation* (New York, NY: Oxford University Press, 1992).
10. Appelbaum, P.S., et al., "False Hopes and Best Data: Consent to Research and the Therapeutic Misconception," *Hastings Center Report* 17:20-24, April 1987.
11. Armstrong, D., and Allen, S., "Task Force Hits Radiation Tests at State Schools," *The Boston Globe* pp. 1,15, Apr. 15, 1994.
12. Arno, P.S., and Feiden, K.L., *Against the Odds: The Story of AIDS Drug Development, Politics & Profit* (New York, NY: HarperCollins, 1992).
13. Arnold, A.J., "Developing, Testing, and Marketing an AIDS Vaccine: Legal Concerns for Manufacturers," *University of Pennsylvania Law Review* 139:1077-1121, 1991.
14. Baier, K. "Moral and Legal Responsibility," *Medical Innovation and Bad Outcomes: Legal, Social, and Ethical Responses,* M. Siegler (ed.) (Ann Arbor, MI: Health Administration Press, 1987).
15. Baynes, T.E., "Liability for Vaccine Related Injuries: Public Health Considerations and Some Reflections on the Swine Flu Experience," *St. Louis University Law Journal* 21:44-75, 1977.
16. Bergen, R.P., "Insurance Coverage for Clinical Investigation," *Journal of the American Medical Association* 201:305-306, 1967.
17. Bixby, L., and Spencer-Molloy, F., "The Struggle for Money to Fuel a Research Mission," *The Hartford Courant,* p. A1, Feb. 8, 1993.
18. Blum, A., "Halcion Stirs Litigation Storm," *National Law Journal,* A1, A23, Apr. 11, 1994.
19. Boston Consulting Group, Inc., "The Changing Environment for U.S. Pharmaceuticals: The Role of Pharmaceutical Companies in a Systems Approach to Health Care," monograph sponsored by Pfizer Inc. (Boston, MA: April 1993).
20. Bovbjerg, R.R., "Legislation on Medical Malpractice: Further Developments and a Preliminary Report Card," *University of California, Davis Law Review* 22:499-556, 1989.
21. Bovbjerg, R.R., "Problems and Solutions in Medical Malpractice: Comments on Chapters Six and Seven." *The Liability Maze: The Impact of Liability Law on Safety and Innovation*, P.W., Huber and Litan R.E. (eds.)(Washington, DC: The Brookings Institution, 1991).
22. Bovbjerg, R.R., et al.,"Valuing Life and Limb in Tort: Scheduling 'Pain and Suffering'," *Northwestern Law Review* 83:908-976, 1989.
23. Braham, D., "No Fault Compensation Finnish Style," *The Lancet* 733-36, Sept. 24, 1988.

24. Burke, D.S., "Human HIV Vaccine Trials: Does Antibody-Dependent Enhancement Pose a Genuine Risk?" *Perspectives in Biology and Medicine* 35:511-530, 1992.
25. Burstin, H.R., et al., "Do the Poor Sue More? A Case-Control Study of Malpractice Claims and Socioeconomic Status," *Journal of the American Medical Association* 270: 1697-1701, 1993.
26. Calabresi, G., *The Cost of Accidents: A Legal and Economic Analysis* (New Haven, CT: Yale University Press, 1970).
27. Cardon, P.V., et al., "Injuries to Research Subjects: A Survey of Investigators," *New England Journal of Medicine* 295:650-654, 1976.
28. Carley, W.M., "Fatal Flaws, Artificial Heart Valves That Fail Are Linked to Falsified Records," *Wall Street Journal,* p. A1, Nov. 7, 1991.
29. Chase, M., "Multiple Mutating HIV Strains Stymie Researchers Seeking a Vaccine for AIDS," *Wall Street Journal*, p. B1, May 26, 1992.
30. Chesebro, K., "Galileo's Retort: Peter Huber's Junk Scholarship," *American University Law Review* 42:1637-1726, 1993.
31. Clayton, E.W., "Liability Exposure When Offspring Are Injured Because of Their Parents' Participation in Clinical Trials," *Women and Health Research: Ethical and Legal Issues of Including Women in Clinical Studies,* A.C. Mastroianni, et al. (eds.) (Washington, D.C.: National Academy Press, 1994).
32. Cohen, J., "Is Liability Slowing AIDS Vaccines?" *Science* 256:168-170, 1992.
33. Cohen, J., "Childhood Vaccines: The R&D Factor," *Science* 259:1528-1529, 1993.
34. Cohen, J., "Jitters Jeopardize AIDS Vaccine Trials," *Science* 262:980-981, 1993.
35. Cohen, J., "AIDS Vaccines: Are Researchers Racing Toward Success, Or Crawling?" *Science* 265:1373-75, 1994.
36. Cohen, J., "AIDS Vaccines: Will Media Reports KO Upcoming Real-Life Trials?" *Science* 264:1660, 1994.
37. Cohen, J., "Bumps on the Vaccine Road," *Science* 265:1371-73, 1994.
38. Cohen, J., "Peer Review Triumphs Over Lobbying," *Science* 263:463, 1994.
39. Cohen, J., "The HIV Vaccine Paradox," *Science* 264:1072-74, 1994.
40. Cohen, J., "U.S. Panel Votes to Delay Real-World Vaccine Trials," *Science* 264:1839, 1994.
41. Cotton, P., "Infants, Science May Lose as Liability Is Blamed for Company Pullout from HIV Prevention Trial," *Journal of the American Medical Association* 268:1987, 1991-1992, 1992.
42. Council for International Organizations of Medical Sciences, *International Ethical Guidelines for Biomedical Research Involving Human Subjects* (Geneva, Switzerland: World Health Organization, 1993).
43. Danaher, E.A., "Products Liability Overhaul: Strict Liability Is Coming to Japan," *The National Law Journal,* pp. 25, 28-29, Feb. 7, 1994.
44. Daniels, S., and Andrews, L., "The Shadow of the Law: Jury Decisions in Obstetrics and Gynecology Cases," *Medical Liability and the Delivery of Obstetrical Care,* Institute of Medicine (Washington, DC: National Academy Press, 1989).
45. Daniels, S., and Martin, J., "Myth and Reality in Punitive Damages," *Minnesota Law Review* 75:1-64, 1990.
46. Danzon, P., *Medical Malpractice: Theory, Practice, and Public Policy* (Cambridge, MA: Harvard University Press, 1985).
47. Dickinson, S.L.J., "Clinical Trial Reversals Forcing Biotech Firms to Refine Strategy," *The Scientist* 8:1, 6-7, 1994.
48. DiMasi, J.A., et al., "New Drug Development in the United States, 1963-90," *Clinical Pharmacology and Therapeutics* 50:471-86, 1991.
49. Dungworth, T., *Product Liability and the Business Sector: Litigation Trends in Federal Courts* (Santa Monica, CA: RAND Institute for Civil Justice, 1987).

50. Eisenberg, T., and Henderson, J.A., "Inside the Quiet Revolution in Products Liability," *UCLA Law Review* 39:731-810, 1992.
51. Englard, I., "The System Builders: A Critical Appraisal of Modern American Tort Theory," *Journal of Legal Studies* 9:27-69, 1980.
52. Epstein, R., "A Theory of Strict Liability," *Journal of Legal Studies* 2:151-204, 1973.
53. Faden, R.R., and Beauchamp, T.L., *A History and Theory of Informed Consent* (New York, NY: Oxford University Press, 1986).
54. Felsenthal, Edward, "Vaccine Injury Claims, *Wall Street Journal*, p. B5, Mar. 29, 1994.
55. Fersko, R.S., and Connolly, M.J., "AIDS Effort Sparks Patent Concerns," *New Jersey Law Journal* July 12, 1993.
56. Fineberg, H.V., and Nustadt, R.E., *The Epidemic That Never Was: Policy Making and the Swine Flu Scare* (New York, NY: Vintage Books, 1983).
57. Fisher, L.M., "Ciba-Geigy Deal with Chiron Set," *New York Times*, pp. D1, D6, Nov. 22, 1994.
58. Flannery, E.F., and Greenberg, S.N., "Liability Exposure for Exclusion and Inclusion of Women as Subjects in Clinical Studies," *Women and Health Research: Ethical and Legal Issues of Including Women in Clinical Studies*, vol. 2., Report of the Committee on the Ethical and Legal Issues Relating to the Inclusion of Women in Clinical Studies, Institute of Medicine, A.C. Mastroianni, et al. (eds.) (Washington, DC: National Academy Press, 1994).
59. Fletcher, G.P., "Fairness and Utility in Tort Theory," *Harvard Law Review* 85:537-573, 1972.
60. Galanter, M., "Reading the Landscape of Disputes: What We Know and Don't Know (and Think We Know) About Our Allegedly Contentious and Litigious Society," *UCLA Law Review* 31:4-71, 1983.
61. Garber, S., *Product Liability and the Economics of Pharmaceuticals and Medical Devices*, R-4285-ICJ (Santa Monica, CA: RAND Institute for Civil Justice, 1993).
62. Gellhorn, W., "Medical Malpractice Litigation (U.S.) Medical Mishap Compensation (N.Z.)," *Cornell Law Review* 73:170-211, 1988.
63. Gilhooley, M., "Learned Intermediaries, Prescription Drugs, and Patient Information," *St. Louis University Law Journal* 30: 633-702, 1985.
64. Grabowski, H.G., and Vernon, J.M., *The Regulation of Pharmaceuticals: Balancing the Benefits and Risks* (Washington, DC: American Enterprise Institute, 1983).
65. Grodin, M.A., and Glantz, L.H. (eds.), *Children as Research Subjects: Science, Ethics and Law* (New York, NY: Oxford University Press, 1994).
66. Groufein, W.P., and Kinney, E.D., "Controlling Large Malpractice Claims: The Unexpected Impact of Damage Cops," *Journal of Health Politics, Policy and Law* 16:441-464, 1991.
67. Hamilton, J., "Biotech: An Industry Crowded with Players Faces an Ugly Reckoning," *Business Week* 84-88,90,92, Sept. 24, 1994.
68. Hansen, R.W., "The Pharmaceutical Development Process: Estimates of Development Costs and Times and the Effects of Proposed Regulatory Changes," *Issues in Pharmaceutical Economics*, R. I. Chien, (ed.) (Lexington, MA: Lexington Books, 1979).
69. Harris, D., et al., *Compensation and Support for Illness and Injury* (New York, NY: Oxford University Press, 1984).
70. Harvard Medical Practice Study, *Patients, Doctors, and Lawyers: Medical Injury, Malpractice Litigation, and Patient Compensation in New York*, The Report of the Harvard Medical Malpractice Study to the State of New York, 1990.
71. Henderson, J.A., Jr., and Eisenberg, T., "The Quiet Revolution in Products Liability: An Empirical Study of Legal Change," *UCLA Law Review* 37:479-553, 1990.
72. Henderson, J.A.Jr., and Twerski, A.D., "Doctrinal Collapse in Product Liability:

The Empty Shell of Failure To Warn," *New York University Law Review* 65:265-327, 1990.

73. Hensler, D., Vaiana, M., and Kakalik, J., *Trends in Tort Litigation: The Story Behind the Statistics* (Santa Monica, CA: RAND Institute for Civil Justice, 1987).
74. Hensler, D., et al., Compensation for Accidental Injuries in the U.S. (Santa Monica, CA: RAND Institute for Civil Justice, 1991).
75. Hilts, P.J., "Agency Faults a U.C.L.A. Study for Suffering of Mental Patients," *New York Times*, pp. A1, B10, Mar. 10, 1994.
76. Hogan, N., "Shielded from Liability," *American Bar Association Journal* 56-59, May 1994.
77. Hoke, F., "Optimistic Report Predicts Rebound for Biotechnology," *The Scientist* 8:1,11, Oct. 31, 1994.
78. Holmes, O.W., *The Common Law* (Boston, MA: Little, Brown, 1881 [1963 edition]).
79. Huber, P.W., "Safety and the Second Best: The Hazards of Public Risk Management in the Courts," *Columbia Law Review* 85:277-337, 1985.
80. Huber, P.W., *Liability: The Legal Revolution and Its Consequences* (New York, NY: Basic Books, Inc., 1988).
81. Huber, P.W., and Litan, R.E. (eds.), *The Liability Maze: The Impact of Liability Law on Safety and Innovation*, (Washington, DC: The Brookings Institution, 1991).
82. Institute of Medicine, *Vaccine Supply and Innovation* (Washington, DC: National Academy Press, 1985).
83. Institute of Medicine, *Medical Liability and the Delivery of Obstetrical Care* (Washington, DC: National Academy Press, 1989).
84. Institute of Medicine, *Developing New Contraceptives: Obstacles and Opportunities*, Report of the Committee on Contraceptive Development (Washington, DC: National Academy Press, 1990).
85. Institute of Medicine, *Adverse Effects of Pertussis and Rubella Vaccines* (Washington, DC: National Academy Press, 1991).
86. Institute of Medicine, *Expanding Access to Investigational Therapies for HIV Infection and AIDS: Summary of a Conference* (Washington, DC: National Academy Press, 1991).
87. Institute of Medicine, *DPT Vaccine and Chronic Nervous System Dysfunction: A New Analysis* (Washington, DC: National Academy Press, 1994).
88. Jones, J.H., *Bad Blood: The Tuskegee Syphilis Experiment* (New York, NY: Free Press, 1981).
89. Kahneman, D., Slovic, P., and Tversky, A. (eds.), *Judgments Under Uncertainty: Heuristics and Biases* (Cambridge, England: Cambridge University Press, 1982).
90. Katz, J., *Experimentation with Human Beings* (New York, NY: Russell Sage, 1972).
91. Katz, J., *The Silent World of Doctor and Patient* (New York, NY: The Free Press, 1984).
92. Katz, J., "Human Experimentation and Human Rights," *St. Louis University Law Journal* 38:7-54, 1993.
93. Keeton, W.P., "The Meaning of Defect in Products Liability Law—A Review of Basic Principles," *Missouri Law Review* 45:579-596, 1980.
94. Keeton, W.P., et al. (eds.), *Prosser and Keeton on the Law of Torts*, 5th Ed. (St. Paul, MN: West Publishing Co., 1984).
95. The Keystone Center, *Final Report of the Keystone AIDS Vaccine Liability Project* (Keystone, CO: The Keystone Center, 1990).
96. The Keystone Center, "Final Report of the Keystone AIDS Vaccine Liability Project," *Vaccine* 9:703-709, 1991.
97. Kitch, E.W., "The Vaccine Dilemma," *Issues in Science and Technology* II(2):108-121, 1986.
98. Koff, W.C., and Hoth, D.F., "Development and Testing of AIDS Vaccines," *Science*, 241:426-42, 1988.
99. Koff, W.C., and Six, H.R. (eds.), *Vaccine Research and Developments* (New York, NY: Marcel Dekker, Inc., 1992).

100. Koff, W.C., "The Next Steps Toward a Global AIDS Vaccine," *Science* 266:1335-1337, 1994.
101. Kong, D., "1,800 Tested in Radiation Experiments," *The Boston Globe,* pp.8, 22, Feb. 20, 1994.
102. Kramer, P., *Listening to Prozac* (New York, NY: Viking, 1992).
103. Ladimer, I., "Clinical Research Insurance," *Journal of Chronic Diseases* 16:1229, 1233, 1963.
104. Landes, W.M., and Posner, R.A., *The Economic Structure of Tort Law* (Cambridge, MA: Harvard University Press, 1987).
105. Lasagna, L., "The Chilling Effect of Product Liability on New Drug Development," *The Liability Maze: The Impact of Liability Law on Safety and Innovation*, Huber, P.W., and Litan, R.E. (eds.) (Washington, DC: The Brookings Institution, 1991).
106. Letvin, N.L., "Vaccines Against Human Immunodeficiency Virus—Progress and Prospects," *New England Journal of Medicine* 329:1400-1405, 1993.
107. Levine, C., "Women and HIV Research: The Barriers to Equity," *Evaluation Review* 14:447-463, 1990.
108. Levine, C., "Women as Research Subjects: New Priorities, New Questions," *Emerging Issues in Biomedical Policy: An Annual Review,* vol. 2., Blank, R.H., and Bonnicksen, A.L. (eds.) (New York, NY: Columbia University Press, 1993).
109. Localio, A.R., et al., "Relationship Between Malpractice Claims and Adverse Events Due to Negligence: Results of the Harvard Medical Practice Study III," *New England Journal of Medicine* 325:245-251, 1991.
110. Lurie, P., et al., "Ethical, Behavioral, and Social Aspects of HIV Vaccine Trials in Developing Countries," *Journal of the American Medical Association* 271:295, 1994.
111. Madge, N., et al., "The National Childhood Encephalophathy Study: A 10-Year Follow-up. A Report of the Medical, Social, Behavioral and Educational Outcomes After Serious, Acute, Neurologic Illness in Early Childhood," *Developmental Medicine & Child Neurology* 35 (suppl. no. 68):1-118, 1993.
112. Mariner, W.K., "Compensation Programs for Vaccine-Related Injury Abroad: A Comparative Analysis," *St. Louis University Law Journal* 31:599-654, 1987.
113. Mariner, W.K., "Informed Consent in the Post-Modern Era," *Law & Social Inquiry* 13:385-406, 1988.
114. Mariner, W.K., "The Ethical Conduct of Clinical Trials of HIV Vaccines," *Evaluation Review* 14:538-564, 1990.
115. Mariner, W.K., "The National Vaccine Injury Compensation Program," *Health Affairs* 11:255-265, 1992.
116. Mariner, W.K., "Compensation for Research Injuries," *Women and Health Research: Ethical and Legal Issues of Including Women in Clinical Studies,* vol. 2., Report of the Committee on the Ethical and Legal Issues Relating to the Inclusion of Women in Clinical Studies, Institute of Medicine, A.C. Mastroianni, et al., (eds.) (Washington, DC: National Academy Press, 1994).
117. Mariner, W.K., and Gallo, R.C., "Getting to Market: The Scientific and Legal Climate for Developing an AIDS Vaccine," *Law, Medicine & Health Care* 15:17-26, 1987.
118. Mastroianni, A.C., Faden, R., Federman, D. (eds.), *Women and Health Research: Ethical and Legal Issues of Including Women in Clinical Studies,* 2 vols., Report of the Committee on the Ethical and Legal Issues Relating to the Inclusion of Women in Clinical Studies, Institute of Medicine (Washington, D.C.: National Academy Press, 1994).
119. McKenna, R.M., "The Impact of Product Liability Law on the Development of a Vaccine Against the AIDS Virus," *University of Chicago Law Review* 55:943-64, 1988.
120. Miller, D.L., et al., "Pertussis Immunization and Serious Acute Neurological Illness in Children," *British Medical Journal* 307:1171-1176, 1993.

121. Mitchell, V.S., Philipose, N., and Sanford, J.P. (eds.), *The Children's Vaccine Initiative: Achieving the Vision, Report of the Committee on the Children's Vaccine Initiative, Institute of Medicine* (Washington, DC: National Academy Press, 1993).
122. National Institute of Allergy and Infectious Diseases, "AIDS Vaccines Contracts Pave Way for Large National and International Studies," *News from NIAID,* Oct. 10, 1993a.
123. National Institute of Allergy and Infectious Diseases Blue Ribbon Panel on Vaccine Research, *Summary* (Bethesda, MD: March 26, 1993b).
124. National Institute of Allergy and Infectious Diseases, "Chimpanzee Vaccine Model Protects Against HIV-1 Infection," *NIAID News,* Aug. 9, 1994a.
125. National Institute of Allergy and Infectious Diseases, "HIV Trials Continue But Without Expansion," *NIAID AIDS Agenda* 1,6, Summer 1994b.
126. National Institute of Allergy and Infectious Diseases, *Conference on Advances in AIDS Vaccine Development—Seventh Annual Meeting of the National Cooperative Vaccine Development Group for AIDS* (Bethesda, MD: 1994c).
127. National Commission for the Protection of Human Subjects of Biomedical and Behavioral Research, *The Belmont Report: Ethical Principles and Guidelines for the Protection of Human Subjects of Research* (Washington, DC: U.S. Government Printing Office, 1978).
128. Naude, A., "Two Worlds: Sales of Adult and Pediatric Vaccines, Pharmaceuticals," *Chemical Marketing Reporter* 245:SR28, March 7, 1994.
129. Neustadt, R.E., and Fineberg, H.V., *The Swine Flu Affair: Decision-Making on a Slippery Disease* (Washington, DC: Dept. of Health, Education, and Welfare, 1978).
130. O'Connell, J., "Offers That Can't Be Refused: Foreclosure of Personal Injury Claims by Defendants' Prompt Tender of Claimants' Net Economic Losses," *Northwestern University Law Review* 77:589-632, 1982.
131. O'Connell, J., and Kelly, C.B., *The Blame Game: Injuries, Insurance, and Injustice* (New York, NY: Basic Books, 1988).
132. Page, J., "'Generic Product Risks': The Case Against Comment k and for Strict Product Liability," *New York University Law Review* 58:853-891, 1983.
133. Palca, J., "Testing Target Date Looms, But Will the Vaccines Be Ready?" *Science* 257:1472-1473, 1992.
134. Peterson, M., *Civil Juries in the 1980's: Trends in Jury Trials and Verdicts in California and Cook County, Illinois* (Santa Monica, CA: The RAND Corporation, 1987).
135. Peterson, M., Sarma, S., and Shanley, M., *Punitive Damages: Empirical Findings* (Santa Monica, CA: RAND Institute for Civil Justice, 1987).
136. Pharmaceutical Manufacturers Association, American Medical Association, *Brief of the Pharmaceutical Manufacturers Association and the American Medical Association, as Amici Curiae in Support of Petitioner,* in *Pacific Mutual Life Insurance Company* v. *Haslip*, Supreme Court of the United States, May 31, 1990.
137. Pharmaceutical Manufacturers Association, *Statistical Fact Book* (Washington, DC: Pharmaceutical Manufacturers Association, 1991).
138. Philipson, T.J., and Posner, R.A., *Private Choices and Public Health: The AIDS Epidemic in an Economic Perspective* (Cambridge, MA: Harvard University Press, 1993).
139. Physicians GenR_X (Smithtown, NY: Data Pharmaceutica Inc., 1994).
140. Presidential Commission on the Human Immunodeficiency Virus Epidemic, *Report,* (Washington, D.C.: The White House, 1988).
141. President's Commission for the Study of Ethical Problems in Medicine and Biomedical and Behavioral Research, *Compensating for Research Injuries: The Ethical and Legal*

Implications of Programs to Redress Injured Subjects, vol. 1 (Washington, DC: U.S. Government Printing Office, 1982).
142. Prosser, W.L., and Keeton, P., *Prosser and Keeton On The Law of Torts* (St. Paul, MN: West Publication Co., 1984).
143. Reuter, P., *The Economic Consequences of Expanded Corporate Liability* (RAND Institute for Civil Justice, 1988).
144. Rheingold, P.D., "Products Liability - The Ethical Drug Manufacturer's Liability," *Rutgers Law Review* 18:947-1018, 1964.
145. Rheingold, P.D., "The MER/29 Story-An Instance of Successful Mass Disaster Litigation," *California Law Review* 56:116-148, 1968.
146. Rheingold, P.D., "The Expanding Liability of the Drug Manufacturer to the Consumer," *Food Drug & Cosmetic Law Journal* 40:135-44, 1985.
147. Robbins, A., and Freeman, P., "Obstacles to Developing Vaccines for the Third World," *Scientific American,* pp. 126-133, Nov. 1988.
148. Rosenberg, R., "Progress on AIDS Vaccine Boosted," *The Boston Globe* p. 47, Sept. 15, 1992.
149. Rosenfeld, "The Strict Products Liability Crisis and Beyond: Is There Hope for an AIDS Vaccine," *Jurimetrics* 31:187, 1991
150. Rosenthal, E., "Debate Fails to Explain Vaccine Costs," *New York Times* p. A8, Mar. 15, 1993.
151. Russell, C., "AIDS Work Is Stern Test of Optimism," *Washington Post* p. A1, April 29, 1984.
152. Rustad, M., *Demystifying Punitive Damages in Products Liability Cases: A Survey of a Quarter Century of Trial Verdicts* (Washington, DC: Rosco Pound Foundation, 1991).
153. Saks, M., "Do We Really Know Anything About the Behavior of the Tort Litigation System—And Why Not?," *University of Pennsylvania Law Review* 140:1147-1292 (1992).
154. Sanders, J., "The Bendectin Litigation: A Case Study in the Life Cycle of Mass Torts," *Hastings Law Journal* 43:301-418, 1992.
155. Schwartz, G.T., "The Character of Early American Tort Law," *UCLA Law Review* 36:641-718, 1989.
156. Schwartz, G.T., "The Beginning and the Possible End of the Rise of Modern American Tort Law," *Georgia Law Review* 26:601-702, 1992.
157. Schwartz, T.M., "Products Liability Law and Pharmaceuticals: New Developments and Divergent Trends," *Food Drug & Cosmetic Journal* 43:33-53, 1988.
158. Schwartz, V., "The Post-Sale Duty to Warn: Two Unfortunate Forks in the Road to a Reasonable Doctrine," *New York University Law Review* 58:892-904, 1983.
159. Schwartz, V.E. "Unavoidably Unsafe Products: Clarifying the Meaning and Policy Behind Comment K," *Washington & Lee Law Review* 42:1139-1148, 1985.
160. Scott, J., "Liability Protection Needed for Vaccines Studies, Experts Say," *Los Angeles Times*, p. A3, July 17, 1992.
161. Shavell, S., *Economic Analysis of Accident Law* (Cambridge, MA: Harvard University Press, 1987).
162. Shaw, Jr., D.C., Vice-President for Medical Affairs, Wyeth Laboratories, "Statement," *Vaccine Injury Compensation,* hearing before Subcommittee on Health and the Environment, Committee on Energy and Commerce, House of Representatives, U.S. Congress, December 19, 1984.
163. Shuck, P.H. (ed.), *Tort Law and the Public Interest* (New York, NY: W.W. Norton, 1991).
164. Shulman, S.R., "The Broader Message of Accutane," *American Journal of Public Health* 79:1565-68, 1989.
165. Shulman, S.R., and Lasagna, L. (eds.), *Trends in Product Liability Law and No-Fault Compensation for Drug-Induced Inju-*

ries (Boston: The Center for the Study of Drug Development, Tufts University, 1990).

166. Sloan, F.A., Mergenhagen, P.M., and Bovbjerg, R.R., "Effects of Tort Reform on the Value of Closed Medical Malpractice Claims: A Microanalysis," *Journal of Health Policy, Politics and Law* 14:663-89, 1989.
167. Slovic, P., "Perception of Risk," *Science* 236:280-285, 1987.
168. Smith, H. William, III, "Vaccinating AIDS Vaccine Manufacturers Against Product Liability," *Case Western Reserve Law Review* 42(1):207-254, 1992
169. Spencer-Molloy, F., "Pregnant Women to be Vaccinated in Pediatric AIDS Trial in State," *The Hartford Courant* p. A1, December 19, 1992.
170. Stark, F.H., "The National AIDS Vaccine Development and Compensation Act of 1992, H.R. 5893," Discussion Draft, August, 1992.
171. Stein, R.E., "The Development of an HIV Vaccine: Legal and Policy Aspects," in Koff, W.C., Six, H.R. (eds.), *Vaccine Research and Developments,* vol. 1, 1992.
172. Stein, R.E., "Insurance and Liability Issues in AIDS Vaccine Development," *AIDS Research and Human Retroviruses*, 9 (suppl. 1), 1993.
173. Stein, R.E., "Selected Issues of AIDS Vaccine Liability," contractor report prepared for the Office of Technology Assessment, U.S. Congress, Washington, DC, 1994.
174. Stratton, K.R., Howe, C.J., and Johnston, R.B.,Jr. (eds.), *Adverse Events Associated with Childhood Vaccines: Evidence Bearing on Causality* (Washington, DC: National Academy Press, 1994).
175. Sturmer, U., Koepke, J.E., and Reischel, B., *New EEC Product Liability: The U.S. in Comparison* (Cologne: Gerling-Konsern Allgemeine Versicherungs-AG, 1988).
176. Sugarman, S.D., *Doing Away with Personal Injury Law: New Compensation Mechanisms for Victims, Consumers, and Business* (New York, NY: Quorum Books, 1989).
177. Sunstein, C.R., *The Partial Constitution* (Cambridge, MA: Harvard University Press, 1993).
178. Swazey, J., "Prescription Drug Safety and Product Liability," *The Liability Maze: The Impact of Liability Law on Safety and Innovation*, Huber, P.W., and Litan, R.E. (eds.) (Washington, DC: The Brookings Institution, 1991).
179. Swazey, J., and Glantz, L.H., "A Social Perspective on Compensation for Injured Research Subjects," *Compensating for Research Injuries: The Ethical and Legal Implications of Programs to Redress Injured Subjects,* President's Commission for the Study of Ethical Problems in Medicine and Biomedical and Behavioral Research, vol. 2 (Washington, DC: U.S. Government Printing Office, 1982).
180. Swine Flu Act (National Swine Flu Immunization Program), Pub. L. 94-380, 90 Stat. 113, 1976, codified at 42 U.S.C. 247b(j)-(l); repealed by Pub. L. 95-626, sec.202, 92 Stat. 3574, 1978.
181. Tancredi, L.R., and Bovbjerg, R.R., "Rethinking Responsibility for Patient Injury: Accelerated-Compensation Events: A Malpractice and Quality Reform Ripe for a Test," *Law & Contemporary Problems* 54:147-78, 1991.
182. Taragin, M.I., et al., "The Influence of Standard of Care and Severity of Injury on the Resolution of Malpractice Claims," *Annals of Internal Medicine* 117:780-84, 1992.
183. Tuskegee Syphilis Study Ad Hoc Advisory Panel, *Final Report* (Washington, DC: U.S. Dept. of Health, Education and Welfare, 1973).
184. U.S. Congress, General Accounting Office, *Medical Malpractice: 6 State Case Studies Show Claims and Costs Still Rise Despite Reforms,* GAO/HRD-87-21 (Washington, DC, December 1986).

185. U.S. Congress, General Accounting Office, *Product Liability: Extent of "Litigation Explosion" in Federal Courts Questioned* (Washington, DC, January 1988).
186. U.S. Congress General Accounting Office, *Product Liability: Verdicts and Case Resolution in Five States,* GAO/HRD-88-99 (Washington, DC, U.S. Government Printing Office, September 1989).
187. U.S. Congress, General Accounting Office, *Medical Malpractice: Maine's Use of Practice Guidelines to Reduce Costs,* GAO/HRD-94-8 (Washington, DC, October 1993).
188. U.S. Congress, General Accounting Office, *Human Experimentation: An Overview on Cold War Era Programs,* Testimony Before the Legislation and National Security Subcommittee, Committee on Government Operations, House of Representatives, U.S. Congress, Sept. 28, 1994, GAO/T-NSIAD-94-266 (Washington, DC: U.S. Government Printing Office, 1994).
189. U.S. Congress, House of Representatives, Committee on Energy and Commerce, Subcommittee on Health and the Environment, *Vaccine Injury Compensation,* hearing, Dec.19, 1984, Serial No. (Washington, DC: U.S. Government Printing Office, 1984).
190. U.S. Congress, House of Representatives, Committee on Energy and Commerce, Subcommittee on Energy Conservation and Power, *American Nuclear Guinea Pigs: Three Decades of Radiation Experiments on U.S. Citizens,* Report, (Washington, DC: U.S. Government Printing Office, 1986).
191. U.S. Congress, Office of Technology Assessment, *Compensation for Vaccine-Related Injuries—Technical Memorandum,* OTA-TM-H-6 (Washington, DC: U.S. Government Printing Office, November 1980).
192. U.S. Congress, Office of Technology Assessment, AIDS-Related Series: #5, "How Has Federal Research on AIDS/HIV Disease Contributed to Other Fields?" Staff Paper, NTIS#PB90-253774 (Washington, DC: U.S. Government Printing Office, 1990).
193. U.S. Congress, Office of Technology Assessment, *Impact of Legal Reforms on Medical Malpractice Costs,* OTA-BP-H-119 (Washington, DC: U.S. Government Printing Office, October 1993a).
194. U.S. Congress, Office of Technology Assessment, *Pharmaceutical R&D: Costs, Risks and Rewards,* OTA-H-522 (Washington DC: U.S. Government Printing Office, February 1993b).
195. U.S. Congress, Office of Technology Assessment, *Defensive Medicine and Medical Malpractice,* OTA-H-602 (Washington, DC: U.S. Government Printing Office, July 1994).
196. U.S. Congress, Senate, S. 1757, *Health Security Act,* (Washington, DC: U.S. Government Printing Office, 1993.
197. U.S. Congress, Senate, S.491, *American Health Security Act of 1993,* (Washington, DC: U.S. Government Printing Office, 1993).
198. U.S. Department of Health and Human Services, Office of Inspector General, *The National Vaccine Injury Compensation Program: A Program Review* (Washington, DC: DHHS, 1992).
199. U.S. Department of Health and Human Services, Public Health Service, National Institutes of Health, Division of Vaccine Injury Compensation, "National Vaccine Injury Compensation Program Monthly Status Report-September 7, 1994," (Washington, DC: DHHS, 1994).
200. U.S. Department of Health, Education, and Welfare, *HEW Secretary's Task Force on the Compensation of Injured Research Subjects, Report* (Washington, DC: DHEW, January 1977).
201. U.S. Department of Health, Education, and Welfare, *Liability Arising Out of Immunization Programs: Final Report to Congress* (Washington, DC: DHEW, May 1978).
202. U.S. Department of State, *Human Immunodeficiency Virus (HIV) Testing Requirements for Entry into Foreign Countries* (Washington, DC: November, 1993).

203. Viscusi, W.K., *Reforming Products Liability* (Cambridge, MA: Harvard University Press, 1991).

204. Wade, J.W., "An Evaluation of the 'Insurance Crisis' and Existing Tort Law," *Houston Law Review* 24:81-96, 1987.

205. Wade, J.W., "On the Effect in Product Liability of Knowledge Unavailable Prior to Marketing," *New York University Law Review* 58:734-764, 1983.

206. Wade, J.W., "On the Nature of Strict Liability for Products," *Mississippi Law Journal,* 44:825-851, 1973.

207. Walker, M.C., and Fast, P.E., "Clinical Trials of Candidate AIDS Vaccines," *AIDS* 8 (Supp.1): S213-S236, 1994.

208. Wiggins, S.N., "The Pharmaceutical Research and Development Decision Process," *Drugs and Health: Economic Issues & Policy Objectives,* Helms, Robert B. (ed.) (Washington, DC: American Enterprise Institute, 1981).

209. Williams, D., Vice-President & General Manager, Connaught Laboratories, Inc., "Statement," *Vaccine Injury Compensation,* hearing before Subcommittee on Health and the Environment, Committee on Energy and Commerce, House of Representatives, U.S. Congress, December 19, 1984.

210. Williams, G., "The Aims of the Law of Tort," *Current Legal Problems* 4:137-176, 1951.

211. Willig, "The Comment k Character: A Conceptual Barrier to Strict Liability," *Mercer Law Review* 29:545-581, 1978.

212. Zoon, K.C., and Beatrice, M.G., *New Directions for FDA's Center for Biologics Evaluation and Research (CBER). New Drug Approvals in 1992* (Washington, DC: Pharmaceutical Manufacturers Association, 1993).

213. Zuckerman, S., Bovbjerg, R.R., and Sloan, F., "Effects of Tort Reforms and Other Factors on Medical Malpractice Insurance Premiums," *Inquiry* 27:167-182, 1990.

Court Cases

214. *Abbott* v. *American Cyanamid Co.,* 844 F.2d 1108 (4th Cir.), cert. denied, 488 U.S. 908 (1988).

215. *Abbott* v. *Secretary,* V 1992 Cl. Ct. LEXIS 473 (1992), rev'd on other grounds, 27 Fed. Cl. 792 (1993).

216. *Adams* v. *G.D. Searle & Co.,* 576 So.2d 728 (Fla. Dist. Ct. App.), review denied, 589 So.2d 290 (Fla. 1991).

217. *Albala* v. *City of New York,* 445 N.Y.S. 2d 108 (1981).

218. *Allen* v. *G.D. Searle & Co.,* 708 F. Supp. 1142 (D. Or. 1989).

219. *Allison* v. *Merck & Company, Inc.,* 110 Nev. 762; 878 P.2d 948; 1994 Nev. LEXIS 112

220. *Anderson* v. *Owens-Corning Fiberglass Corp.,* 53 Cal.3d 987, 810 P.2d 549 (1991).

221. *Ayers* v. *Johnson & Johnson Baby Products Co.,* 117 Wash.2d 747, 818 P.2d 1337 (1991).

222. *Berkovitz* v. *United States,* 486 U.S. 531 (1988).

223. *Beshada* v. *Johns-Manville Products Corp.,* 90 N.J. 191, 447 A.2d 539 (1982).

224. *Brochu* v. *Ortho Pharmaceutical Corp.,* 642 F.2d 652 (1st Cir. 1981).

225. *Brown* v. *Superior Court,* 44 Cal.3d 1049, 245 Cal. Rptr. 412, 751 P.2d 470 (1988).

226. *Canterbury* v. *Spence,* 464 F.2d 772 (D.C. Cir. 1972).

227. *Carlenstope* v. *Merck,* 819 F.2d 33-37 (2nd Cir. 1987).

228. *Carmen* v. *Eli Lilly & Co.,* 32 N.E.2d 729 (Ind. App. 1941).

229. *Castrignano* v. *E.R. Squibb & Sons, Inc.,* 546 A.2d 755 (R.I. 1988); district court verdict aff'd, 900 F.2d 455 (1st Cir. 1990).

230. *Chan Tse Ming* v. *Cordis Corp.,* 704 Fed. Supp. 217-220 (S.D. Fl. 1989).

231. *Cobbs* v. *Grant,* 8 Cal. 3d 229, 104 Cal. Rptr. 505, 502 P.2d 1 (1972).

232. *Collins* v. *Eli Lilly Co.,* 116 Wis.2d 166, 342 N.W.2d 37, cert. denied, 469 U.S. 826 (1984).

233. *Corrigan* v. *Bjork Shiley Corp.*, 182 Calif. Appellate Reports 166-183 (1986).
234. *Daubert* v. *Merrell Dow Pharmaceuticals*, 113 S.Ct. 2786 (1993).
235. *Davis* v. *Wyeth Laboratories*, 399 F.2d 121 (9th Cir. 1968).
236. *DeMelo* v. *Lederle Laboratories*, 801 F.2d 1058 (8th Cir. 1986).
237. *Dowling* v. *Hyland Therapeutics*, 767 F. Supp 57 (S.D.N.Y. 1991)
238. *Dunn* v. *Lederle Laboratories*, 121 Mich. App. 73, 328 N.W.2d 576 (1983).
239. *Escola* v. *Coca Cola Bottling Co. of Fresno*, 24 Cal.2d 453, 150 P.2d 436 (1944) (Traynor, J., dissenting).
240. *Ezagui* v. *Dow Chemical Corp.*, 598 F.2d 727 (2d Cir. 1979).
241. *Falk* v. *Keene Corp.*, 113 Wash.2d 645, 782 P.2d 974 (1989).
242. *Feldman* v. *Lederle Laboratories*, 97 N.J. 429, 479 A.2d 374 (N.J. 1984) (Feldman I), rev'd after remand, 561 A.2d 288 (N.J. Super. Ct. App. Div. 1989), rev'd, 125 N.J. 117, 592 A.2d 1176 (N.J. 1991) (Feldman II), cert. denied, 112 S.Ct. 3027 (1992).
243. *Finn* v. *G.D. Searle & Co.*, 35 Cal. 3d 691; 677 P.2d 1147; 200 Cal. Rptr. 870 (1984).
244. *Flood* v. *Wyeth Laboratories*, 183 Cal. App. 3d 1272, 288 Cal. Rptr. 700 (1986).
245. *Fraley* v. *American Cyanamid*, 589 F. Supp. 826 (D. Col. 1984).
246. *Garside* v. *Osco Drug, Inc.*, 764 F.Supp. 208 (D. Mass. 1991).
247. *Gassman* v. *United States*, No. 79-314-ORL-CIV-06, Slip opinion (M.D. Fla. June 27, 1984).
248. *Gaston* v. *Hunter*, 588 P.2d 326 (Ariz. Ct. App. 1978).
249. *Givens* v. *Lederle*, 556 F.2d 1341 (5th Cir. 1977).
250. *Gottsdanker* v. *Cutter Laboratories*, 182 Cal. App. 2d 602, 6 Cal. Rptr. 320 (1960).
251. *Graham* v. *Wyeth Laboratories*, 906 F.2d 1399 (10th Cir. 1990), cert. denied, 498 U.S. 981 (1990).
252. *Grant* v. *Parke-Davis & Co.*, 544 F.2d 521 (7th Cir. 1976).
253. *Greenman* v. *Yuba Power Products, Inc.*, 59 Cal. 2d 67, 377 P.2d 897 (1963).
254. *Griffin* v. *United States*, 500 F.2d 1949 (3d Cir. 1974).
255. *Grundberg* v. *Upjohn Co.*, 813 P.2d 89 (Utah 1991).
256. *Haddad* v. *Richardson-Merrell, Inc.* 588 Fed. Supp. 1158-1164 (N.D. Ohio 1984).
257. *Hahn* v. *Richter*, 427 Pa. Super. 130, 628 A.2d 860 (1993).
258. *Hill* v. *Searle Laboratories*, 884 F.2d 1064 (8th Cir. 1989).
259. *Hillsborough County* v. *Automated Medical Laboratories*, 471 U.S. 707 (1985).
260. *Hockett* v. *United States*, 730 F.2d 709 (11th Cir. 1984).
261. *Hodson* v. *A.H. Robins Co., Inc.*, 528 Fed. Supp. 809-824 (E.D. Va. 1981).
262. *Hopkins* v. *Dow Corning Corporation*, 1994 U.S. App. LEXIS 23097 (9th Cir. 1994).
263. *Hunt* v. *Hoffman-LaRoche, Inc.*, 785 F. Supp. 547 (D. Md. 1992).
264. *Hurley* v. *Lederle Labs*, 863 F.2d 1173 (5th Cir. 1988).
265. *Hyman* v. *Jewish Chronic Disease Hospital*, 15 N.Y.2d 317, 206 N.E.2d 338 (1965).
266. In re Sabin Oral Polio Vaccine Products Liability Litigation, 743 F.Supp. 410 (D.Md. 1990).
267. In re Tetracycline Cases, 747 F. Supp. 543 (W.D. Mo. 1989).
268. In re Union Carbide Corporation, 634 F. Supp. 842-867 (S.D.N.Y. 1986), affirmed and modified, 809 F.2d 195-206 (2nd Cir. 1987), cert denied, 484 U.S. 871 (1987).
269. Incollingo v. Ewing, 444 Pa. 299, 282 A.2d 206 (1971).
270. *Johnson* v. *American Cyanamid*, 239 Kan. 279, 718 P.2d 1318 (1986).
271. *Jones* v. *Lederle Laboratories*, 785 F.Supp. 1123 (S.D.N.Y. 1992).
272. *Keane* v. *Lederle Laboratories*, 1994 U.S. Dist. LEXIS 4305 (1994).

273. *Kearl* v. *Lederle Laboratories,* 172 Cal. App. 3d 827, 218 Cal. Rptr. 453 (1985).
274. *King* v. *Collagen Corp.,* 983 F.2d 1130 (5th Cir. 1993), cert. denied, 114 S.Ct. 84 (1993).
275. *Larsen* v. *Pacesetter Systems, Inc.,* 837 P.2d 1273 (Haw. 1992).
276. *Mazur* v. *Merck & Co., Inc.,* 742 F. Supp. 239 (E.D. Pa. 1990) (Mazur I), 767 F. Supp. 697, aff'd, 964 F.2d 1348 (3d Cir. 1992) (Mazur II).
277. *McKee* v. *Moore,* 648 P.2d 21 (Okla. 1982).
278. *Mitchell* v. *Iolab Corp.,* 700 F. Supp. 877 (E.D. La. 1988).
279. *Moore* v. *Kimberly-Clark,* 867 F.2d 243 (5th Cir. 1989).
280. *Morris* v. *Parke-Davis & Co.,* 667 F.Supp. 1332 (C.D. Cal. 1987).
281. *Natanson* v. *Kline,* 186 Kan. 393, opinion on denial of motion for rehearing, 187 Kan. 186 (1960).
282. *Oresman* v. *Searle & Co.,* 321 F. Supp. 449 (R.I. 1971).
283. *Pacific Mutual Life Insurance Company* v. *Haslip,* 499 U.S. 1 (1991).
284. *Parke-Davis & Co.* v. *Stromsodt,* 411 F.2d 1390 (8th Cir. 1969).
285. *Pease* v. *American Cyanamid Co.,* 795 F. Supp. 755 (D. Md. 1992).
286. *Petty* v. *United States,* 740 F.2d 1428 (8th Cir. 1984).
287. *Piper Aircraft Co.,* v. *Reyno,* 454 U.S. 235 (1981), rev'g 630 F.2d 149 (3rd Cir. 1980) rev'g 479 F. Supp. 727 (M.D. Pa. 1979).
288. *Plummer* v. *Lederle Laboratories,* 819 F.2d 349 (2d Cir.) cert. denied, 484 U.S. 898 (1987).
289. *Pollard* v. *Ashby,* 793 S.W.2d 394 (Mo. Ct. App. 1990).
290. *Reyes* v. *Wyeth Laboratories,* 498 F.2d 1264 (5th Cir.), cert. denied, 419 U.S. 1096 (1974).
291. *Roberts* v. *Patel,* 620 F. Supp. 323 (N.D. Ill. 1985).
292. *Rohrburgh* v. *Wyeth Laboratories, Inc.,* 719 F. Supp. 470 (N.D.W. Va. 1989), aff'd, 916 F.2d 970 (4th Cir. 1990).
293. *Salgo* v. *Leland Stanford Jr. University,* 317 P.2d 170 (Cal. Ct. App. 1957).
294. *Samuels* v. *American Cyanamid Co.,* 130 Misc.2d 175, 495 N.Y.S.2d 1006 (1985).
295. *Sandel* v. *State,* 126 S.C.1, 119 S.E. 776, appeal dismissed, 269 U.S. 532 (1922).
296. *Savina* v. *Sterling Drug, Inc.,* 247 Kan. 105, 795 P.2d 915 (1990).
297. *Schackil* v. *Lederle Laboratories,* 116 N.J. 155, 561, A.2d 511 (1989).
298. *Schafer* v. *American Cyanimid Co.,* 1994 U.S. App. LEXIS 5477 (1st Cir. 1994).
299. *Schindler* v. *Lederle Laboratories,* 725 F.2d 1036 (6th Cir. 1984).
300. *Senn* v. *Merrill-Dow Pharmaceuticals, Inc.* 850 F.2d 611 (9th Cir. 1988).
301. *Shanks* v. *Upjohn Co.,* 835 P.2d 1189 (Alaska 1992).
302. *Sheffield* v. *Eli Lilly & Co.,* No. A013100, Cal. Ct. App. 1st Dist. 1983 .
303. *Singer* v. *Sterling Drug, Inc.,* 461 F.2d 288 (7th Cir. 1972).
304. *Slater* v. *Optical Radiation Corp.,* 961 F.2d 1330 (7th Cir.), cert. denied, 113 S.Ct. 327 (1992).
305. *Spencer* v. *United States,* 569 F. Supp. 325 (W.D. Mo. 1983).
306. *Stamps* v. *Collagen Corp.,* 1993 U.S.App. LEXIS 2745 (1st Cir. 1993), cert. denied, 114 S.Ct. 86 (1993).
307. *Stanback* v. *Parke, Davis & Co.,* 657 F.2d 642 (4th Cir. 1981).
308. *Sulesky* v. *United States,* 545 F. Supp. 426 (S.D. W. Va. 1982).
309. *Taggart* v. *Richards Medical Company, Inc.,* 677 F. Supp. 1102 (Col. 1988).
310. *Thomas* v. *Hoffman La-Roche, Inc.,* 949 F.2d 806 (5th Cir. 1992).
311. *Tinnerholm* v. *Parke-Davis & Co.,* 411 F.2d 48 (2d Cir. 1969).
312. *Toner* v. *Lederle Laboratories,* 112 Idaho 328, 732 P.2d 297 (1987).
313. *Tracey* v. *Merrell Dow Pharmaceuticals, Inc.* 569 N.E.2d 875 (Ohio 1991).

314. *Tremaine* v. *H.K. Mulford Co.,* 317 Pa. 97, 176 A.2d 212 (1935).
315. *Unthank* v. *United States,* 732 F.2d 1517 (10th Cir. 1984).
316. *Vincent* v. *Thompson,* 79 Misc.2d 1029, 361 N.Y.S.2d 282 (1974), rev'd in part, 50 App. Div. 211, 377 N.Y.S.2d 118 (1975).
317. *Walker* v. *Merck & Co.,* 648 F. Supp. 931 (M.D.Ga. 1986), aff'd without opinion, 831 F.2d 1069 (11th Cir. 1987).
318. *West* v. *G.D. Searle & Co.,* 305 Ark. 33, 806 S.W.2d 608 (1991).
319. *White* v. *Wyeth Laboratories,* 40 Ohio St. 3d 390, 533 N.E.2d 748 (1988).
320. *Whitlock* v. *Duke University,* 637 F. Supp. 1463 (M.D.N.C. 1986), aff'd, 829 F.2d 1340 (4th Cir. 1987).
321. *Williams* v. *Lederle,* 591 F. Supp. 381 (S.D. Ohio 1984).
322. *Wyeth Labs, Inc.* v. *Fortenberry,* 530 So.2d 688 (Miss. 1988).

Appendix A
A Technical Review of the Evidence for Adverse Reactions to HIV Vaccines

A

This appendix reviews the various theoretical risks that have been proposed by various investigators to be potentially associated with HIV vaccines for prophylactic and/or therapeutic use. The theoretical basis for these risks, as well as their proposed mechanisms and experimental support are also examined. As is explained below, some of the risks reviewed here are unlikely or are entirely theoretical (i.e., are currently without experimental support). Suggestions for research initiatives to uncover clues to potential adverse reactions from HIV vaccines are provided.

A key point to remember throughout this analysis is the high rate of genetic mutation of HIV (2, 5, 7, 25, 32, 58); these mutations may allow the virus to become resistant to antiviral drugs and to escape immune surveillance. On average, the virus makes one genetic "mistake" every time it replicates. This is because the unique enzyme that allows the virus to turn RNA genetic information into DNA genetic informationa process called reverse transcriptionis a *low fidelity* enzyme that makes many errors. Such errors are called mutations, and may be lethal (i.e., incompatible with viral replication) or may be tolerated.

Unfortunately, HIV appears to tolerate an extraordinary number of mutations throughout the length of its genome. Under certain conditions these mutations even confer a selective advantage to the virus. This is the basis for the high rate of evolution of new viral mutants (or *quasispecies*). For example, if the mutation interferes with the ability to bind active metabolites of the antiviral drug AZT (zidovudine), the resulting mutant virus may be resistant to AZT. If the infected patient (the host) is treated with AZT, the mutant virus will have a selective advantage and over a period

by
David Schwartz
Johns Hopkins University School of Hygiene and Public Health, Baltimore, MD

of months to years become the predominant type of virus in the patient (the *dominant quasispecies*) (12, 56).

Similarly, if a mutation occurs at a site previously recognized by the patient's neutralizing antibodies, the virus carrying this mutation (the *escape mutant*) may evade immune detection and emerge as the dominant quasispeciesat least until a new set of antibodies are formed that can recognize and block the mutant virus (20, 46). Thus, HIV is continually evolving under the selective pressure from the host's immune response and from antiviral drugs. This evolution occurs not only at the level of the overall population of infected people, but also within a single infected individual over the course of disease.

Enhancing Antibodies

The possibility that HIV vaccination could induce antibodies that facilitate viral entry into immune phagocytic cells has been studied in the laboratory using a variety of cell types[143]. Results have been inconsistent among studies, and the evidence for this phenomenon has recently been comprehensively reviewed by a study group sponsored by the National Institutes of Health (NIH) (39). Some have suggested that anti-HIV antibodies that are protective or inactive at one concentration may be enhancing at a lower concentration (50). To date, there has been little laboratory evidence of antibody dependent enhancement in the sera of HIV vaccine recipients, but this may be due to the limited number of laboratories that are examining this potential problem. More importantly, the activity of HIV in humans may not be adequately approximated by laboratory studies. Investigators have presented evidence that macaques that were vaccinated with SIV protein subunit vaccine (17) or transfused with anti-SIV antibodies (26) showed enhanced rates of infection and disease progression when subsequently exposed at mucosal membranes to SIV.

Original Antigenic Sin

HIV infection induces an abundance of antibodies, including neutralizing antibodies; however several groups have shown that the generation of neutralizing antibodies tends to lag behind the generation of viral escape mutants by several months or even years. One explanation for this observation involves the phenomenon of *original antigenic sin* (OAS), the fixing of an immune response in a nonadaptive pattern.

OAS was first observed in immune responses to sequential influenza A virus infections. Investigators observed that, in some instances, exposure of an individual to one strain of influenza A virus triggered the production of antibodies that were predominantly directed at another strain of influenza A virus that had infected the individual in the past. The antibodies that were produced had weak affinity for the newly encountered strain of influenza A virus. OAS is a particularly important problem with organisms that mutate frequently. OAS has also been observed in some bacterial infections as well, but its mechanism has never been fully elucidated.

Some investigators have argued that, during the course of HIV infection, an OAS pattern occurs with respect to antibodies recognizing the V3 loop and other variable regions of HIV envelope proteins (31, 44).

In infected individuals, there may emerge a predominance of neutralizing antibodies directed against HIV species present at some earlier time of infection, but not to the contemporaneous HIV species.[144] While this may simply reflect a delay in the development of measurable titers of anti-

---

[143] This antibody dependent enhancement may occur in the presence (50) or absence (15) of complement.

[144] The mechanism by which OAS occurs has been investigated. The current hypothesis is that previously stimulated B lymphocyte clones bearing surface receptors with high affinity for previously circulating strains of virus may be sufficiently cross-reactive (due to membrane surface-arrayed multivalent binding) to be triggered by new viral strains; but the B lymphocytes secrete antibody that, in soluble monomeric form, have only low affinity for the new strains.

body directed against the more recent circulating strain of HIV, this delay may have potentially significant immunologic consequences, and its mechanism remains unclear. There is also some recent laboratory evidence that an OAS pattern can be observed in B and T lymphocytes from uninfected volunteers following vaccination with recombinant HIV protein subunit vaccines (54).

Related to the observation of a lagging antibody response to HIV escape mutants is that of a limited and relatively fixed diversity of antigenic specificity seen among antibodies created in response to HIV antigens (14, 31, 43, 44, 45, 61). Whether this is a cause or effect of the delayed antibody response to emergence of new strains of virus is unclear. In either case, this low diversity antibody response to HIV is probably detrimental to the host's ability to suppress infection.

It should be emphasized, however, that the evidence supporting the view that there is a limited diversity in antibody response to HIV rests largely on the finding that certain antibody *variable region* genes, the genes that code for an antibody's antigenic specificity, are used disproportionately for the immune response to the dominant antigenic regions of the virus. This still allows for greater diversity to be generated during the course of the immune response by a process called *somatic mutation*, as demonstrated by Andris and colleagues (1). Thus, studies showing that only a restricted number of variable region genes are used for the production of anti-HIV antibodies probably underestimate the true diversity of the antibody response.

Vaccine-induced OAS may occur when a vaccinated individual is exposed to a noncross reactive strain of HIV that induces the production of antibodies specific for the vaccine strain that are unable to neutralize the newly encountered strain. When exposed to HIV, however, vaccinated individuals exhibiting OAS may be no worse off than unvaccinated individuals because unvaccinated individuals also have a lag in generation of antibody to HIV because their immune response has not been "primed" by vaccination. It is not known whether the lag in antibody production in unvaccinated individuals is greater than the lag in the production of antibody directed to contemporaneous HIV strains in vaccinated individuals exhibiting OAS.

Expansion of V_3H family or other families of B lymphocytes

Investigators have found that certain genes for a particular family of antigen receptors on B lymphocytes (the V_3H family) are expressed much more frequently among HIV-infected individuals than uninfected individuals. Because more than half of all HIV-infected individuals express these antibodies, which bind to viral proteins, we know that the virus induces their expression (43, 61). Muller and colleagues have shown that such antibodies were even further elevated in 40 of the 44 HIV-infected patients with B cell lymphomas (24). Because these antibodies are not necessarily protective and seem to be associated with lymphomas, their presence may not be desirable.

Recently Schwartz and colleagues examined the sera of vaccinees receiving various HIV envelope-based vaccines for the presence of these antibodies. They found that many vaccinees made them at some point after immunization, generally at times of peak total antibody response (unpublished data). Thus, envelope based-vaccines are, at least transiently, inducing antibodies that mimic this aspect of the host response to HIV infection.

Recently, a group of investigators presented evidence that HIV-envelope (gp120) protein can function as a superantigen for B lymphocytes carrying another family of antigen receptors (4). By binding to a common portion of the surface immunoglobulin receptors of B lymphocytes, gp120 -envelope protein initially induces stimulation and then exhaustive depletion of those B lymphocytes carrying surface receptors from that family of genes. Other investigators (34) believe such B lymphocytes can support infectious replication of HIV and also may contribute to B cell lymphomas in HIV-infected patients. Hence, a concern that most HIV envelope vaccines in development could expand this pool of B lymphocytes and induce B cell lymphomas exists.

Expansion of "Double Jeopardized" CD4+ (T Helper) Cells, Leading to Increased HIV Replication

There may be subsets of CD4+ T lymphocytes that are particularly susceptible to HIV infection early in disease. All CD4+ T lymphocytes can be infected by HIV by virtue of their surface membrane CD4 molecules, which serves as the site of attachment of the virus. However, it has long been appreciated that immune-activated CD4+ lymphocytes are better hosts for HIV entry, integration, and replication than are resting CD4+ cells. Further, cells cannot become infected unless they are brought into proximity either with infected cells or virus. At the earliest stages of HIV infection, the number of infected cells limits the cell-to-cell spread of the virus, and therefore there is a low likelihood that a random CD4+ lymphocyte will come into contact with an infected cell. By contrast, CD4+ lymphocytes with specificity for HIV are constantly "searching" for HIV infected cells to bind to, and thus are at increased risk of coming into close proximity to virus and becoming infected. If HIV undergoes a burst of replication in such cells, this would contribute to early dissemination of virus and poorer long-term prognosis.

Circumstantial evidence supporting the early destruction of HIV-specific CD4+ lymphocytes comes from the results of in vitro *lymphoproliferation assays*, which measure the magnitude of the proliferative response of lymphocytes to a series of *recall antigens* to which the lymphocytes have previously been exposed. These experiments have shown that HIV envelope protein was unable to induce the proliferation of CD4+ lymphocytes obtained from asymptomatic HIV-infected individuals, even though the responses of these CD4+ lymphocytes to other recall antigens were intact.

Experimental evidence also exist for the special ability of antigen-presenting immune cells pulsed with HIV to activate and destroy CD4+ lymphocytes with which they come in contact (8, 38). At the same time, these activated cells can become infected with HIV and support a burst of HIV replication prior to destruction of the infected cells. This might be expected to happen with vaccine-induced CD4+ lymphocytes, which would seek out and proliferate in response to HIV at the earliest stages of infection. A mathematical model this scenario has recently been published (55).

Priming for T Helper 2 (TH2) and T Helper 1 (TH1) Patterns of Cytokine Response

Cytokines are cell-to-cell communication and growth molecules, which can be thought of as short-range hormones. The distinct and to some degree antagonistic cytokine profiles of TH1 and TH2 responses have received increasing attention from HIV researchers. TH1 responses are characterized by the production of the cytokines interleukin-2 (IL-2), IL-12, and Interferon gamma. These cytokines are important in the induction of cytotoxic T lymphocytes. TH2 responses produce IL-4, IL-5, and IL-10—cytokines crucial for the induction and amplification of various antibody responses. Furthermore, the cytokine IL-12, produced by the TH1 response, suppresses TH2 cytokine production, while IL-10, produced by the TH2 response, suppresses TH1 cytokine production. This negative feedback inhibition between TH2 and TH1 responses can accentuate the differences between them.

Although TH1 and TH2 responses were first described in mice, similar though less clearly distinct cytokine profiles have been demonstrated in human cells in vitro, with mitogens (cytokines that induce cell division) and recall antigens inducing predominantly TH1 responses in PBMCs of normal donors and a TH2 profile in PBMCs of HIV-infected individuals (10, 11, 41).

To the extent that TH2 responses in HIV-infected individuals are not protective and are antagonistic to desirable TH1 responses, some researchers have argued that priming for TH2 responses is an inappropriate, counterproductive goal for vaccination, and a likely consequence of recombinant protein subunit vaccines (51).

Schwartz and colleagues at Johns Hopkins University are currently testing the cytokine profiles of vaccinees' PBMCs restimulated in vitro with HIV or HIV antigen. Unpublished preliminary results suggest that the TH1 response remains dominant, thus assuaging some of the concerns that vaccines may prime for TH2 responses.

Induction of Autoimmunity

Any pathogen that binds to or mimics the structure of self-antigens is capable of inducing antibodies directed against the self (autoantibodies). HIV both binds to CD4 receptors of T lymphocytes via it's gp120 -envelope protein and bears sequence homology with several human antigens. There have been several autoantibodies among HIV-infected and envelope vaccinated individuals found, albeit of questionable significance (13, 18, 19, 33, 47, 52). Most intriguing has been the transient, episodic appearance of anti-CD4 antibodies in HIV-infected individuals and in uninfected recipients of rgp160- or rgp120-envelope vaccines (28, 29, 30). Originally a concern because of the potentially immune suppressive effects of such antibodies on CD4+ lymphocytes, the transient appearance of anti-CD4 antibodies has not had detectable effects on healthy vaccinees as judged by their CD4+ lymphocyte counts and the results of in vitro lymphoproliferation assays against recall antigens. Furthermore, Neurath and colleagues have recently demonstrated that hyperimmune rabbit anti-gp120/gp160 antisera had negligible binding activity against a variety of CD4, HLA-I and HLA-II cell surface antigens (30). These authors concluded that detrimental effects from envelope vaccines are improbable.

Interestingly, Letvin and colleagues have shown that the purposeful induction of anti-CD4 antibodies in chimpanzees (63) or administration of anti-CD4 monoclonal antibodies in macaques (48) can protect their cells in vitro from infection with HIV or SIV upon subsequent challenge. Furthermore, immunization of SIV-infected macaques with soluble recombinant RCD4 receptors resulted in both an anti-CD4 and an antiviral response (63). The significance of the low and intermittent anti-CD4 antibody titers seen in the sera of HIV-infected patients is unknown. The possibility of autoimmunity is frequently invoked in discussions of HIV immunosuppression and the destruction of uninfected CD4+ lymphocytes, but there is presently no evidence that anti-CD4 antibodies play a role.

Induction of Endogenous Retroviruses or Oncogenes by HIV Genes or Proteins

In mice, various mammary tumor viruses encode superantigens that can activate dysfunctional lymphocyte proliferation (see discussions of clonal expansion above). Gallo and colleagues were able to induce Kaposi sarcoma-like lesions in male mice transgenically engineered to express only the HIV tat gene (16). Recently, Sekaly and colleagues have shown that transfection of only the HIV gag gene into mice carrying latent mouse mammary tumor virus (MMTV) can cause the induction of active expression of the MMTV viruses, with detrimental MMTV-induced immune consequences. Humans may also carry latent endogenous retroviruses or retrovirus related cellular oncogenes with pathogenic potential. It is possible that introduction of even partial HIV genomes in live vectors carrying, for example, the gag and tat genes, could activate harmful endogenous retroviral genes.

There is a high frequency of tumors in HIV-infected individuals, and in most cases these cells do not harbor HIV. Therefore, secondary effects of HIV infection must be invoked, and these effects may not be dependent on the presence of the complete viral genome. Recently, McGrath and colleagues have identified the HIV genome at constant chromosomal location in the genome of non-B cell lymphoma cells obtained from several unrelated patients with this cancer (57). This further supports the notion that HIV genes may have oncogenic potential.

Induction of Short-Term Immunosuppression

Luban and colleagues have shown that HIV gag proteins bind to cyclophilins (37). These cyclophilins are also targeted by the potent immunosuppressive drugs cyclosporin A and FK506. Thus, production of significant amounts of gag gene product for any extended length of time, which may occur as a result of vaccination with a live vector coding for HIV gag gene, might induce immune suppression by the same mechanism as cyclosporin A. Presumably, the vaccine-induced immune response would then eliminate this source of gag.

Cross-linking of CD4 by HIV envelope gp120 or gp160 proteins sends an incomplete signal leading to immune exhaustion (anergy) or subsequent programmed cell suicide (apoptosis) (3, 35, 41, 62). This is thought by some to be a major mechanism of immunosuppression in HIV disease. It is unlikely that the amounts of gp120 used or produced by HIV vaccines would be sufficient to induce any serious immunosuppression, but subtle short-term effects might be induced, especially if anti-gp120 antibodies have also been induced by vaccination (36). Similarly, while apparently not a long-term problem, it is possible that the vaccine-induced production of anti-CD4 antibodies, as described above, could also cause transient immunosuppression.

Short-term immunosuppression following vaccination may occur due to temporary dysregulation of cytokine responses. This is observed after measles vaccination (21) and mimics the more severe immunosuppression accompanying measles infection (22).

The detrimental consequences of transient acute post-vaccination immunosuppression may be much greater in developing countries and other settings where there are high pathogenic burdens (due to other viruses, bacteria, and parasites) found in many third world countries. Subtle immunosuppression of selected T lymphocyte clones—even some HIV specific clones—may not be detected on current routine tests of immune function. Limited data on the course of HIV infection is acquired from several volunteers who became infected during or following immunization with experimental vaccines. It is too soon to know if disease progression will be accelerated in these individuals.

Recombination in HIV Infected Vaccinees: Retroviruses are capable of genetically recombining with themselves, other viruses, and with host-cell genes (27, 59). This raises the possibility that even multiply deleted, replication incompetent, live vector or naked DNA vaccines might conceivably recombine in the vaccinated host with preexisting or newly acquired HIV or other viruses. There is also the possibility of integration of the HIV genome at a site that has oncogenic (cancer inducing) potential, as is noted above. This is likely to be a rare event, and not readily predicted by preclinical studies.

Activation of HIV from Latently Infected Cells

It has been a goal of HIV vaccine developers to generate protective cytotoxic T lymphocyte responses to HIV. Many other viral infections are thought to be controlled by the constant surveillance and appropriate activation of cytotoxic T lymphocytes recognizing viral antigens in the context of histocompatibility antigens on the surface of infected cells. Recently, however, some studies have raised the possibility that, at least under some conditions, activated cytotoxic T lymphocytes may release cytokines such as TNF-alpha and GM-CSF that can stimulate HIV production in infected cells (6, 23). This concern has caused at least one biotechnology company to discontinue a program of ex vivo expanded autologous anti-HIV cytotoxic T lymphocyte reinfusion, following what they perceived to be a downhill course during treatment of their first patient. However, similar Phase I clinical trials under the direction of Dr. Judy Lieberman at Boston University/New England Medical Center appear to be moving forward with encouraging results.

Possible Adverse Immunological Consequences At The Population Level

There is a possibility that widespread immunization with vaccines could select for more virulent strains of HIV at the population level. Some of the same mutations that permit HIV to avoid neutralization by the immune system may also select for greater virulence. There is some evidence for this occurring naturally during the course of HIV infection in individuals, in that HIV recovered from patients in later stages of infection is generally more rapidly growing, has a more pathogenic effect, and attacks a wider variety of cells, than HIV isolated from patients in early stages of infection (9, 53, 60). Empirical evidence exists, as well as theoretical reason, to consider these late stage viruses as mutants that escaped host immune defenses. If the effect of vaccination programs were to select for the these late stage viruses early in disease, they might become the dominant circulating strains in the population, leading to more acute disease progression among infected individuals. It is also theoretically possible that large scale vaccination could select for the most infectious strains of HIV[145].

Current studies of early seroconverting cohorts suggest that macrophage tropic, non-syncytium inducing (NSI) HIV strains are the most readily transmitted (40, 65, 64). These also tend to be the strains associated with better health and longer term survival. By contrast, syncytium-inducing (SI) strain emergence is correlated with a downhill course in the host (49). Because of the apparent role of NSI strains in HIV transmission, there has been discussion of focusing vaccine efforts against such strains. If this selective pressure favors transmissible SI strains, it might result in increased prevalence of those more pathogenic strains.

No firm evidence has developed that HIV has evolved toward greater pathogenicity at the population level since the onset of the global pandemic. One reason for this may be the relatively early stage of worldwide host-virus equilibrium in a plague that is still spreading exponentially through many populations. Also because of the high rate of mutation intrinsic to HIV, only the most strongly and consistently selected mutations will remain constant, with reversions occurring as soon as specific selective pressures are removed. Some evidence for population-based selective pressure has come from the reported recovery of AZT-resistant strains in recently infected individuals who had never received AZT, but lived in areas where the use of AZT in infected individuals was high.

Vaccination for particular HIV strains or epitopes would create the conditions for constant and widespread selective pressures that may affect the genotype and phenotype of HIV in the population. If enough members of a population were vaccinated, selection pressures would favor the predominance of escape mutants in the population, resistant to vaccine-induced immune responses. Because of the long-lived nature of successful immunizations, and the fact that a large percentage of uninfected high-risk individuals may have been vaccinated within a given community, the long-term selective effects of vaccination on the circulating strains of HIV may be more difficult to reverse than those of an antiviral drug such as AZT, which can be stopped completely, allowing for rapid reversion to drug sensitivity in the circulating strains of virus.

APPENDIX A REFERENCES

1. Andris, J., et al., "Molecular Characterization of Five Human Anti-Human Immunodeficiency Virus Type 1 Antibody Heavy Chains Reveals Extensive Somatic Mutation Typical of an Antigen-Driven Immune Response," *Proceedings of the National Academy of Science USA* 88:7783-7787, 1991.
2. Balfe, P., et al., "Concurrent Evolution of Human Immunodeficiency Virus Type 1 Patients Infected From the Same Source: Rate of Sequence Change and Low Frequency of Inactivating Mutations," *Journal of Virology* 64: 6221-6233, 1990.
3. Banda, N.K., et al., "Crosslinking CD4 by Human Immunodeficiency Virus Gp120 Primes T Cells for Activation-Induced Apop-

[145]The most infectious strains are capable of causing infection with the least number of input virions or infected cells.

tosis," *Journal of Experimental Medicine* 176:1099-1106, 1992.

4. Berberian, L., et al., "Immunoglobulin V_h3 Gene Products: Natural Ligands for HIV gp120," *Science* 261:1588-1591, 1993.
5. Boeri, E., et al., "In Vivo Genetic Variability of the Human Immunodeficiency Virus Type 2 V3 Region," *Journal of Virology* 66:4546-4550, 1992.
6. Bollinger, R.C., et al., "Cytokine Production by HIV-1 Specific Human Cytolytic T Lymphocytes Induced by Vaccination: Potential Effects on HIV-1 Replication and the Clearance of Infected Cells," *Journal of Immunology*, in press.
7. Burger, H., et al., "Evolution of Immunodeficiency Virus Type 1 Nucleotide Sequence Diversity Among Close Contacts," *Proceedings of the National Academy of Sciences USA* 88:11236-11240, 1991.
8. Cameron, P., et al., "Infection and Apoptotic Cell Dearth of CD4+ T Cells During an Immune Response to HIV-1 Pulsed Dendritic Cells," *AIDS Research and Human Retroviruses* 10:61-71, 1994.
9. Cheng-Mayer C., et al., "Biologic Features of HIV-1 that Correlate with Virulence in the Host," *Science* 240:80-82, 1988.
10. Clerici, M., et al., "Changes in T-Helper Function in Human Immunodeficiency Virus Infected Children During Didanosine Therapy as a Measure of Antiretroviral Activity," *Blood* 80:2196-2202, 1992.
11. Clerici, M., and Shearer, G. A., "TH1—>TH2 Switch Is a Critical Step in the Etiology of HIV Infection," *Immunology Today* 14: 107-111, 1993.
12. Conlon, C.P., et al., "Heterosexual Transmission of Human Immunodeficiency Virus Type 1 Variants Associated with Zidovudine Resistance," *Journal of Infectious Diseases* 169:411-415, 1994.
13. Corre, J.P., et al., "Anti-Idiotypic Antibodies to Human Anti-gp120 Antibodies Bind Recombinant and Cellular Human CD4," *European Journal of Immunology* 21: 743-751, 1991.
14. D'amelio, R., et al., "Spectrotype of Anti-gp120 Antibodies Remains Stable During the Course of HIV Disease," *Journal of AIDS* 5:930-935, 1992.
15. Eaton A, et al., "An Anti-gp41 Human Monoclonal Antibody That Enhances HIV-1 Infection in the Absence of Complement," *AIDS Research and Human Retroviruses* 10:13-18, 1994.
16. Ensoli, B., Barillari, G., and Gallo, R.C., "Pathogenesis of AIDS-associated Kaposi's Sarcoma," *Hematology, Oncology Clinics of North America* 5:281-295, 1991.
17. Gardner, M., et al., "Passive Immunization of Rhesus Macaques Against SIV Infection and Disease," *AIDS Research and Human Retroviruses*, in press.
18. Golding, H., et al., "Identification of Homologous Regions in Human Immunodeficiency Virus I gp41 and Human MHC Class II Beta 1 Domain. I. Monoclonal Antibodies Against the gp41-Derived Peptide and Patients' Sera React with Native HLA Class II Antigens, Suggesting a Role for Autoimmunity in the Pathogenesis of Acquired Immune Deficiency Syndrome," *Journal of Experimental Medicine* 167:914-923, 1988.
19. Golding, H., et al., "Common Epitope in Human Immunodeficiency Virus (HIV) 1-gp41 and HLA Class II Elicits Immunosuppressive Autoantibodies Capable of Contributing to Immune Dysfunction in HIV-1-Infected Individuals," *Journal of Clinical Investigation* 83:1430-1435, 1989.
20. Goudsmit, J., Back, N.K.T., and Nara, P.I., "Genomic Diversity and Antigenic Variation of HIV-1: Links Between Pathogenesis, Epidemiology and Vaccine Development," *FASEB Journal* 5:2427-2436, 1991.
21. Griffin, D.E., and Ward, B.J., "Changes in Cytokine Production After Measles Virus Vaccination: Predominant Production of IL-4 Suggests Induction of a TH2 Response,"

Clinical Immunology and Immunopathology 67:171-177, 1993.

22. Griffin, D.E., and Ward, B.J., "Differential CD4 T Cell Activation in Measles," *Journal of Infectious Diseases* 168:1-7, 1993.
23. Harrer, T., et al., "Induction of HIV-1 Replication in a Chronically Infected T-Cell Line by Cytotoxic T Lymphocytes," *Journal of Acquired Immune Deficiency Syndrome* 6:865-871, 1993.
24. Herndier, B., et al., "A Non-lymphoma Idiotype Is Indicative and Predictive for B Cell Malignancies in AIDS," *Hybridoma* 12:529-537, 1993.
25. Holmes, E.C., et al., "Convergent and Divergent Sequence Evolution in the Surface Envelope Glycoprotein of Human Immunodeficiency Virus Type 1 Within a Single Infected Patient," *Proceedings of the National Academy of Sciences USA* 89: 4835-4839, 1992.
26. Jennings, M., et al., "Limitations of Inactivated Whole SIV Vaccine," *IXth International Conference on AIDS*, PO-A30-0712, Berlin, Germany 1993.
27. Katz, R., and Skalka, A., "Generation of Diversity in Retroviruses," *Annual Review of Genetics* 24:409-445, 1990.
28. Keay, S., "Anti-CD4 Anti-Idiotype Antibodies in Volunteers Immunized with rgp160 of HIV-1 or Infected with HIV-1," *AIDS Research and Human Retroviruses* 8:1091-1097, 1992.
29. Keay, S. and Schwartz, D., Department of Immunology and Infectious Diseases, School of Hygiene and Public Health, Johns Hopkins University, Baltimore, MD. Report unpublished, 1994.
30. Keiser, P., et al., "Anti-CD4 Antibodies Are Associated with HIV-1 Seroconversion and May Be Detectable before Anti-HIV-1 Antibodies," *AIDS Research and Human Retroviruses* 8:1919-1927, 1992.
31. Kohler, H., Goudsmit, J., and Nara, P., "Clonal Dominance: Cause for a Limited and Failing Immune Response to HIV-1 Infection and Vaccination," *Journal of AIDS* 5:1158-1168, 1992.
32. Kuiken, C.L., et al., "Evolution of the V3 Domain in Proviral Sequences and Isolates of Human Immunodeficiency Virus Type 1 During Transition of the Viral Biological Phenotype," *Journal of Virology* 66:4622-4627, 1992.
33. Kulberg, A., "Structural Homology Between HIV-1 *tat* Protein and Various Human Proteins," *AIDS Research and Human Retroviruses* 6:1059-1060, 1990.
34. Laurence, J., et al., "A Model System for Regulation of Chronic HIV-1 Infection in Peripheral B Lymphocytes," *Virology* 196:433-441, 1993.
35. Laurent-Crawford, A.G., et al., "Membrane Expression of HIV Envelope Glycoproteins Triggers Apoptosis in CD4 Cells," *AIDS Research and Human Retroviruses* 9:761-773, 1993.
36. Liegler, T.J., and Stites, D.P., "HIV-1 gp120 and Anti-gp120 Induce Reversible Unresponsiveness in Peripheral CD4 Lymphocytes," *Journal of Acquired Immune Deficiency Syndrome* 7:340-348, 1994.
37. Luban, J., et al., "Human Immunodeficiency Virus Type 1 Gag Protein Binds to Cyclophilins a and B," *Cell* 73:1067-1078, 1993.
38. Manca, F., Habeshaw, J.A., and Dalgleish, A., "HIV Envelope Glycoprotein, Antigen Specific T- Cell Responses, and Soluble CD4," *Lancet* 335:811-815, 1990.
39. Mascola, J.R., et al., "Summary Report: Workshop on the Potential Risks of Antibody-Dependent Enhancement in Human HIV Vaccine Trials," *AIDS Research and Human Retroviruses* 9:1175-1184, 1993.
40. McNeary, T., et al., "Relationship of Human Immunodeficiency Virus Type 1 Sequence Heterogeneity to Stage of Disease," *Proceedings of the National Academy of Sciences USA* 89:10247-10251, 1992.
41. Meyaard, L., et. al., "Dysfunction of TH1 Cells and Outgrowth of TH2 Cells After HIV

Infection" (abstract), Keystone Symposium on Lymphocyte Activation Keystone, CO. April 10 - 17, 1994.

42. Meyaard, L., et al., "Programmed Death of T Cells in HIV-1 Infection," *Science* 257:217-219, 1992.
43. Muller, S., et al., "Generation and Specificity of Monoclonal Anti-Idiotypic Antibodies Against Human HIV-Specific Antibodies," *Journal of Immunology* 147:933-941, 1991.
44. Muller, S., et al., "Clonal Patterns in the Human Immune Response to HIV-1 Infection," *International Review of Immunology* 9:1-13, 1992.
45. Muller, S., et al., "B Cell Abnormalities in AIDS: Stably and Clonally-Restricted Antibody Response in HIV-1 Infection," *Scandinavian Journal of Immunology* 38:327-334, 1993.
46. Nowak, M.A., et al., "Antigenic Diversity Thresholds and the Development of AIDS," *Science* 254:963-969. 1991.
47. Reiher, W.E., Blalock, J.E., and Brunck, T.K., "Sequence Homology Between Acquired Immunodeficiency Syndrome Virus Envelope Protein and Interleukin 2," *Proceedings of the National Academy of Science USA* 83:9188-9192, 1986.
48. Reimann, K.A., et al., "In Vivo Administration to Rhesus Monkeys of a CD4-Specific Monoclonal Antibody Capable of Blocking AIDS Virus Replication," *Journal of AIDS* 9:199-207, 1993.
49. Richman, D., and Bozzette, S., "The Impact of Syncytium-Inducing Phenotype of Human Immunodeficiency Virus on Disease Progression" *Journal of Infectious Diseases* 169:968-974, 1994.
50. Robinson, W., Montefiore, D., and Mitchell, W., "Complement-Mediated, Antibody-Dependent Enhancement of HIV-1 Infection in Vitro Is Characterized by Increased Protein and RNA Synthesis and Infectious Virus Release," *Journal of AIDS* 2:33-42, 1989.
51. Salk, J., et al., "A Strategy for Prophylactic Vaccination Against HIV," *Science* 260:1270-1272, 1993.
52. Schneider, T., et al., "The HIV-1 *nef* Protein Shares an Antigenic Determinant with a T-Cell Surface Protein," *AIDS* 7:647-654, 1993.
53. Schuitemaker, H., et al., "Biological Phenotype of Human Immunodeficiency Virus Type 1 Clones at Different Stages of Infection: Progression of Disease Is Associated with a Shift from Monocytotropic to T-Cell Tropic Virus Populations," *Journal of Virology* 66:1354-1360, 1992.
54. Schwartz, D., et al., "Antibody Responses to Neutralizing Domains of gp120 in HIV(-) Vaccinees Boosted with Homologous Or Heterologous rgp120," *IXth International Conference on AIDS,* PO-A29-0690, Berlin, Germany 1993.
55. Schwartz, D., "Potential Pitfalls on the Road to an Effective HIV Vaccine," *Immunology Today* 15:54-57, 1994.
56. Shafer, R.W., et al., "Combination Therapy with Zidovudine and Didanosine Selects for Drug-Resistant Human Immunodeficiency Virus Type 1 Strains with Unique Patterns of *pol* Gene Mutations," *Journal of Infectious Diseases* 169:722-729, 1994.
57. Shiramizu, B., Herndier, B., and McGrath, M., "Identification of a Common Clonal Human Immunodeficiency Virus Integration Site in Human Immunodeficiency Virus-Associated Lymphomas," *Cancer Research* 54:2069-2072, 1994.
58. Simmonds, P., et al., "Analysis of Sequence Diversity in Hypervariable Regions of the External Glycoprotein of Human Immunodeficiency Virus Type 1," *Journal of Virology* 64:5840-5850, 1990.
59. Tan, W., et al., "Cotransfection of HIV-1 Molecular Clones with Restricted Cell Tropism May Yield Progeny with Altered Phenotype," *AIDS Research and Human Retroviruses* 9:321-329, 1993.

60. Tersmette, M., et al., "Differential Syncytium-Inducing Capacity of Human Immunodeficiency Virus Isolates: Frequent Detection of Syncytium-inducing Isolates in Patients with Acquired Immunodeficiency Syndrome (AIDS) and AIDS-related Complex," *Journal of Virology* 62:2026-2032, 1988.
61. Wang, H., et al., "Human Monoclonal and Polyclonal Anti-human Immunodeficiency Virus-1 Antibodies Share a Common Clonotypic Specificity," *European Journal of Immunology* 22:1749-1755, 1992.
62. Ward, B.J., and Griffin, D.E., "Changes in Cytokine Production After Measles Virus Vaccination: Predominant Production of IL-4 Suggests Induction of a TH2 Response," *Clinical Immunology and Immunopathology* 67:171-177, 1993.
63. Watanabe, M., et al., "Immunization of Simian Immunodeficiency Virus Infected Rhesus Monkeys with Soluble Human CD4 Elicits an Antiviral Response.," *Proceedings of the National Academy of Science USA* 88:4616-4620, 1991.
64. Zhang, L.Q., et al., "Selection for Specific Sequences in the External Envelope Protein of Human Immunodeficiency Virus Type 1 Upon Primary Infection," *Journal of Virology* 67:3345-3356, 1993.
65. Zhu, T., et al., "Genotypic and Phenotypic Characterization of HIV-1 in Patients with Primary Infection." *Science* 261:1179-1181. 1993.

Appendix B Acknowledgments

B

Arthur J. Ammann
Pediatric AIDS Foundation
Novato, CA

Larry Arthur
Program Resources Incorporated
Frederick, MD

Alberto Avendano
National Association of People with AIDS
Washington, DC

Nancy K. Bannon
American Medical Association
Chicago, IL

Lewellys F. Barker
Division of AIDS
National Institute of Allergy and Infectious Diseases
National Institutes of Health
Bethesda, MD

Ronald Bayer
School of Public Health
Columbia University
New York, NY

David Beier
Genentech, Inc.
Washington, DC

Robert Belshi
Infectious Diseases Division
St. Louis University Health Sciences Center
St. Louis, MO

David Benor
Office of the General Counsel
U.S. Department of Health and Human Services
Rockville, MD

Raoul E. Benveniste
Division of Cancer Etiology
National Cancer Institute
National Institutes of Health
Bethesda, MD

Robert C. Bollinger
Division of Infectious Diseases
School of Medicine
Johns Hopkins University
Baltimore, MD

Dani P. Bolognesi
Department of Surgery
Duke University Medical Center
Durham, NC

Randall Bovbjerg
The Urban Institute
Washington, DC

Kenneth Bridbord
International Studies Branch
Fogarty International Center
National Institutes of Health
Bethesda, MD

Baruch Brody
Center for Ethics
Baylor College of Medicine
Houston, TX

Colonel Donald S. Burke
Division of Retrovirology
Walter Reed Army Institute of Research
Rockville, MD

Margaret A. Chesney
Prevention Sciences Group
University of California at San Francisco
San Francisco, CA

Thomas Christoffel
School of Public Health
University of Illinois at Chicago
Chicago, IL

Mary Lou Clements
School of Hygiene and Public Health
Johns Hopkins University
Baltimore, MD

John Coffin
Department of Molecular Biology and Microbiology
School of Medicine
Tufts University
Boston, MA

James D. Cross
The Travelers Insurance Company
Hartford, CT

John G. Curd
Genentech, Inc.
South San Francisco, CA

James Curran
Division of HIV/AIDS
National Center for Infectious Diseases
Centers for Disease Control and Prevention
Atlanta, GA

Suzanne Dandoy
Virginia Department of Health
Richmond, VA

Paul De Stefano
Pennie & Edmunds
Menlo Park, CA

Abby P. Dilley
The Keystone Center
Washington, DC

Linda Distlerath
Merck & Company, Inc.
Whitehouse Station, NJ

Lynda Doll
Division of HIV/AIDS
National Center for Infectious Diseases
Centers for Disease Control and Prevention
Atlanta, GA

Gordon Douglas
Merck Vaccine Division
Merck & Company, Inc.
Whitehouse Station, NJ

Gary B. Ebbert
Connaught Laboratories Inc.
Swiftwater, PA

Emilio Emini
Research Laboratories
Merck & Company, Inc.
West Point, PA

Patricia Fast
Division of AIDS
National Institute of Allergy and Infectious Diseases
National Institutes of Health
Bethesda, MD

Genoveffa Franchini
Division of Cancer Etiology
National Cancer Institute
National Institutes of Health
Bethesda, MD

Donna Freeman
Division of Antiviral Drugs
Center for Drug Evaluation and Research
Food and Drug Administration
Rockville, MD

L. Patrick Gage
Genetics Institute, Inc.
Cambridge, MA

Murray B. Gardner
Department of Pathology
School of Medicine
University of California at Davis
Davis, CA

Helene Gayle
Office of the Director
Centers for Disease Control and Prevention
Washington, DC

Karen L. Goldenthal
Office of Vaccine Research and Review
Division of Vaccines and Related Products Application
Food and Drug Administration
Rockville, MD

Allan L. Goldstein
Department of Biochemistry and Molecular Biology
George Washington University Medical Center
Washington, DC

Barney S. Graham
Department of Infectious Diseases
School of Medicine
Vanderbilt University
Nashville, TN

Olga A. Grinstead
Preventive Sciences Group
University of California at San Francisco
San Francisco, CA

Ronald W. Hansen
School of Business Administration
University of Rochester
Rochester, NY

Deborah Harnesberger
Wunder, Diefenderfer
Washington, DC

Leslie Hardy
Institute of Medicine
Washington, DC

John Hoff
Swidler and Berlin
Washington, DC

Harold Jaffe
National Center for Infectious Diseases
Centers for Disease Control and Prevention
Atlanta, GA

Michael Jacobs
School of Law
DePaul University
Chicago, IL

Edward Kantongole-Mbidde
Uganda Cancer Institute
Kampala, Uganda

Ted Kirsch
Wyeth-Ayerst Laboratories
Radnor, PA

Wayne C. Koff
United Biomedical, Inc.
Hauppauge, NY

Peter Lamptey
The AIDS Project
Family Health International
Arlington, VA

Jeffrey Laurence
Department of Medicine
The New York Hospital-Cornell Medical Center
New York, NY

Carol Levine
The Orphan Project
New York, NY

Robert J. Levine
Department of Internal Medicine
School of Medicine
Yale University
New Haven, CT

Peter Lurie
Institute for Health Policy Studies
Center for AIDS Prevention Studies
University of California at San Francisco
San Francisco, CA

Mary Lyons
MicroGeneSys, Inc.
Meriden, CT

William Lyons
Ciba-Geigy Corporation
Washington, DC

Jonathan Mann
Center for Health and Human Rights
Harvard University
Cambridge, MA

Bonnie J. Mathieson
Division of AIDS
National Institute of Allergy and Infectious Diseases
National Institutes of Health
Bethesda, MD

Captain Douglas L. Mayers
Division of Retrovirology
Walter Reed Army Institute of Research
Rockville, MD

Janet W. McGrath
Department of Anthropology
Case Western Reserve University
Cleveland, OH

Richard P. McGuire
Merck & Company Inc.
Whitehouse Station, NJ

Lieutenant Colonel John McNeil
HIV Prevention Program
Walter Reed Army Institute of Research
Rockville, MD

Donald N. Medearis
Children's Service
Massachusetts General Hospital
Cambridge, MA

Peter Nara
National Cancer Institute
National Institutes of Health
Frederick, MD

Phillip Nieburg
Division of HIV/AIDS
National Center for Infectious Diseases
Centers for Disease Control and Prevention
Atlanta, GA

Jeffrey O'Connell
School of Law
University of Virginia
Charlottesville, VA

June E. Osborn
School of Public Health
University of Michigan
Ann Arbor, MI

Jean W. Pape
Cornell University Medical College,
New York, NY
and Medical School of Haiti
Port Au Prince, Haiti

Paul Parkman
Parkman Associates
Kensington, MD

William Paul
Office of AIDS Research
National Institutes of Health
Bethesda, MD

Sallie Perryman
AIDS Institute
New York State Department of Health
New York, NY

John C. Petricciani
Genetics Institute
Cambridge, MA

Jane Pitt
Department of Pediatrics
College of Physicians and Surgeons
Columbia University
New York, NY

Philip A. Pizzo
National Cancer Institute
National Institutes of Health
Bethesda, MD

Stanley A. Plotkin
Pasteur-Merieux Serums and Vaccines
Marnes-La Coquette, France

Joan Porter
Office for Protection from Research Risks
National Institutes of Health
Bethesda, MD

Moses Pounds
Office of Science and Epidemiology
Bureau of Health Resources Development
Health Resources and Services Administration
Rockville, MD

Albert T. Profy
Procept, Inc.
Cambridge, MA

William Randolph
Bethesda, MD

Richard Reisberg
Office of General Counsel
Public Health Division
Department of Health and Human Services
Rockville, MD

Jerry M. Rice
Division of Cancer Etiology
National Cancer Institute
National Institutes of Health
Bethesda, MD

H. Alexander Robinson
American Civil Liberties Union
Washington, DC

Helen Rodriguez-Trias
Brookdale, CA

Martin Rose
Alpha 1 Biomedicals, Inc.
Bethesda, MD

Philip Russell
School of Hygiene and Public Health
Johns Hopkins University
Baltimore, MD

Gerald Schochetman
Division of HIV/AIDS
National Center for Infectious Diseases
Centers for Disease Control and Prevention
Atlanta, GA

Teresa Schwartz
School of Law
George Washington University
Washington, DC

Belinda Seto
Office of Extramural Research
National Institutes of Health
Bethesda, MD

Amy R. Sheon
Division of AIDS
National Institute of Allergy and Infectious Diseases
National Institutes of Health
Bethesda, MD

Merrill Singer
Hispanic Health Council
Hartford, CT

Jane E. Sisk
School of Public Health
Columbia University
New York, NY

Herbert B. Slade
Rhone-Poulenc Rorer Central Research
Children's Hospital of Philadelphia
Collegeville, PA

William Snow
ACT UP Golden Gate
San Francisco, CA

Joy Stevens
Office of Legislative Affairs
Food and Drug Administration
Rockville, MD

Jeff Stryker
Center for AIDS Prevention Studies
University of California at San Francisco
San Francisco, CA

Jeremy Sugarman
Division of General Internal Medicine
Duke University Medical Center
Durham, NC

Martin Teicher
Ciba-Geigy Corporation
Ardsley, NY

Eugene A. Timm
Rochester Hills, MI

Ramon A. Torres
St. Vincent Hospital and Medical Center
New York, NY

Beth L. P. Ungar
Vaccine Trials and Epidemiology Branch
National Institute of Allergy and Infectious Diseases
National Institutes of Health
Bethesda, MD

Robert Vasquz-Pacheco
The National Latino/a Lesbian & Gay Organization
Washington, DC

David Vlahov
School of Hygiene and Public Health
Johns Hopkins University
Baltimore, MD

Paul A. Volberding
AIDS Program and Department of Clinical Oncology
San Francisco General Hospital
San Francisco, CA

Franklin Volvovitz
MicroGeneSys, Inc.
Meriden, CT

Catherine M. Wilfert
Department of Pediatrics
Duke University Medical Center
Durham, NC

Ann Wion
Office of the General Counsel
U.S. Department of Health and Human Services
Rockville, MD

Kathryn Zoon
Center for Biologics, Evaluation, and Research
Food and Drug Administration
Bethesda, MD

References and Glossary C

ABBREVIATIONS

ADR	alternative dispute resolution
AIDS	acquired immunodeficiency syndrome
ALI	American Law Institute
ARAC	AIDS Research Advisory Committee (NIAID)
AVCTN	AIDS Vaccine Clinical Trials Network
AVEU	AIDS Vaccine Evaluation Unit (NIH)
AVEG	AIDS Vaccine Evaulation Group (NIH)
AZT	Zidovudine
CDC	Centers for Disease Control and Prevention, (PHS)
CIOMS	Council for International Organizations of Medical Sciences
CTL	cytotoxic T lymphocytes
DAIDS	Division of AIDS (NIAID)
DES	diethylstilbestrol
DHHS	U.S. Department of Health and Human Services
DNA	deoxyribonucleic acid
DOD	U.S. Department of Defense
DTP	diphtheria, tetanus, and pertussis
ELISA	enzyme-linked immunosorbent assay
EIA	enzyme immunoassay
FDA	Food and Drug Administration, U.S. (PHS)
GPA	Global Programme on AIDS (WHO)
HAV	hepatitis A virus
HBV	hepatitis B virus
Hib	*Haemophilus influenza* type B
HIV	human immunodeficiency virus
HIV-1	human immunodeficiency virus, type 1
HIV-2	human immunodeficiency virus, type 2
HIVIG	human immunodeficiency virus immune globulin
HIVNET	HIV Trial Network (NIH)
IND	investigational new drug
IOM	Institute of Medicine
IPV	injected polio vaccine
NCI	National Cancer Institute (NIH)
NIAID	National Institute of Allergy and Infectious Diseases (NIH)
NIH	National Institutes of Health, (PHS)
OIG	Office of the Inspector General (DHHS)
OPV	oral polio vaccine
PAHO	Pan American Health Organization
PCR	polymerase chain reaction
PHS	Public Health Service (DHHS)
R&D	research and development
RNA	ribonucleic acid
SIV	simian immunodeficiency virus
UNICEF	United Nations Children's Emergency Fund
WHO	World Health Organization

GLOSSARY

Acquired immunodeficiency syndrome
see *AIDS*.

Adenovirus
Any of a group of DNA-containing viruses originally identified in human adenoid tissue, causing respiratory diseases, and including some capable of inducing malignant tumors in experimental animals. See also *virus*; compare *reovirus* and *retrovirus*.

Adjuvant
A substance or treatment given in conjunction with another treatment. In immunology, a substance, such as alum, added to a vaccine which non-specifically enhances its antigenicity.

ADR
See *alternative dispute resolution*.

AIDS (acquired immunodeficiency syndrome)
A disease caused by infection with HIV (human immunodeficiency virus) and characterized by impaired immune function. The primary defect in AIDS is an acquired, persistent, quantitative functional depression within the T4 subset of lymphocytes. This depression often leads to infections caused by microorganisms that usually do not produce infections in individuals with normal immunity. HIV infection can be transmitted from one infected individual to another by means that include the sharing of contaminated, intravenous needles and engaging in unprotected sexual intercourse (i.e., intercourse without condoms), as well as transmission from infected mother to newborn (vertical transmission).

Alternative dispute resolution (ADR)
A process outside the judicial system for resolving legal claims. Decisions are made by dispute resolution professionals. ADR can be binding or nonbinding. See *arbitration*.

Amino acid
Any of a group of 20 molecules that join together in various combinations to form proteins. A protein's shape, properties, and biological functions are determined in part by the specific sequence of its constituent amino acids.

Anaphylaxis
An uncommon potentially life-threatening allergic reaction that occurs immediately (within minutes) following exposure to a previously encountered antigen, such as from an insect bite or vaccine injection. It can be manifested as either a localized response (an allergic attack) or as an extreme and generalized reaction (anaphylactic shock) in which difficult breathing, pallor, hypotension, loss of consciousness, and possibly heart failure may result if untreated. Anaphylaxis is has not been observed with HIV vaccine candidates studied.

Annuity
A set sum is paid at maturity.

Antibiotic
A chemical substance that is administered to inhibit the growth of bacterial and fungal infections in humans or animals. Examples are penicillin, tetracycline, erythromycin, and cephalosporins.

Antibody
A blood protein (immunoglobulin) produced by B lymphocytes, a type of white blood cell, in response to the introduction of a specific antigen (e.g., vaccine antigen, invading bacteria, incompatible red blood cells, inhaled pollen grains, or foreign tissue grafts). Once produced, the antibody has the ability to combine, a process called neutralization with the specific antigen that stimulated antibody production, and thereby render the antigen harmless. This reaction to foreign substances is part of the immune response. The production of neutralizing antibody is one important biological measure of vaccine protection.

Appeasement
Assuaging the victim's desire for vengeance through compensation.

Antigen
A substance that elicits an immune response. Vaccine antigen is protein, derived from a microbe, which can induce a protective immune response when administered to a recipient.

Arbitration
A form of alternative dispute resolution in which the parties agree to have one or more trained arbitrators hear the evidence of the case and make a determination on liability or damages. The rules of evidence and other procedural matters may often be specified by the parties. There are two types of arbitration: binding and nonbinding. In binding arbitration the arbitration decision is subject to every limited judicial review. If arbitration is nonbinding, the parties may proceed to trial if they are not satisfied with the outcome of the

arbitration. Some states require paries to submit a claim to nonbinding arbitration before trial.

Assumption of risk

A person is aware of risks of harm inherent in a decision, and accepts responsibility for the consequences of the decision.

Attenuated vaccine

A vaccine derived from pathogenic organisms that has been altered or weakened so that it is incapable of producing disease, but still capable of causing an inapparent infection and inducing immunity.

Attorney fee limits

Legislation that either limits a plaintiff's attorney fees to a set percentage of the award or allows for court review of the proposed fee and approval of what it considers to be a "reasonable fee."

Autoantibody

An antibody that is formed by an individual against the individual's own tissues. See *antibody.*

Autoimmune

Referring to an abberent response of the immune system directed against an individual's own tissues, an abnormal reaction (the immune system is designed to respond to foreign tissue) believed to contribute to a number of chronic diseases (e.g., rheumatoid arthritis, diabetes mellitus type I). Some traditional vaccines may cause diseate by this mechanism

Autonomous choice

Refers to an individual's ability to independently make choices in his or her own interests.

Avirulent

Lacking virulence (the ability to produce a significant infection or disease); used to refer to mutant strains of ordinarily pathogenic organisms.

Awarding costs, expenses, and fees

Statutes that provide that the losing party in a frivolous suit may be required to pay the other party's reasonable attorney and expert witness fees and court costs. These provisions are designed to deter the pursuit of frivolous medical injury claims.

AZT

See *Zidovudine.*

B lymphocytes (or B cells)

An immune lymphocyte that can produce antibody in response to an antigen. B indicates its bone marrow origin. See *lymphocyte.*

Beneficence

Mercy, kindness, or charity. In ethics, it is the principle that one has a duty to confer benefits or to help others to further their legitimate interests.

Beyond a reasonable doubt

A standard of evidence typically used in criminal cases, that means fully satisfied, entirely convinced, satisfied to a moral certainty; and phrase is the equivalent of the words clear, precise, and indubitable.

Biologics

Drug products made from living organisms and their products, including viruses, serums, vaccines, antigens, antitoxins, allergenic, or analogous products.

Biotechnology

Commercial techniques that use living organisms or substances from those organisms to make or modify a product for use in medicine and industry. Biotechnology includes the use of novel biological techniques such as recombinant DNA and cell fusion.

Blinded trial

Clinical trial in which the investigator and/or the subjects are not made aware of whether the subject has been assigned to the treatment group or a comparison group. In a single-blind trial, only the investigator knows to which group the subject has been assigned. In a double-blind trial, both the investigator and the subject are not aware of which group the subject has been assigned. The investigator and/or the subject is kept unaware of which group the subject has been assigned in order to minimize bias.

Blood cells

Cells found in whole blood, including red blood cells (erythrocytes) and various types of white blood cells (such as granulocytes, monocytes, and lymphocytes).

Blood plasma

See *plasma.*

Blood serum

The clear liquid that separates from blood after the red blood cells, fibrin, and clotting factors are removed by centrifugation or vigorous stirring.

Blood
A liquid (plasma) containing red blood cells (erythrocytes), white blood cells (leukocytes), and platelets (thrombocytes) that circulates through the heart, arteries, veins, and capillaries, carrying oxygen and nutrients to body tissues, removing carbon dioxide and other wastes, transferring hormonal messages between organs, carrying substances that prevent excessive bleeding and protect injury sites with clots, and transporting antibodies and infection-fighting cells to sites of infection.

Caps on damages
Legislative limits on the amount of money that can be awarded to the plaintiff for economic or noneconomic damages in a personal injury claim, such as medical malpractice or product liability. The limit is imposed regardless of the actual amount of economic and noneconomic damages.

Cause-based compensation
A system of compensation where one's entitlement to compensation for injury depends on its cause.

CDH-receptor
The target receptor for HIV infection.

CD4+ binding site
Domain on the HIV-1 envelope protein that attaches to the CD4+ cell receptor. See *CD4+ cell.*

CD4+ cell
A type of helper T lymphocyte that bears CD4 receptors on its surface. The CD4+ cell is a target for HIV infection. The virus binds to the CD4 receptor in the process of cell entry.

CD8+ cell
A type of cytotoxic T lymphocyte that bears CD8 receptors on its surface; CD8+ lymphocytes are able to lyse infected cells that are otherwise hidden from antibody. See *cytotoxic T lymphocytes.*

Cell-mediated immunity
Immune protection provided by a network of white blood cells in the blood and tissues; immune protection provided directly by the direct action of immune cells, without the intermediation of antibodies.

Cell-mediated immunity
Immunity resulting from an increase of activity by living cells in the blood and other tissues (e.g., T lymphocytes, cytotoxic T lymphocytes) that directly and nonspecifically destroys infected cells and other foreign material. Compare *humoral immunity.*

Challenge
In immunology, administration of an antigen to assess the state of immunity. In vaccine testing, a vaccinated animal or person is challenged with an infectious agent or antigen to determine whether the vaccine has increased the animal or person's ability to fight infection.

Children's Vaccine Initiative
See *National Vaccine Injury Compensation Program.*

Clade
A major subgroup of viral strains; for HIV, at least five clades have been identified. Clade B is predominant in the Americas and Western Europe.

Claimant
Person who is requesting compensation for injury.

Classic prophylactic vaccination
Vaccination of uninfected individuals to prevent infection or disease. Compare *second order prophylactic vaccination.*

Clear and convincing proof
Proof beyond a reasonable (i.e., well founded) doubt.

Clinical trial
Experimental research in which preventive, diagnostic, or therapeutic agents, devices, regimes, and procedures are given to human subjects under controlled conditions in order to define their safety and effectiveness. In a randomized clinical trial, subjects are assigned at random to one or more treatment groups or to a control group that is given a placebo or a comparison treatment. See *phase I, II, III, and IV studies.*

Collateral source offsets
Reduce the amount of awards to the plaintiffs by prohibiting plaintiffs from collecting payment for insured losses, such as medical expenses.

Compensation
In personal injury, refers to replacing a victim's losses.

Compensatory damages
In personal injury, refers to money awarded to the plaintiff to compensate the plaintiff for losses incurred as a result of an injury.

Compensatory justice

Principle of fairness in compensation for harms.

Confidentiality (of the physician/patient relationship)

The state or quality of being confidential, that is intended to be held in confidence or kept secret. Courts and legislatures have established a physician-patient privilege to protect the confidentiality of communications between physicians and their patients and have established similar privileges to ensure the confidentiality of communications between other types of health care providers and their patients or clients.

Contingency fee

Legal fees that are dependent on the plaintiff's recovery.

Contract

A legally binding agreement between two or more parties.

Contractors

A person entering a contract, often seen as a businessperson striking a bargain. As long as the bargaining process is fair, contractors may be entitled to no more than what they bargained for, and may be seen as seeking an unfair advantage if they later demand more.

Control group

In a randomized clinical trial, the group receiving no treatment or some treatment with which the group receiving experimental treatment is compared. The control treatment is generally a standard treatment, a placebo, or no treatment. Compare *experimental group*.

Core antigens

Proteins that make up the internal structure or core of a virus. The core proteins of HIV are the products of the genes *gag* and *pol*. Compare *envelope antigens*.

Cross-protection

The ability of immunization for one strain of virus to provide protection against infection against another strain of virus.

Cross-reactivity

The property of an organism to be able to provoke an immunological reaction against a different organism. The tuberculosis vaccine BCG, for example, is an attenuated strain of *Mycobacterium bovis* (a bovine tuberculosis) that provokes the immune reaction against *M. tuberculosis*, the cause of human tuberculosis.

CTL

See cytotoxic T lymphocytes.

Cyclophilins

Proteins that function in immune modulation; acted on by Cyclosporin A, a potent immunosuppressant drug.

Cytokines

Molecules secreted from cells that affect growth or other activity in closely proximate cells. Cytokines are often thought of as short-range hormone, accomplishing cell to cell communications.

Cytotoxic T lymphocytes (CTL)

T lymphocyte characterized by its ability to recognize and destroy cells producing HIV-1; see *$CD8^+$ lymphocytes*.

ddC (zalcitabine)

An inhibitor of HIV replication by interfering with viral DNA synthesis, indicated in combination with Zidovudine, is used in patients with advanced HIV infection and immunosuppression.

ddI (didanosine)

An inhibitor of the replication of HIV, used in HIV infected patients who are intolerant or nonresponsive to Zidovudine. Also known by its brand name Videx (Bristol-Myers).

Damages

In personal injury litigation, refers to money that is awarded by the court to the plaintiff for injuries for which the defendant is legally responsible.

Defendant

In personal injury litigation, refers to the party that is alleged to be responsible for the injury.

Denaturation

The separation of double-stranded DNA into its single strands or of protein into its constituent peptides through treatment with chemicals, heat, or extremes of pH. Denaturation also results in loss or reduction of the biological properties of the substance.

Deoxyribonucleic acid

See *DNA*.

Design defect

When an object is lacking in some particular that is essential to its completeness, rendering it not fit for the purpose for which it was sold and used. A design is defective if the product could have been developed so as to reduce its inherent danger to the user without significantly decreasing its effectiveness.

Deterrence

The creation of disincentives for socially undesirable activities.

Developmental risk

The danger or hazard of incurring financial losses through litigious action resultant from research, development, and trials of a vaccine.

Diagnostic test

A medical test administered to those asymptomatic but high-risk individuals identified by a screening test, or a test used to identify the cause of abnormal physical signs or symptoms. Compare *predictive test* and *screening test.*

Diethylstilbestrol (DES)

A white, crystalline, synthetic non-steroidal estrogen having estrogenic activity similar to but greater than that of estrone. Diethylstilbestrol is one of several drugs that have been withdrawn from the market in the United States because of adverse reactions.

Diphtheria

An acute infectious disease affecting primarily the membranes of the nose, throat, or larynx, characterized by the formation of a gray white pseudomembrane; attended by fever and pain of varying degree and aphonia and respiratory obstruction in the laryngeal form; caused by the toxigenic gram-positive bacillus *Corynebacterium diphtheriae.*

Diphtheria, tetanus, pertussis (DTP) vaccine

A combination vaccine composed of two toxoids (diphtheria and tetanus) and one inactivated whole-cell bacterial vaccine (pertussis). Included among vaccines recommended in childhood.

Disability insurance

Insurance that provides payments to insured people should they be unable to work due to physical or mental incapacitation.

Disease

Any deviation from or interruption of the normal structure or function of any part, organ, or system (or combination thereof) of the body that is manifested by a characteristic set of symptoms and signs whose etiology, pathology, and prognosis may be known or unknown.

Distributive justice

Fairness in the distribution of benefits and burdens among members of society.

DNA

(deoxyribonucleic acid) The genetic material of most living things (exceptions include some RNA viruses, such as HIV) that determines the hereditary characteristics by directing protein synthesis in the cells. DNA is composed of two strands of nucleotide bases that are linked and wound around each other to form a spiral-shaped molecule. Compare *RNA.*

Double-jeopardized $CD4^+$ T cells

Vaccine-activated $CD4^+$ T cells with specificity for HIV. One theoretical risk is that vaccination may facilitate HIV infection by "activating" $CD4^+$ T cells. Active $CD4^+$ T cells are better hosts for HIV entry, integration, and replication. In addition, $CD4^+$ T cells activated by HIV vaccine will search for HIV-infected cells to bind to, increasing the rate of dissemination of HIV infection among $CD4^+$ T cells.

DT vaccine

Combined vaccine against diphtheria and tetanus.

DTP vaccine

See *diphtheria, tetanus, pertussis vaccine.*

Economic damages

Monetary damages that compensate the plaintiff for his or her actual economic losses—i.e., past and future medical expenses, lost wages, rehabilitation expenses, and other tangible losses.

Economic efficiency

The state in which the greatest direct and indirect gains (benefits) are derived from the resources expended (costs) to achieve a stated objective.

Effectiveness

Same as efficacy (see below) except that it refers to "...average or actual conditions of use." Compare *efficacy.*

Efficacy

The probability of benefit to individuals in a defined population from a medical technology applied for a given medical problem under ideal conditions of use. Efficacy is generally evaluated in controlled trials of an experimental therapy and a control condition. Compare to *effectiveness.*

Efficiency
See *economic efficiency.*

Encephalitis
Inflammation of the brain.

Encephalopathy
Any degenerative disease of the brain.

Endogenous retroviruses
Genes present in the host genome that code for retroviruses. One theoretical risk is that HIV vaccines could activate latent disease-causing retroviruses present in the host genome.

env gene
Gene coding for HIV *env* envelope protein.

Envelope (*env*) antigens
Proteins that constitute the envelope or surface of a virus. For HIV, these include the gp 160, gp 120, and gp 41 proteins. Compare *core antigens.*

Enzyme immunoassay (EIA)
An assay based on antigen-antibody interactions, which uses enzymes to measure the reaction.

Enzyme-linked immunosorbent assay (ELISA)
A type of enzyme immunoassay for determining the amount of protein or other antigen in a given sample by means of an enzyme-catalyzed color change. ELISA is used as a screening test to detect the presence of antibodies to HIV in human sera. ELISA tests that are positive for HIV are confirmed by the Western blot test. See *enzyme immunoassay.*

Enzymes
Proteins that are produced by living cells and that mediate and promote the chemical processes of life without themselves being altered or destroyed.

Episome
The genome of a virus that remains free in the nucleus of the host cell. Compare *provirus.*

Epitope
A structural part of an antigen that is responsible for an antibody response against that antigen. Also known as an "antigenic determinant."

Equity
The concept of fairness or justice.

Erythrocytes
Red blood cells. These cells contain hemoglobin and are adapted for the transport of oxygen in the blood.

Excise tax
A tax imposed on the performance of an act, the engaging in an occupation, or the enjoyment of a privilege.

Experimental group
In a randomized clinical trial, the group receiving the treatment being evaluated for safety and efficacy.

Federal Tort Claims Act (FTCA)
Enacted in 1946 (28 U.S.C.A. sec. 1346(b)(Supp. 1988)), the FTCA allows an injured party to sue the U.S. government.

forum non conveniens
Motion to dismiss a case brought by foreign plaintiffs in U.S. courts on the basis that a more suitable alternative forum exists (usually the home country of the victim, or the place where the injury occurred).

Fraud
An intentional perversion of truth for the purpose of inducing another in reliance upon it to part with some valuable thing belonging to him or to surrender a legal right.

Free virus
Virus that resides outside of cells.

gag gene
A gene that codes for HIV structural core (internal) proteins p18, p24, and p15. See *core antigens.*

Gene
The basic unit of genetic information. Each gene codes for a specific antigen.

Genome
The total genetic information or collection of genes in an organism, composed of RNA or DNA subunits.

gp 120
An HIV surface glycoprotein that bears the principle sites for induction of neutralizing antibody and binding to the host CD4 receptor. These are sites where vaccine-induced antibody can block viral replication.

gp 160
A membrane-bound surface glycoprotein that projects through the virus envelope surface. Also termed "envelope" or *env* protein, the gp160 protein is comprised of an external portion (gp120) protein, and a transmembrane region (gp 41 protein).

Gross negligence
The intentional failure to perform a manifest duty in reckless disregard of the consequences as affecting the life or property of another.

Haemophilus influenzae type b (Hib)
A parasitic bacterium that occurs in an encapsulated form. In children and debilitated older adults, infection may result in destructive inflammation of the larynx, trachea, and bronchi, and may also cause subacute bacterial endocarditis and purulent meningitis. Immunization against Hib is available through inoculation with anti-*Haemophilus influenzae* serum.

Haemophilus influenzae type B (Hib) vaccine
Vaccine included among those recommended in childhood. See *Haemophilus influenzae* type b.

Hepatitis A
Viral hepatitis, type A. An acute inflammation of the liver caused by infection with hepatitis A virus, which is transmitted by fecal contamination of food or water (e.g., through infected people handling food), or through parenteral infection (by contaminated needles or administration of blood products). Formerly known as "infectious hepatitis."

Hepatitis B
Viral hepatitis, type B. An acute inflammation of the liver caused by infection with hepatitis B virus, which is transmitted mainly by sexual contact, parenteral exposure (contaminated needles or administration of blood products), and from carrier mother to baby. In some cases, infection may be severe and result in prolonged illness, destruction of liver cells, cirrhosis, and death. Formerly known as "serum hepatitis."

Herd immunity
Resistance of a population to spread of infection. Vaccines can induce herd immunity by decreasing the transmission of infection among members of the population. The immunity to infection of some members of the population may reduce the likelihood of spread of infection to other members of the population, including spread to members who are not immune. Models for herd immunity include the worldwide smallpox vaccination program and the U.S. childhood vaccination program. Compare *individual immunity.*

Heroes
Willing volunteers who assume risks in order to accomplish a goal, ordinarily for someone else's sake.

HIV-1
Human immunodeficiency virus, type 1; a virus found in most of the world that causes the immune deficiency leading to AIDS; a member of the retrovirus subfamily that includes HIV-2 and SIV.

HIV-2
Human immunodeficiency virus, type 2; a retrovirus that is found in West Africa; in the same virus subfamily as HIV-1 and SIV.

HIV
See *human immunodeficiency virus.*

HIV-related diseases
Diseases that occur more frequently in persons who are infected with the human immunodeficiency virus (HIV).

Horizontal justice
The concept that similarly situated individuals should be treated in a like manner.

Host
In virology, the organism used for growth and reproduction of viruses.

Human immunodeficiency virus (HIV)
A retrovirus that is the etiologic agent of AIDS and whose infection has been associated with depression of the immune system and various opportunistic diseases. HIV infects and disables the CD4+ subset of T lymphocytes, which are key elements of the immune system. See *AIDS.*

Humoral immunity
Immunity associated with antibodies that circulate in the blood.

Hypersensitivity
In immunology, a state of heightened reactivity to a previously encountered antigen; may cause mild allergy or severe anaphylactic shock.

Idiotype (or idiotope)
An antigenic determinant specific for an individual immunoglobulin molecule; idiotypes are regions near the antigen binding site of an antibody that act as anti-

gens themselves by stimulating the production of antibodies.

Immediate post-exposure vaccination

Vaccination of individuals immediately after infection to prevent the infection from becoming permanently established. An example is rabies vaccine, which is administered immediately after being bitten by a rabies-infected animal.

Immune deficiencies

Any number of disorders, including AIDS, resulting from a failure or malfunction of the bodily defense mechanisms, or immune system.

Immune enhancement

The facilitation of infection and disease progression by the immune system. One theoretical risk of an HIV vaccine is that vaccination may induce the production of antibodies that may facilitate entry of HIV into phagocytic cells (cells such as macrophages that ingest microorganisms or other substances), and thereby increase dissemination of HIV infection in those cells.

Immune response

A defensive reaction of the body in response to exposure to certain substances not recognized as normal body components (pathogenic microorganisms, transplanted tissue, etc.). Immune responses may involve the production of antibodies that react with antigens on the surface of the foreign substances to render them harmless, as well as a variety of physical and chemical responses from other cells of the immune system.

Immune system

The group of organs, specialized cells, and cell products that protect the body from harmful microorganisms, contribute to allergy and hypersensitivity reactions, are involved in the rejection of transplanted tissue and organs, and may play a role in the development of cancer.

Immune

Protected against disease by innate or acquired resistance to specific foreign or pathogenic substances or organisms. See *immunity.*

Immunity

The condition of being immune, or being protected against disease by the action of the immune system. Immunity may be either innate or acquired; innate immunity is present from birth having been passed to the baby from the mother during pregnancy; acquired immunity may be active (resulting from either previous exposure to the disease-causing agent or vaccination) or passive (resulting from the injection of preformed antibodies derived from an individual already immune to a particular antigen).

Immunization

The deliberate introduction of an antigenic substance (vaccination, or active immunization) or antibodies (passive immunization) into an individual, with the aim of inducting immunity or resistance to disease. Compare *vaccination.*

Immunocompetence

The capacity to respond immunologically to an antigen.

Immunodeficient

A defect in the host's ability to mount an effective immune response.

Immunogenic

Able to cause an immune response.

Immunogenicity

The ability to generate an immune response in the host.

Immunoglobulin

Any of a group of specific proteins (produced by white blood cells) that react to the presence of a foreign antigen, react more quickly to a previously encountered antigen than to a new one, and under normal circumstances, do not respond to components of its own body. They are found in the blood plasma and lymph and in other body tissues and fluids. There are five basic classes of immunoglobulins—IgA, IgD, IgE, IgG, and IgM. See *antibody.*

Immunology

The scientific study of the ability of organisms to identify and attack foreign substances, to distinguish self from nonself, to form antibodies and antigen-reactive lymphocytes, and to become hypersensitive to common allergens.

Immunopathogenesis

A process in which the course of a disease is altered or affected by an immune response (either the cellular (T-cell) or humoral (B-cell) response) or by products of an immune reaction, such as the antigen-antibody-complement complexes deposited in renal glomeruli.

Immunosuppression
Inhibition or suppression of the immunologic response (e.g., by infection, as in AIDS, or by the administration of drugs to prevent rejection of tissue grafts or transplanted organs, or by irradiation or biochemical agents).

Immunosuppressive
Pertaining to or inducing the artificial prevention or diminution of the immune response. See *immunosuppression.*

Implied warranty of merchantability
An implied contract between seller and purchaser of consumer goods that the goods meet each of the following: 1) pass without objection in the trade under the contract description; 2) are fit for the ordinary purposes for which such goods are used; 3) are adequately contained, packaged, and labeled; 4) conform to the promises or affirmations of fact made on the container or label.

Influenza
A viral disease that is characterized by prominent systemic symptoms, such as weakness, fever, and malaise; usually occurs in epidemics.

In vitro test
Experimentation using cells, tissues, or explants grown in a nutritive medium rather than using living animals or human subjects.

In vivo
Literally, "in the living," pertaining to a biological process or reaction taking place in a living organism. In biomedical research, used to describe the experiments or processes in whole animals (e.g., mice, rats, humans), as opposed to those in a test tube or other experimental system.

Individual immunity
A person's ability to resist infection and disease. Compare *herd immunity.*

Infectivity
The ability or propensity to transmit infection.

Informed consent
As applied to human research, the agreement of a person (or his/her legally authorized representative) to serve as a research subject, in full knowledge of all anticipated risks and benefits of the experiment. Informed consent requires that the researcher impart to the prospective subject any information that might influence the subject's decision to participate or not participate in the research, including an explanation of the methodology to be used, the availability of alternative therapies, and the prospective subject's freedom to withdraw from the experiment at any time, without prejudice.

Informed consent
As applied to clinical care, a patient's agreement to allow a medical procedure based on full disclosure of the material facts needed to make an informed decision. The required elements of disclosure differ from state to state, but generally include the duty of health care providers to inform patients of the risks and benefits of medical tests or treatments, and to the patient's right to refuse medical care.

Institutional Review Board (IRB)
A group established by an institution conducting medical research to assess the legal, ethical, and scientific aspects of that research on human subjects. IRB approval is required by the Department of Health and Human Services before proposals can receive federal funding. IRBs must review research protocols on a regular basis, but not less than once a year.

Internal protein
Protein found inside the cell.

Investigational New Drug (IND) application
An application submitted by a sponsor to the Food and Drug Administration (FDA) before beginning human testing on an unapproved drug or on an approved drug for an unapproved use.

Joint and several liability
A rule under which each of the defendants in a tort suit can be held liable for the total amount of damages, regardless of his or her individual responsibility. In other words, even if a defendant was only 20 percent responsible, he or she could be held liable for 100 percent damages if other defendants are unable to pay. Several states have eliminated joint and several liability so that defendants are liable only in proportion to their responsibility.

Jurisdiction
In law, refers to the authority of a court to decide the case that is before it.

Justice
In liability for personal injury, refers to imposing the costs of injury on the one who causes it.

Learned intermediary Rule

A manufacturer of prescription drugs or vaccines need only provide product warnings to the prescribing physician, not the patient receiving the product.

Leukocyte

White blood cells (WBCs), including lymphocytes, monocytes, neutrophils, basophils, and eosinophils. WBCs are formed in lymph nodes and bone marrow and are present in the blood and lymphatic circulation. Their main function is to protect the body against infection and to fight infection when it occurs.

Liability

Legal responsibility.

Litigation

A lawsuit. Legal action, including all proceedings therein.

Lump sum payment

In tort, refers to an award, the entirety of which is to be made in a single payment.

Lymphocytes

Specialized white blood cells involved in one type of immune response that does not depend directly on antibody attack (cell-mediated immunity). Lymphocytes originate from fetal stem cells and develop in the bone marrow. They normally comprise about 25 percent of the total white blood cell count and increase in number in response to infection. They occur in two forms: B cells and T cells. B cells, which circulate in an immature form and secrete antibodies that are carried on their surface membranes, search out, identify, and bind with specific antigens. T cells mature in the thymus gland and differentiate into thymocytes when exposed to an antigen; they divide rapidly and produce large numbers of new T cells sensitized to that antigen.

Lymphoma

A neoplastic disorder of the lymphoid tissue. Malignant lymphomas are classified based on their predominant cell type. B cell lymphomas have predominantly B-lymphocyte-type cells.

Lyse

To damage or rupture a cell membrane, allowing the release of cell contents into the extracellular medium.

Macrophage

A large, specialized immune cell in the circulation or tissues that is an important intermediary in many stages of the immune response, including engulfing bacteria and other foreign particles; the macrophage is one target of HIV infection.

Manufacturing defects

Something other that the product intended by the manufacturer is produced; the manufacturing process fails to conform to the manufacturer's own specifications; generally limited to particular units or batches of the product.

Maternal-fetal HIV transmission

Transmission of the human immunodeficiency virus across the placenta from the mother to the fetus.

Measles, mumps, rubella (MMR) vaccine

A combination vaccine composed of the three live, attenuated virus vaccines providing long-term immunity against measles, mumps, and rubella; given by injection in a two-dose schedule, usually at 15 months of age and again at school entry.

Measles

A highly contagious viral disease involving primarily a hacking cough with steadily mounting fever followed by the eruption of red papules on the skin. It is spread by respiratory contact, primarily airborne droplets of nasal secretions containing the virus.

Microbe

A minute living organism; the term especially applies to those minute forms of life that are capable of causing disease in animals and man, including bacteria, protozoa, viruses, and fungi.

Model

A disease in animals used to study an analogous disease in man. SIV infection of chimpanzees and Asian monkeys has been used as a model for HIV infection and disease progression in man.

Molecular biology

The study of biology at the level of individual molecules, such as proteins and DNA.

Mucosa

The thin membrane lining various tubular structures of the body, including the colon, small and large intestine, mouth, nasal cavity, pharynx, and esophagus. The mucosal surfaces of the vagina, anus, and rectum are common sites of sexual transmission of HIV.

Mucosal immunity

Immune protection provided by antibody and immune cells located in the surface of mucous membranes.

Mumps
An acute, viral infection that produces painful inflammation and swelling of the salivary glands in the face and neck; occurs most commonly in school-aged children.

Mutation
A change in the structure or amount of genetic material (DNA, or in RNA viruses, RNA), either by changes in the base sequence of DNA or RNA, by changes affecting larger portions of a chromosome, or by the loss or addition of an entire chromosome. Mutations can be induced (e.g., caused by exposure of genetic material to a physical or chemical agent), spontaneous (occurring in the absence of any known causative agent), or heritable (changes in genetic material passed from parent to offspring). The human immunodeficiency virus (HIV) is characterized by frequent spontaneous mutations. This, in combination with selection, allows HIV to evade immune control.

National Childhood Vaccine Injury Act
Enacted by Congress in 1986 (42 U.S.C. SCCS. 3000aa *et seq.*), this Act sets up a program of administrative hearings to review claims for adverse reactions resulting in injury or death from taking a childhood vaccine. The amount of compensation for adverse reactions to these vaccines is determined by reference to a vaccine injury table. Currently, MMR, DPT and polio vaccines are covered under the Program.

National Vaccine Development and Compensation Act of 1992
Introduced by Congressman Fourtney (Pete) Stark, This Act (H.R. 5893)sought to provide the framework, based on the 1986 National Childhood Vaccine Injury Act, for dealing with AIDS vaccine liability concerns both during the period of research and development phase, as well as in the marketing phase.

National Vaccine Injury Compensation Program
This program sets up administrative hearings to review claims that injuries or deaths resulted from adverse reactions to approved childhood vaccines.

Natural killer cell
A type of lymphocyte that attacks cancerous or virus-infected cells without previous exposure to the antigen.

Natural selection
The process by which simpler ancestral species of animals and plants evolve into new species, based on variations among traits in populations and differential reproductive success that selects for certain of those traits; described by Charles Darwin in 1858 in *On the Origin of Species.*

Negligence
The doing of some act that a person of ordinary prudence would not have done under similar circumstances or failure to do what a person of ordinary prudence would have done under similar circumstances. In product liability law, negligence is conduct by the product maker that deviates from standards of acceptable conduct adhered to by the ordinary manufacturer of similar products and that results in harm to the product user.

Neutralizing antibody
Antibody with capacity to inactivate virus directly. The capacity of antibody to neutrialize virus is tested in vitro by mixing the antibodyand virus, and then assaying residual viable virus in sensitive cells. It is a biologically significant measure of protection, i.e., when compared to antibody that can physically bind viral antigen but cannot neutralize.

New Drug Application
An application to the FDA for approval to market a new chemical (non-biological) drug for human use in U.S. interstate commerce.

NK cell
See natural killer cell.

No-fault compensation
A system of compensation where one's entitlement to compensation is not contingent upon establishing who is at fault for an injury; claimants must merely establish that they were injured and that the injury arose from a specified cause.

Non-economic damages
In personal injury litigation, refers to claims for harms from the injury that cannot be expressed in sums certain of money, such as pain and suffering.

Nucleic acid
Macromolecules composed of sequences of nucleotides that carry genetic information. Two kinds of nucleic acids exist, occurring as double-or single-stranded molecules *DNA*, which contains the coded instructions for an organism's development in the chromosomes and is transferred to daughter cells; and *RNA*, which helps transport, translate, and implement

the DNA instructions, particularly the biosynthesis of proteins.

Nucleotide

A subunit of DNA or RNA, consisting of a nitrogenous base (adenine, guanine, thymine, cytosine, or uracil), a phosphate molecule, and a sugar molecule (deoxyribose in DNA or ribose in RNA). The linkage of thousands of these subunits forms the DNA or RNA molecule.

Nucleus

The membrane-enclosed structure in eukaryotic cells that contains the genetic material (DNA).

Oncogenes

Genes present in the host genome that, if activated, have the potential to cause cancer. One theoretical risk is that HIV vaccines could, upon integration into the host genome, activate latent oncogenes.

Oncogenic

Cancer inducing.

Original antigenic sin

Fixing of an immune response in a non-adaptive pattern. One theory is that HIV vaccination may induce a non-adaptive immune response that, in response to infection with a closely related strain of HIV, produces antibodies that are directed to the vaccine strain of HIV, but that weakly bind to the infecting strain of HIV.

Peptide

A compound consisting of two or more amino acids linked together by chemical bonds. Peptides are the building blocks of proteins.

Per capita

According to the number of individuals; in the law of descent and distribution, that method of dividing an intestate estate by which an equal share is given to each of a number of persons, all of whom stand in equal degree to the decedent, without reference to their stocks or the right of representation.

Periodic payment

In tort, refers to an award of damages that are to be paid in portions over a specified time interval; contrast *lump sum payment.*

Personal injury action

A suit brought in court based on a hurt or damage done to a man or woman's person, such as a cut or bruise, a broken limb or the like, as distinguished from an injury to property or reputation. In statutes the term "personal injury" is also used in a much wider sense, including any injury that is an invasion of personal rights, and in this signification it may include such injuries to the person as libel or slander, criminal conversation, malicious prosecution, false imprisonment, and mental suffering.

Pertussis

An acute, infectious inflammatory respiratory disease of children caused by the bacterium *Bordetella pertussis*. The disease is characterized by explosive attacks of coughing ending in an inspiratory whoop or choking on mucus and occurs in infants and children who have not been immunized against the disease. Also known as "whooping cough."

Petition

A written request to a court officer, legislature, or other body for the exercise of its authority in the redress of some wrong, or the grant of some favor, privilege, or license.

Petitioner

One who presents a petition to a court, officer, or legislative body.

Phase I, II, III, IV studies

Specific phases of the clinical (human) testing of new drug or vaccine products. Phase I studies of vaccines are small trials usually involving only healthy uninfected volunteers to document the safety and immune response it produces. Phase II studies further test the vaccine's safety and immunogencityand note any adverse reactions in vaccinated individuals. Phase III studies assess the vaccines effectiveness and risks among a large number of volunteers under conditions of ordinary use. These trials are randomized, placebo-controlled, and double-blind in design. Phase IV studies refer to surveilllance conducted after a vaccine is already approved for marketing, to further determine its safety and efficacy.

Placebo

A drug or procedure with no intrinsic therapeutic value. In a randomized clinical trial, a placebo is given to patients in control groups as a means to blind investigators and patients as to whether the patient is receiving the experimental or control treatment.

Plaintiff

In personal injury litigation, refers to the injured party.

Plasma
The liquid portion of blood, excluding blood cells but including a large number of dissolved substances (e.g., salts, hormones, glucose, amino acids, fats, vitamins, and waste products). Compare *blood serum*.

***pol* gene**
In HIV, a gene coding for three enzymes, including polymerase reverse transcriptase. See *core antigens*, *reverse transcriptase*.

Poliomyelitis
An acute, infectious, viral disease, occurring sporadically and in epidemics. The disease is caused by three strains of poliovirus, which attack the central nervous system, leading to the selective destruction of motor neurons of the spinal cord and brain stem, followed by extensive paralysis. The disease is preventable through use of the oral polio vaccine.

Polymerase chain reaction (PCR)
A very sensitive laboratory test to detect the presence of HIV RNA or DNA in the circulating blood.

Postmarketing surveillance
Surveillance for adverse reactions occurring after the drug or biologic has been approved by the FDA and placed on the market.

Preclinical research
Laboratory and animal research conducted prior to the clinical testing of a new chemical entity. Preclinical research may include basic research and applied nonclinical research.

Predictive test
A medical test generally applied to asymptomatic individuals to provide information regarding the future occurrence of disease. Compare *diagnostic test* and *screening test*.

Preemption
Doctrine adopted by U.S. Supreme Court holding that certain matters are of such a national, as opposed to local, character that federal laws preempt or take precedence over state laws. As such, a state may not pass a law inconsistent with federal law.

Premarket testing
Testing of pharmaceuticals and medical devices that occurs before a product can be introduced into the market. The FDA requires clinical evidence of safety and efficacy before a drug or medical device can be sold in the United States.

Premium
A reward for an act done.

Preponderance of the evidence
Standard of evidence, typically used in civil litigation, that means more likely than not, or a majority of the evidence.

Presumption
A rule of law, statutory or judicial, by which finding of a basic fact gives rise to existence of presumed fact, until presumption is rebutted.

Product liability
Refers to the legal liability of manufacturers and sellers to compensate buyers, users, and even bystanders, for damages or injuries suffered because of defects in goods purchased.

Prophylactic vaccine
Vaccine to prevent infection or disease in uninfected individuals (classic prophylaxis), or to reduce their infectivity should they subsequently become infected (second order prophylaxis).

Prophylaxis
The prevention of disease and preservation of health.

Protein
A molecule composed of many linked amino acids in a specific sequence, which is, in turn, determined by the sequence of nucleotides in DNA in the gene coding for the particular protein. Proteins are required for the structure, function, and regulation of the various cells, tissues, and organs in the body.

Provirus
The genome of a virus integrated into the chromosome of the host cell, and thereby replicated in all of the host's daughter cells. Compare *episome*.

Punitive damages
Money that is awarded to the plaintiff to punish the defendant for wrongful (usually intentional) activity.

Quasispecies
New viral mutants that have evolved from initial infecting strains of virus.

Randomized clinical trial (RCT)
An experiment designed to test the safety and efficacy of a medical technology in which people are randomly allocated to experimental or control groups, and outcomes are compared.

Rebuttable presumption
A legal presumption that can be rebutted upon presentation of sufficient evidence. See *presumption.*

Recklessness
The state of mind accompanying an act, which either pays no regard to its probably or possibly injurious consequences, or which, though foreseeing such consequences, persists in spite of such knowledge.

Recombinant DNA (rDNA) technology
Techniques involving the incorporation of DNA fragments, generated with the use of restriction enzymes, into a suitable host organism's DNA (a vector). The host is then grown in culture to produce clones with multiple copies of the incorporated DNA fragment. The clones containing this particular DNA fragment can then be selected and harvested. Also called genetic engineering.

Recombinant DNA
Genetic material that contains DNA from different sources that have been combined by genetic engineering methods. Rearrangement of the genes is artificially induced using enzymes to break DNA into fragments, allowing recombination in different sequences.

Recombinant technology
Scientific knowledge of the process of forming new combinations of genes as a result of crossing over between homologous chromosomes.

Recombination
In genetics, the formation of new combinations of genes as a result of crossing over between homologous chromosomes. One theoretical risk is that genetic material from a live vector or naked DNA HIV vaccine could recombine in the vaccinated host with preexisting or newly acquired HIV or other viruses.

Red blood cells
see *erythrocytes.*

Reovirus
Any group of relatively large, widely distributed, and possibly tumor-causing viruses with double-stranded RNA. Unlike retroviruses, which also contain RNA, reoviruses replicate in the cytoplasm of the cells they invade and do not produce DNA analogs to their RNA for incorporation into the host cell's genome. The genus name "reovirus" is derived from the term *r*espiratory *e*nteric *o*rphan virus, to denote both respiratory and enteric trophism and isolation of the virus in the absence of known disease. See also *virus*; and compare *adenovirus* and *retrovirus.*

Replication
In genetics, the synthesis of new DNA from existing DNA.

Respondent
In equity practice, the party who makes an answer to a bill or other proceeding in equity. In appellate practice, the party who contends against an appeal (i.e., the appellee). In the civil law, one who answers or is security for another.

Restatement of Torts
American Law Institute's treaties that summarize several fields of law. Widely considered to be the most authoritative statement of tort law in the country. Most states have adopted its provisions, albeit not uniformly, and some states have interpreted its technical requirements somewhat differently.

Retributive justice
Assuaging the victim's and society's desire for vengeance or retribution through punishment.

Retrovirus
A familly of viruses with an RNA genome and an intermediary DNA stage, which is persistently integrated into the genome of the host cell chromosome. A retrovirus contains two identical single strands of RNA, not DNA, and that reproduces by making a double-stranded DNA transcription of itself in a process catalyzed by a virally encoded enzyme known as a "reverse transcriptase." The resulting DNA product may integrate into the cell genome (as a provirus) or may remain free in the nucleus (as an episome). Either way, it remains as a latent infection to be activated later (by a variety of factors) to a virus-producing form. Retroviruses are found widely in nature and are associated with a variety of diseases, including cancer, neurologic disorders, and immune deficiency syndromes, notably AIDS. Four well-characterized retroviruses are HIV-1 and HIV-2 (major causative agents of AIDS), and HTLV-I and HTLV-II (associated with T-cell leukemia and lymphoma). See also *provirus* and *virus*; and compare *adenovirus* and *retrovirus.*

Reverse transcriptase

Also called RNA-dependent DNA polymerase. Enzyme present in HIV and other retroviruses that allows the virus to turn RNA genetic information into DNA genetic information. See *retrovirus* and *reverse transcription.*

Reverse transcription

The creation of DNA genetic information using RNA genetic information as a template. HIV and other retroviruses are unique in their RNA genetic information into DNA, which is subsequently integrated into the DNA genome of the host. This process is accomplished by the enzyme "reverse transcriptase."

RGB

Purified recombinant glycoprotein expressed in a host cell.

Ribonucleic acid

See *RNA*.

Right of subrogation

A provision typically found in health and disability insurance contracts that requires a plaintiff to reimburse the insurance company for any payments received from the tort system that were for services reimbursed by the insurer.

Risk-benefit analysis

A determination of whether the risks to health and the environment of using a chemical, drug, or vaccine exceed the economic benefits that accrue from its use. In the case of drugs and vaccines, benefits are measured in terms of therapeutic efficacy.

Risk deterrence

The prevention or deterrence of avoidable risk.

RNA

Ribonucleic acid. A type of nucleic acid that carries genetic instructions and assists in the assembly of proteins. RNA is a single-stranded chain of repeating units of adenine, cytosine, guanine, and uracil. Specialized types of RNA include: messenger RNA (mRNA), which carries a transcript of a DNA sequence to be used as a template for protein synthesis; transfer RNA (tRNA), which attaches the correct amino acid to the protein chain being synthesized at a ribosome; and ribosomal RNA (rRNA), a structural constituent of ribosomes. In some viruses, RNA contains the instructions for viral replication. The HIV-1 genome is composed of RNA. However, HIV-1 assmes a DNA form when persistantly integrated into host cell (e.g. CD4+ lymphocytes) genetic material as part of its replication cycle.

Rubella (German measles)

An acute viral illness that causes a diffuse reddish rash and swollen lymph glands. Infection during pregnancy, especially in early stages, can cause miscarriage or congenital rubella syndrome, a potentially fatal disorder involving deafness, cataracts, mental retardation, and/or heart lesions (depending on when infection occurred in gestation). The disease is preventable through vaccination.

Schedule of damages

A set of guidelines for juries to use in deciding appropriate awards for noneconomic damages in malpractice cases.

Screening test

Generally, a test used to sort out apparently well persons who probably have disease from those who probably do not. A screening test is not intended to be diagnostic. Compare *diagnostic test* and *predictive test.*

Second order prophylactic vaccination

Vaccination of uninfected individuals to reduce their ability to transmit subsequently acquired infections. Compare *classic prophylactic vaccination.*

Section 402A liability

Section 402A of the Restatement of Torts (2nd) makes manufacturers of drugs and vaccines strictly liable for adverse reactions in the absence of warnings.

Selection

In combination with mutation, a source of rapid genetic change of HIV. See *Natural selection.*

Selective advantage

In biology, an organism's increased probability of reproduction and producing offspring, conferred by its genetic characteristics.

Selective pressure

In biology, the influence of factors extrinsic to an organism (i.e., environmental factors) on its ability to compete with other organisms for reproductive success.

Sequelae

Aftereffects or secondary consequences of a disease, disorder, or injury.

Seroconversion
The initial development of antibodies specific to a particular agent.

Seropositive
In the context of HIV, the condition in which antibodies to the virus are found in the blood.

Serum
See *blood serum.*

Settlement
In the context of a civil suit, refers to a private agreement of a plaintiff not to further pursue a court judgment in return for compensation from the defendant.

Simian immune deficiency virus (SIV)
A retrovirus from the same virus subfamily as HIV-1 and HIV-2 that infects chimpanzees and Asian monkeys; SIV infection of chimpanzees and Asian monkeys has been used as a model for HIV infection in man.

SIV
See *Simian immunodeficiency virus.*

Spontaneous mutation
In the absence of any known causative agent, a change in the structure DNA or in the number of chromosomes. Also called a "background" mutation. HIV is characterized by frequent spontaneous mutations. See *mutation.*

Statute of limitations
A statute prescribing limitations to the right of action on certain described causes of action or criminal prosecutions; that is, declaring that no suit shall be maintained on such causes of action, nor any criminal charge be made, unless brought within a specified period of time after the right accrued.

Strain
A group of organisms of the same species having a distinctive quality or characteristic (biochemical, pathogenic, or other) that can be differentiated, but is not different enough to constitute a separate species.

Strict liability
A legal concept that states liability lies with the party best able to prevent injury or absorb its costs even if that party was not responsible for causing the specific injury in question through negligence or intent. See *malpractice.*

Subrogation
See *right of subrogation.*

Subunit vaccine
A vaccine that contains only portions of an antigenic molecule from a pathogen. Subunit vaccines can be prepared by using recombinant DNA technology to produce all or part of the antigenic molecule or by artificial (chemical) synthesis of short peptides.

Sunset clause
Clause that provides for the automatic expiration of legislation.

Swine Flu Act
Enacted in 1976, the Act held harmless manufacturers of the swine flu vaccine from claims of individuals injured by the vaccine. The Act also permitted claimants to file suit against the U.S. government under the Federal Tort Claims Act for compensation for injuries from the swine flu vaccine.

Swine flu vaccine
Vaccine against the swine flu, an especially virulent strain of influenza that spread throughout the United States during the fall and winter of 1976.

Systemic
Pertaining to or affecting the body as a whole.

T4 cell
See *CD4+ cell.*

T8 cell
See *cytotoxic T lymphocyte.*

T helper cell
See CD4+ cell.

T lymphocyte (T cell)
A lymphocyte produced in the bone marrow that matures in the thymus and is integral to cell-mediated immunity. T cells regulate the growth and differentiation of other lymphocytes and are involved in antibody production. See *lymphocytes.*

Teratogen
Physical or chemical agents, (e.g. thalidomide, radiation, alcohol, and certain viruses) that act on the fetus in utero to cause congenital malformations.

Teratogenic
Capable of inducing the formation of developmental abnormalities in a fetus.

Tetanus
An acute, potentially fatal disease of the central nervous system caused by infection of a wound with spores of the bacterium *Clostridium tetani*; these spores release a poisonous neurotoxin (tetanus toxoid) that causes trismus ("lockjaw"), generalized muscle spasm, arching of the back, glottal spasm, seizures, respiratory spasms, and paralysis. Short-term immunity can be derived through vaccination. Tetanus vaccine is among vaccines recommended for children. See *DTP vaccine.*

Therapeutic vaccine
Vaccine to prevent or reduce disease progression in infected individuals, or to reduce disease transmission to persons who come in contact with infected individuals.

Tort law
A body of law that provides citizens a private, judicially enforced, remedy for injuries caused by another person. Legal actions based in tort have three elements: existence of a legal duty from defendant to plaintiff, breach of that duty, and injury to the plaintiff as a result of that breach.

Tort liability
Liability imposed by a court for breach of a duty implied by law, contrasted with contractual liability, which is breach of duty arising from an agreement. A legal basis for compensation when property has been damaged or a person has been injured. The tort liability system determines fault and awards compensation for civil wrongs, including medical malpractice and product liability.

Tort reform
A legal reform that changes the way tort claims are handled in the legal system or removes claims from the civil judicial system.

Transaction costs
In personal injury, refers to the administrative costs associated with transferring compensation to the injured.

Transcription
In genetics, the process by which RNA is formed from a DNA template during protein synthesis. Compare *translation, reverse transcription.*

Translation
The process in which the genetic code contained in the nucleotide base sequence of messenger RNA directs the synthesis of a specific order of amino acids to produce a protein. Compare *transcription.*

Transmission
In infectious disease, the passage of a pathogen from one host to another host or from vector to host.

Vaccination
The deliberate introduction of an antigenic substance (vaccine) into an individual, with the aim of producing active immunity to a disease. Compare *immunization.*

Vaccine
A preparation of living, attenuated, or killed bacteria or viruses, fractions thereof, or synthesized antigens identical or similar to those found in the disease-causing organisms that is administered to produce or increase immunity to a particular disease.

Vaccinia virus
The organism that causes cowpox; its injection into humans results in immunity to the related smallpox virus.

Varicella
Virus that causes chickenpox.

Vector
In HIV vaccines, refers to a live attenuated virus or bacterum carrying selected HIV genes, which produces desired antigenic proteins when administered to a recipient. Proteins produced in a living microorganism are generally capable of inducing cytotoxic T lymphocyle responses in addition to antibody.

Victims
Persons misused or injured without their consent.

Virology
The study of viruses and the diseases they cause; also, the isolation and identification of viruses associated with specific infection.

Virus
Any of a large group of submicroscopic agents infecting plants, animals, and bacteria and characterized by a total dependence on living cells for reproduction and by a lack of independent metabolism. A fully formed

virus consists of nucleic acid (DNA or RNA) surrounded by a protein or protein and lipid coat. See also *adenovirus, provirus, reovirus*, and *retrovirus*.

Warning defects

There are two types of warning defects: 1) a failure to provide warnings of risks inherent in the use of the product (failure to warn); and 2) providing directions and warnings that fail to adequately describe product risks (inadequate warning).

Western Blot

A laboratory technique used to detect the presence of antibodies to specific antigens, including those specific for HIV infection. The method is often used to check the validity of a positive ELISA screening test for HIV. It is also used to clinical trials to detect vaccine induced antibody. Electrophoresis is used to separate proteins by their molecular weights, and each protein is identified through combining with its respective antibody or antigen. For example, in Western Blot testing for HIV antibodies, the protein components of HIV are first separated electrophoretically, transferred to blots, then mixed with sera suspected of containing HIV antibodies. The presence of antibodies to specific proteins of HIV is revealed by the combination of antibodies with their specific protein components of HIV.

White blood cells

Cells in the blood stream and tissues, including lymphocytes, macrophages, and neutrophils, that provide immune protection. See *leukocyte*.

Whole, killed-virus vaccine

Vaccine formed from virulent virus that has been altered so that the virus is no longer able to replicate.

Workers compensation

System that provides compensation for work-related injuries, regardless of the fault of the employer.

Zidovudine (AZT)

An inhibitor of the replication of some retrovirses including HIV, used in the treatment of persons with HIV infection who have evidence of impaired immunity. Also known by its brand name, Retrovir (Burroughs Wellcome).

Superintendent of Documents **Publications** Order Form

P3

Telephone orders (202) 512-1800
(The best time to call is between 8-9 a.m. EST.)
To fax your orders (202) 512-2250
Charge your order. It's Easy!

☐ **YES**, please send me the following:

________ copies of ***Adverse Reactions to HIV Vaccines: Medical, Ethical, and Legal Issues (208 pages),*** S/N 052-003-01429-7 at $14.00 each.

The total cost of my order is $_________. International customers please add 25%. Prices include regular domestic postage and handling and are subject to change.

(Company or Personal Name) (Please type or print)

(Additional address/attention line)

(Street address)

(City, State, ZIP Code)

(Daytime phone including area code)

(Purchase Order No.)

Please Choose Method of Payment:

☐ Check Payable to the Superintendent of Documents

☐ GPO Deposit Account ☐☐☐☐☐☐☐ — ☐

☐ VISA or MasterCard Account

☐☐☐☐☐☐☐☐☐☐☐☐☐☐☐☐☐☐☐☐

☐☐☐☐ (Credit card expiration date)

Thank you for your order!

(Authorizing Signature) (9/95)

May we make your name/address available to other mailers? **YES** ☐ **NO** ☐

Mail To: New Orders, Superintendent of Documents, P.O. Box 371954, Pittsburgh, PA 15250-7954

THIS FORM MAY BE PHOTOCOPIED

Superintendent of Documents **Publications** Order Form

P3

Telephone orders (202) 512-1800
(The best time to call is between 8-9 a.m. EST.)
To fax your orders (202) 512-2250
Charge your order. It's Easy!

☐ **YES**, please send me the following:

________ copies of ***Adverse Reactions to HIV Vaccines: Medical, Ethical, and Legal Issues (208 pages),*** S/N 052-003-01429-7 at $14.00 each.

The total cost of my order is $_________. International customers please add 25%. Prices include regular domestic postage and handling and are subject to change.

(Company or Personal Name) (Please type or print)

(Additional address/attention line)

(Street address)

(City, State, ZIP Code)

(Daytime phone including area code)

(Purchase Order No.)

Please Choose Method of Payment:

☐ Check Payable to the Superintendent of Documents

☐ GPO Deposit Account ☐☐☐☐☐☐☐ — ☐

☐ VISA or MasterCard Account

☐☐☐☐☐☐☐☐☐☐☐☐☐☐☐☐☐☐☐☐

☐☐☐☐ (Credit card expiration date)

Thank you for your order!

(Authorizing Signature) (9/95)

May we make your name/address available to other mailers? **YES** ☐ **NO** ☐

Mail To: New Orders, Superintendent of Documents, P.O. Box 371954, Pittsburgh, PA 15250-7954

THIS FORM MAY BE PHOTOCOPIED